GIOVANNA **PERROTTI** TIZIANO **TESTORI** MASSIMILIANO **POLITI**

3D IMAGING AND DENTISTRY

From Multiplanar Cephalometry to Guided Navigation in Implantology

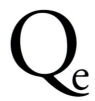

Quintessenza Edizioni

Milan, Berlin, Chicago, Tokyo, Barcelona,
Istanbul, London, Moscow, New Delhi, Paris,
Beijing, Prague, São Paulo, Seoul, Warsaw

Copyright © 2016 by
Quintessenza Edizioni S.r.l.
via Ciro Menotti, 65 - 20017 Rho (MI) Italy
Tel.: +39.02.93.18.08.21 - Fax: +39.02.93.18.61.59
E-mail: info@quintessenzaedizioni.it
www.quintessenzaedizioni.com

ISBN   88-7492-018-0
        978-88-7492-018-1

All rights reserved.
The book and all its parts are protected by copyright. Any use or marketing beyond the scope of copyright without the publisher's prior consent is unlawful and legally prosecutable. This applies in particular to photostats, copies, circular letters, duplications, translations, microfilms, electronic processing and data collection.

Printed in Italy

We dedicate this work to all those who feel like perpetual students, living their work with passion.

*Giovanna Perrotti,
Tiziano Testori,
Massimiliano Politi*

FOREWORD

I am glad to present the book *3D Imaging and Dentistry*, the latest intellectual effort of the University School of Dentistry at Istituto Ortopedico Galeazzi in Milan.

Our discipline has extraordinary merits over the history of medicine; in more recent times, dentists have discovered several etiopathogenic mechanisms while investigating periodontal disease, found new bacteria, and developed tissue regeneration techniques.

Moreover, in the area of radiology, dentistry has been one of the first disciplines to understand the potential of computed tomography and the use of the algorithms derived from it.

While tomography was evolving in the field of three-dimensional reconstructions, odontostomatology immediately seized upon the great potential offered by these techniques, devoting to them in-depth clinical research and using the images thus obtained in orthodontics, surgery, implantology, and endodontics.

This volume guides the reader to a systemic approach to 3D imaging: the subject matter is introduced to students and specialists step by step, and its various branches are investigated in detail. The authors of this book have achieved a phenomenon in the field of translational medicine: starting from basic research, they transfer these concepts to a complete analysis of the stomatognathic system and then to the clinical application of the data gathered.

Reading this book allows one to understand that the authors have transformed what used to be considered as a technique into a true discipline, with all the dignity this term confers to a set of information and concepts—a cultural operation of which we are all very proud, and one which we now defer to the judgment of the reader.

Roberto Weinstein

FOREWORD

During the past few decades dentistry has continued to evolve in many areas to improve patient care based upon multispecialty treatment modalities that traditionally have included orthodontics, endodontics, periodontics, oral surgery, occlusion, prosthodontics, oral and maxillofacial radiology, bone grafting, and implantology. However, regardless of the patient presentation and need for treatment, the foundation must always be the same: proper diagnosis. Wherever clinicians practice dentistry throughout the world, it is of utmost importance that they have the necessary information to assess each individual patient presentation to develop the proper plan of treatment and to avoid potential complications. Advances in technology have provided clinicians with new and innovative tools, but no modality in my opinion has had more impact on patient care than three-dimensional diagnostic imaging and interactive treatment planning software. Therefore as more and more clinicians become educated about these new state-of-the-art modalities, a higher quality of care can be provided for our patients.

However, the progression from two-dimensional (2D) panoramic and periapical radiography to the three-dimensional (3D) world of computed tomography (CT) and cone beam computed tomography (CBCT) is often confusing to many clinicians who were not initially exposed to the technology while in dental school or who are currently in private practice. It is critical that clinicians appreciate how to assess the relationship between hard and soft tissue and vital structures, to interpret, and to evaluate the many views and images made possible by this expansive technology for a wide variety of applications. Giovanna Perrotti, Tiziano Testori, and Massimiliano Politi have presented clinicians with an extremely comprehensive exploration into the world of three-dimensional imaging modalities with their new textbook appropriately entitled *3D Imaging and Dentistry: From Multiplanar Cephalometry to Guided Navigation in Implantology*. The textbook is well organized, bringing the reader through the basic principles of radiology as it applies to dental anatomy in an easy-to-understand illustrative format. The meticulous attention to detail demonstrated throughout each chapter, with excellent photography and clinical documentation, helps to guide the clinician to first understand normal anatomy and then to appreciate variations in anatomical presentations, which confirm that each patient is different. Through side-by-side comparisons with dry skull and cadaver specimen illustrations, the inherent limitations of 2D imaging and the benefits of 3D imaging have been made crystal clear. The authors educate the readers in understanding the new "language" of cross-sectional, coronal, sagittal, axial, and 3D reconstructed images for the identification of anatomical landmarks and the crucial assessment of vital adjacent anatomy, such as the location of an impacted tooth, the path of the inferior alveolar nerve, or intraosseous vessels in the lateral wall of the sinus, to avoid potential complications.

Perhaps the most impressive aspect of this book is consideration for the wide variety of clinical applications afforded CT/CBCT–derived 3D images. Of course, most clinicians consider the utilization of 3D as an aid to assessing dental implant receptor sites and for guided surgery applications to improve accuracy and reduce patient morbidity as the authors have beautifully illustrated. Beyond guided surgery are other uses such as the evaluation of the temporomandibular joint, which can be dramatically improved and better appreciated with an interactive 3D reconstruction seen on the computer screen. Even endodontic treatment can be better served with a 3D analysis—especially with multirooted teeth and the need to determine multiple canals or the exact location of root lesions and bone loss. The book examines the need for a proper 3D assessment of the maxillary sinus for grafting procedures and the many variations of pathological presentations that could not be visualized with conventional 2D radiography. General pathologic findings for both the maxilla and mandible are reviewed in detail with actual clinical presentations. There are additional chapters devoted to the application of 3D imaging in the field of forensic dentistry and the growing area of airway analysis, which can be beneficial with sleep apnea disorders.

As a student of 3D imaging for almost 30 years, I have found that each patient presentation and CT/CBCT scan is a new opportunity to learn more about human anatomy. I would never assume that after examining thousands of scans that there is nothing else left to see ... or to interpret, or discover. The case illustrations in this magnificent textbook provided me with new insights and helped me to continue on my own path of learning and appreciation of hard and soft tissues of the head and neck region. There is a great need to educate the world about the utilization and benefit of 3D imaging, interactive treatment planning software, and the fundamental tools for proper diagnosis. I am very proud and honored to have been asked to write a foreword to a much-needed textbook and congratulate all three authors and other contributors for their dedication, hard work, and efforts in creating a most wonderful contribution to the dental literature. I am certain that every reader, novice to expert, will benefit from each and every page.

With great appreciation and admiration—

Dr Scott D. Ganz

INTRODUCTION

Three-dimensional (3D) digital radiology has given clinicians the opportunity to perform diagnoses and to plan-treatments in dentistry and maxillofacial surgery with greater awareness and accuracy than with conventional two-dimensional radiology. The use of the third dimension and the feasibility of reconstructing the volume of a skeletal area under investigation has opened new frontiers, not only in diagnosis and treatment, but also in education, allowing one to computer-simulate the steps of future surgical procedures.

This textbook aims to provide basic information in volumetric radiology, which is necessary for its correct and rational use, following well-defined internationally acknowledged protocols. The various chapters outline the indications for prescribing 3D scans and explain the wealth of information available from proper image processing. There is a clear and synthetic overview of all dental fields in which cone beam computed tomography (CBCT) can be applied, from orthodontics to implantology, periodontology, endodontics, and temporomandibular disorders, so as to provide the reader with useful guidance in clinical practice.

Great attention has been devoted to the quality of images so as to reproduce as truly as possible the resolution of radiologic images obtained by using dedicated software to process Digital Imaging and Communication in Medicine (DICOM) files. This is an important aspect, as the reader can understand how the use of DICOM files is closely linked to the application of technical processing tools from simple viewers to more complex software products. Starting from DICOM files, images are processed and used for planning treatment as it happens in 3D cephalometry, in programming osteotomy procedures, and in guided implant surgery.

A considerable part of the textbook is devoted to cephalometric diagnostics and the outlining of a new approach in the anthropometric and esthetic analysis. 3D cephalometry is made possible because of the in-depth knowledge of the anatomy provided by 3D radiologic scans. The textbook also includes an anatomical-radiologic atlas with detailed points in bones and soft tissues so as to develop a cephalometric project.

Broad space has been given to investigating the anatomy of the airways for clinical applications: a section describes the structure of the maxillary sinus and its relation to clinical surgery. An extensive chapter covers implant planning and guided surgery, themes that are very topical and of great clinical interest.

This publishing project reconciles the objectives of a textbook for students and a valuable tool for continuous education of professionals with clinical experience. I hope this book can be a useful educational tool, helping clinicians to better treat their patients after they have been entrusted with their oral health.

Giovanna Perrotti,
Massimiliano Politi,
Tiziano Testori

NOTE
All images published in this volume have been personally processed by the authors with dedicated 3D imaging software tools.

COAUTHORS

FRANCESCA BIANCHI, DMD, graduated with a degree in dentistry and dental prosthetics from the University of Milan (1995). Dr Bianchi teaches oral implantology at the Istituti di Ricovero e Cura a Carattere Scientifico (IRCCS) Istituto Ortopedico Galeazzi in Milan. She also teaches the Associazione Nazionale Dentisti Italiani (ANDI) course for chairside assistants. A frequent speaker at Italian congresses, Dr Bianchi is a senior lecturer at the Lake Como Institute and has published papers on implantology and periodontology. She maintains a private practice in Como, Italy.

MASSIMO DEL FABBRO, MD, manages the Oral Physiopathology Unit of the Odontostomatology Service at the IRCCS Istituto Ortopedico Galeazzi in Milan and is the director of the Research Center for Oral Health at the University of Milan. With a PhD in human physiology, Dr del Fabbro is a tenured researcher at the University of Milan, where his work focuses on physiopathology of periodontal and peri-implant tissues, biology of osseointegration, and tissue engineering and regeneration techniques. He is the author of over 240 scholarly papers.

GIULIA FERRARA, DMD, graduated with honors in dentistry and dental prosthetics from the University of Milan. She went on to complete postgraduate clinical training in dentistry and endodontics at Paris Diderot University and now specializes in endodontics and bonded restorations. Dr Ferrara was a former tutor in the Department of Endodontics at the IRCCS Istituto Ortopedico Galeazzi. She has written several papers on endodontics.

SILVIA FERRARIO, DMD, is an attending physician at the Orthognatodontic Hospital Unit within the Dental Clinic at the IRCCS Istituto Ortopedico Galeazzi. She has a degree in dentistry and dental prosthetics from the University of Milan and is currently completing a postdoctoral orthodontics program at the University of Milan.

LUCA FUMAGALLI, DMD, is a tutor of implantology and oral rehabilitation at the Dental Clinic at IRCCS Istituto Ortopedico Galeazzi at the University of Milan, from which he also received his degree in dentistry and dental prosthetics (2001). He is a member of both the Italian Society of Oral Surgery and Implantology (SICOI) and the European Academy of Osseointegration (EAO). Dr Fumagalli serves on the review board for *Quintessenza Internazionale* and the *International Journal of Oral & Maxillofacial Implants* and is the author of over 50 papers and books on implantology and implant prosthetics.

FABIO GALLI, MD, is a medical doctor and surgeon, odontostomatologist, and expert in oral surgery and implant prosthetics. Since 2004, he has been a professor of implantology as well as the head of the Prosthetics Unit within the Implantology and Oral Rehabilitation Department at the University of Milan. An active member of the Italian Society of Osseointegrated Implantology (SIO) and a founding member of both the Advanced Implantology Study Group (AISG) and the Italian Association for the Study of Bisphosphonates in Dentistry (SISBO), Dr Galli is a member of the review board for *Quintessenza Internazionale* and the *International Journal of Oral & Maxillofacial Implants*, and the author of over 100 articles.

FRANCESCO GRECCHI, MD, has served as the first-level health care manager at the Maxillofacial Surgery Unit of Ospedale Niguarda in Milan since 1995 as well as head of the Operating Unit of Maxillofacial Surgery at IRCCS Istituto Ortopedico Galeazzi in Milan since 2000. As unit manager, he is a consultant in maxillofacial traumatology at the Luigi Sacco Hospital at the University of Milan, Ospedale Fatebenefratelli, Ophthalmic Institute, Istituto Clinico Città Studi di Milano, and Ospedale Clinicizzato in San Donato Milanese, as well as maxillofacial reference specialist of the Italian National Association for Ectodermic Dysplasia (ANDE). Dr Grecchi received a degree in medicine in surgery (1981) and completed specialties in general surgery (1986) and maxillofacial surgery (2001) from University of Milan. He has also been a surgical assistant since 1984. He is the author and coauthor of 92 papers in scientific journals.

COAUTHORS

GIULIANA LORÈ, DMD, is an attending physician at the Orthognatodontics Unit and CROME unit of the Dental Clinic at the IRCCS Istituto Ortopedico Galeazzi in Milan. She received her degree in dentistry and dental prosthetics from the University of Milan (2013) and is completing a postdoctoral program in orthodontics. Dr Lorè maintains a private practice in orthodontics and conservative dentistry with a focus on smile esthetics and periodontology.

MARIO MANTOVANI, MD, is a professional collaborator at the Otorhinolaryngological Clinic of the University of Milan, where he first worked as an otorhinolaryngological specialist. He received his degree in medicine and surgery from the University of Pavia (1975) and has since completed specialties in otorhinolaryngology and neck and face pathologies (1975), plastic surgery (1981), and maxillofacial surgery (1986) at the University of Milan. Prof Mantovani is an active member of the Italian Society of Otorhinolaryngology and Neck and Face Surgery and the American Academy of Otolaryngology-Head and Neck Surgery. He is a member of the review board for Italian Oral Surgery as well as the author of over 100 scientific papers.

JOANNA KATARZYNA NOWAKOWSKA, MD, PhD, is a private practitioner in orthognatodontics, pedodontics, and preventive dentistry in Milan and Monza-Brianza, and has been an attending physician at the IRCCS Istituto Ortopedico Galeazzi since 2004. Author of various scientific papers, Dr Nowakowska received her degree in dentistry and dental prosthetics at Danzig Medical Academy (2003), followed by a PhD in innovative techniques in oral implantology and implant-prosthetic rehabilitation (2008), and a second PhD in orthognatodontics (2012), both from the University of Milan.

ANDREA PARENTI, MD, is a tutor in the Implantology and Oral Rehabilitation Unit at the Dental Clinic in the IRCCS Istituto Ortopedico Galeazzi. He received his degree in dentistry and dental prosthetics from the University of Milan (2001). Dr Parenti is a member of both SICOI and SIO, serves on the review board for *Quintessenza Internazionale* and the *International Journal of Oral & Maxillofacial Implants*, and is the author of several scientific articles.

LORENZO PIGNATARO, MD, is the director of Otorhinolaryngology Department Fondazione IRCCS Cà Granda Ospedale Maggiore Policlinico in Milan and a professor in the Department of Clinical Sciences and Community Health at the University of Milan. A prolific writer and well-known speaker, Prof Pignataro is the author of more than 350 scientific papers since he received his degree in medicine and surgery from the University of Milan (1986).

GRAZIA POZZI, MD, is a radiologist at IRCCS Istituto Ortopedico Galeazzi in Milan. Dr Pozzi received both her degree in medicine and surgery (2004) and her PhD in radiodiagnostics (2008) from the University of Milan–Bicocca. She was a contract professor at the University of Milan until 2010 and is the author and coauthor of scientific papers indexed in PubMed.

MARCO SCARPELLI, MD, is a contract professor in Regulatory and Deontological Foundations at Corso di Laurea in Odontoiatria e Protesi Dentaria in Florence and an expert/referee for the Italian Ministry of Health and has served as a professional mediator since 2010. He has a degree in medicine and surgery and a specialization in odontostomatology, both from the University of Milan, and is registered as a specialist in forensic medicine, as well as in the Board of Technical Experts of the Court in Milan. Dr Scarpelli coordinates masters courses in forensic odontology at the Institute for Forensic Medicine at the University of Florence and serves as vice president of the Italian Association Forensic Odontology Project at the Department of Forensic Medicine in Florence. He is the author of over 130 scientific papers and texts.

SILVIO TASCHERI, MD, is a researcher in the Department of Biomedical, Surgical, and Dental Sciences at the Dental Clinic of the IRCCS Istituto Ortopedico Galeazzi at the University of Milan, where he also works as an on-site tutor at the Laboratory of Biological Structural Mechanics in the Polytechnic. Dr Tascheri is a reviewer of the Cochrane Oral Health Group in the School of Dentistry at the University of Manchester. He is also an active member of the European Society of Endodontology, the Italian Society of Endodontics, the Academy of Non-Transfusional Haemo-Components, and the Italian Society of Oral Surgery and Implantology.

ALBERTO ZERBI, MD, is the director of the Hospital Unit of Diagnostic and Interventional Radiology at the IRCCS Instituto Ortopedico Galeazzi in Milan. He received his degree in medicine and surgery from the University of Milan (1982) and returned for a specialty in radiology (1986). Dr Zerbi teaches the Radiology Course at the University of Milan–Bicocca. He is the author of 31 indexed scientific papers and also an active member of the Italian Society of Spine Surgery, Italian Scoliosis Group, and the Eurospine Society and serves on the editorial board of *Eurospine Journal*.

	Foreword by Roberto Weinstein	V
	Foreword by Scott D. Ganz	VI
	Introduction	IX

1 Basic Principles for the Use of CBCT in Dentistry — 1

Principles of Digital Radiology — 2
Computed Tomography — 9
Image Postprocessing — 17
References — 30

2 Changes in Basal Bones from Infancy to Senescence — 33

Growth and Development of Facial Bones in 3D Images — 34
Theories on Control of Craniofacial Growth — 45
Bone Resorption and Atrophy of the Basal Bone — 47
Implant Therapy and Craniofacial Growth — 61
References — 64

3 Systematic CBCT Analysis of the Maxilla and Mandible — 65

Radiologic and Clinical Anatomy of the Maxilla — 66
Radiologic and Clinical Anatomy of the Mandible — 82
Clinical Examples — 96
References — 162

4 Evolution of Cephalometry — 165

Concepts of Cephalometry — 166
Dysgnathic Presentations in 3D — 188
References — 202

5 Atlas of Cephalometric Landmarks — 205
Introduction to Cephalometry — 206
Atlas of Skeletal Landmarks — 211
Atlas of Soft Tissue Landmarks — 244
References — 288

6 3D Analysis of Soft Tissues — 289
Esthetic Analysis of Soft Tissues Using 3D Cephalometry — 290
Diagnostic 3D Analysis of Soft Tissues with Multiplanar
 Cephalometric Analysis: Clinical Cases — 332
References — 350

7 3D Analysis of the Temporomandibular Joint — 353
Anatomy and Pathology of the TMJ — 354
Radiologic Examinations of the TMJ — 357
References — 369

8 3D Analysis of Airway Spaces — 371
Obstructive Sleep Apnea — 372
Risk Factors for Obstruction of the Airways and Development of OSA — 372
References — 380

9 3D Analysis of Impacted Teeth — 381
Impaction of the Permanent Maxillary Canine — 382
3D Imaging and Diagnosis of Impacted Mandibular Third Molars — 422
References — 447

10 CBCT in Periodontology — 453
References — 462

11 CBCT in Endodontics — 463
Imaging in Endodontics — 464
Cone Beam Computed Tomography in Endodontics — 467
References — 485

12 Computer-Assisted Guided Surgery: Indications and Limitations — 491
Analysis of Guided-Surgery Systems — 501
References — 535

13 CBCT: Medicolegal Issues — 537

Basic Principles for the Use of CBCT in Dentistry

G Perrotti
M Politi

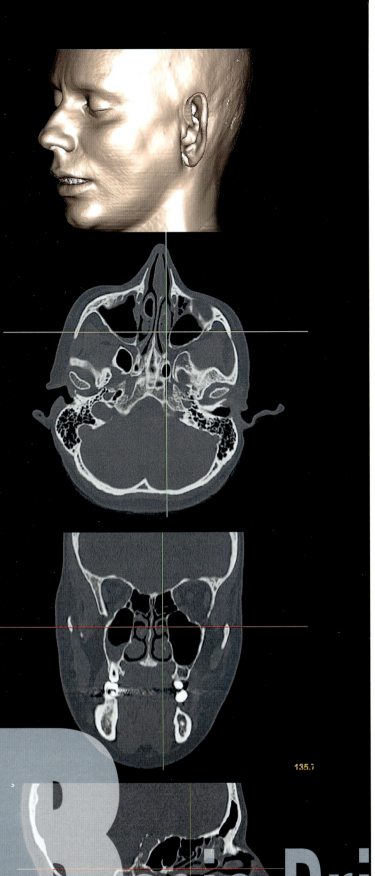

Three-dimensional radiologic examinations in dentistry are performed using computed tomography (CT) and cone beam computed tomography (CBCT). The American Dental Association Council on Scientific Affairs has recently published guidelines on higher radiosensitivity in pediatric patients. The recommendations include the following general strategies: *(1)* assessing the patient's history, clinical examination, already-available radiographs, and clinical status to ascertain that the diagnostic benefits outweigh radiation risks, thus justifying this test on a case-by-case basis; *(2)* prescribing CBCT only in patients whose clinical needs cannot be adequately addressed using conventional radiographs with a lower radiation dose (eg, intraoral or panoramic radiographs) and never as a screening or routine exam; *(3)* avoiding additional two-dimensional (2D) radiographs when a recent CBCT image of the same area is available; *(4)* quantifying the radiation risk by comparing the dose delivered by CBCT with other types of radiographs (eg, panoramic or CT images) and with equivalent environmental radiation and explaining risks and benefits to patients; *(5)* minimizing exposure by knowing how the scanner and patient protection devices operate; *(6)* acquiring adequate skills to perform and interpret CBCT with training and refresher courses as needed by the operator so as to interpret the whole volume displayed. These six items have guided the authors in writing the following chapters, starting with the basic principles and technical skills in three-dimensional (3D) radiology.

Principles of Digital Radiology

Diagnosis is an essential requirement in orthodontics to develop a complete, individualized treatment plan. An accurate and exhaustive diagnosis includes, besides the collection of the patient's history and clinical examination, the acquisition of optimal radiologic images to assess the various treatment options and to monitor and document treatment progress, final results, and the stability of the results over time.

In 1931 Broadbent[1] introduced cephalometric analysis as a tool for qualitative and quantitative assessment of patients and, in his article "A New X-ray Technique and Its Application to Orthodontia," he stated that it is important to analyze dental and dentofacial structures with two cephalometric projections, posteroanterior and lateral, to get the best possible vision of skull anatomy. He also introduced for the first time a craniostat capable of reducing distortion and standardizing the radiologic procedure.

Even though over time they have become the gold standard in diagnosis and evaluation of results, conventional radiographs cannot display anatomical and anatomopathologic structures very accurately, as these structures are always three-dimensional and, lacking the third dimension, plane geometry is not suitable for visualizing solid structures.

2D diagnostic images such as skull radiographs in various projections, cephalometric tracings, and intra- and extraoral clinical pictures have been part of orthodontic patients' records for decades. The limitations in the analysis of these images are well known; they include geometric distortions, enlargements, overlapping of structures, and projection dislocation (which can lengthen or distort the dimensions of the object perceived).

The possibility of acquiring radiologic images in three spatial planes—sagittal, coronal, and axial—has revolutionized the medical-diagnostic field. Over the last 10 years the introduction of CBCT devoted to specific imaging has made 3D imaging applicable to many fields, broadening the range of patients who can undergo this radiologic exam in the fields of implant dentistry, surgery, otorhinolaryngology, and maxillofacial and orthodontic medicine.

The aim of this book is to assess clinically and statistically a 3D system of cephalometric analysis to verify the linear measures obtained with images derived from a CBCT and CT file dataset and to compare them with a conventional 2D cephalometric system based on cephalometric images in lateral projection obtained by synthesizing Digital Imaging and Communications in Medicine (DICOM)[2] files from the same dataset.

X-Rays

Wilhelm Roentgen discovered x-rays by chance on a November evening in 1895. Roentgen was studying the phenomena that happen when electricity passes through gas at a very low pressure. He was working in a dark room and had fully wrapped the discharge tube in a thick sheet of black cardboard to eliminate any light when a sheet of paper covered with a phosphorescent substance on one side placed on a table nearby just by chance suddenly became fluorescent.

He explained the phenomenon as being due to the emission of invisible rays exciting fluorescence from the discharge tube. X-rays are a form of electromagnetic radiation, a category that also includes visible light, radio waves, microwaves, cosmic rays, and some other varieties. They are all made of "energy packets" called photons that have certain properties, the most important being wavelength and frequency. Electromagnetic rays can have different wavelengths, ranging from 10^{-13} to 10^3 m; X-rays are within the 10^{-13} to 10^{-9} m range. Very importantly, the shorter the wavelength the greater the energy they contain, the deeper they penetrate into matter, and the more energy they transfer to matter itself. When x-rays with this energy hit atoms, they trigger atomic ionization. When patients undergo radiologic investigations, millions of photons cross their bodies, which can damage some molecules, noticeably DNA, because of ionization. Most of the DNA is immediately repaired; only very seldomly is a chromosome section damaged permanently. When this happens, it can lead to altered cell duplication and permanent alterations, inducing neoplastic degeneration. The latency period between exposure to x-rays and clinical diagnosis of a neoplastic condition is several years. The risk of neoplasm, of course, depends on the dose of x-rays to which people are exposed.

Units of Measurement and X-Ray Exposure

The dose of x-rays absorbed can be measured for specific tissues or organs (skin, eyes, bones, marrow, etc) or for the whole body. Exposure refers to the machine setup (time, mA, kV). A commonly used unit is the dose delivered measured in grays (Gy; usually measured in mGy), which is estimated by applying dosimeters on the skin of patients.

The radiation dose is commonly expressed as an effective dose, measured in units of energy delivered per unit of mass (joules/kg) and called a sievert (Sv; usually measured as μSv). The effective dose is calculated for each x-ray technique by measuring the energy delivered to a number of key tissues or organs. The dose for each organ is then multiplied by a charge factor, which is defined as a specific function of its radiosensitivity. All of these values are combined to calculate the total detrimental effect. It is not possible to clinically calculate the effective dose in vivo; it can only be inferred from laboratory studies. Many investigations have been carried out to measure the dosage of x-rays in dental radiographs, but only some have estimated the effective dose, and most did not use charge factors. The radiation damage can be considered as the total damage suffered by an individual exposed to x-rays. In addition to tissue damage, stochastic effects of radiation include the nominal risk of tumors and inheritable effects. The likelihood that radiation induces stochastic effects in the entire population is 5.7×10^{-2} Sv^{-1}. The risk estimate is defined as nominal because it refers to exposure of a nominal population of men and women with a predefined age distribution, calculated from mean values for the various age brackets and both genders.

The risk is age-dependent; it is higher for the young and lower for the old. For persons aged 80 years and older, the risk becomes negligible because the latency period between x-ray exposure and clinical presentation of tumors is likely to be longer than the patient's residual life. Conversely, the tissues of the young are more radiosensitive, and their life expectancy is likely to be longer than the latency period.

The data in Table 1-1 are derived from International Commission on Radiological Protection (ICRP) 1990 recommendations and reflect a relative risk of 1 at age 30 years (population average risk).[3]

In medicine, especially in diagnostic radiology, the acronym ALARA (as low as reasonably achievable)[4] is used to refer to the minimum useful dose of radiation that must be delivered to acquire the information necessary for the diagnosis and treatment of patients.

To optimize the performance of radiodiagnostic exams, reference diagnostic levels (RDL) should be considered according to the guidelines (Table 1-2). Among many risks, we are all exposed to normal background radiation (on average about 2,400 µSv every year according to the European Commission 2001 worldwide average values).

Patients do not benefit at all from receiving the excessive quantity of radiation associated with conventional CT scans, but the development of CBCT has allowed the delivered radiation dose[5–7] to be reduced considerably.

Table 1-1 Age-related risk[3]	
Age (years)	Risk-factor multiplier
<10	X 3
10-20	X 2
20-30	X 1.5
30-50	X 0.5
50-80	X 0.3
80+	Negligible risk

Table 1-2 Reference diagnostic levels of skull cephalometric radiographs[4]

	Exam	Absorbed dose (mGy)
Adult patients	Skull, AP view	5
	Skull, PA view	5
	Skull, lateral view	3
Pediatric patients (5 years)	Skull, PA/AP views	1.5
	Skull, lateral view	1

AP = anteroposterior; PA = posteroanterior.

Volumetric CBCT, because of the higher resolution of its detectors and the high intrinsic contrast of bone structures, allows the clinician to obtain good-quality images of these structures while delivering lower doses to patients than those usually administered by CT machines with standard setups (5 to 20 times lower doses for the same radiated volume). The dosages and radiation risks arising from CBCT are usually higher than with conventional dental (intraoral, panoramic, and cephalometric) radiographs, but they are nevertheless lower than that of conventional CT. Table 1-3 shows the effective dose for conventional imaging and multislice CT (MSCT).

Most of the studies in Table 1-3 were based on thermoluminescent dosimetry (TLD) using standard dummies. They differed greatly in methodology, most of all with reference to the type of dummies used and the number and position of TLD dosimeters applied. Furthermore, the effect of the number and position of TLD dosimeters placed was not well documented.

Table 1-3 Effective dose in conventional dental exams[3,8,9]

Type	Effective dose (in μSv)	References
Intraoral radiograph	≤ 8.3	
Panoramic radiograph	2.7–2.3	Ludlow et al 2006, Okano et al 2009, Silva et al 2008, Palomo et al 2008, Garcia-Silva et al 2008
Lateral radiograph	30	Compagnone et al 2006
Posteroanterior radiograph	40	Compagnone et al 2009
CT, full head		
Somatom Volume Zoom 4 (Siemens)	1,100	Ludlow et al 2009
Somatom Sensation 16 (Siemens)	995	
Mx-8000 IDT (Philips)	1,160	
CT, maxillomandibular	180–2,100	Ludlow et al 2009, Okano et al 2009, Silva et al 2008, Loubele et al 2005
CT, maxilla	1,400	Ludlow et al 2006

The dose fundamentally depends on two things:

- Exposure settings, in particular the field of view (FOV) selected
- The type of equipment

The exposure to radiation in CBCT scans is markedly lower than in spiral CT, but image resolution[3,10,11] is definitely worse. A review of the literature performed by the SEDENTEXCT Project includes 11 papers in which CBCT dosimetry was obtained by calculating the effective dose using tissue charge factors given by ICRP (2007)[3] (Table 1-4). Projection radiographs provide a 2D representation of 3D cranial structures and, for each projection, only allow a 2D assessment (Fig 1-1).

CBCT scans must nevertheless be justified for each patient, proving that benefits outweigh risks; they should add new information to 2D exams[12,13] to improve planning of the patient's treatment.

Table 1-4 Range of effective dose of the various CBCT machines in μSv*

CBCT unit	Effective dose (μSv) Dentoalveolar	Craniofacial	References Dentoalveolar	Craniofacial
NewTom 3G (Quantitative Radiology)	41–75	30–78	Ludlow et al 2003	
Accuitomo/Veraviewepocs (Morita)	11–102		Okano et al 2009 Loftag-Hanese et al 2008 Hirsh et al 2008 Loubele et al 2008	
Galileos (Sirona)		70–128		Ludlow et al 2008
ProMax (PlanMeca)	488–652		Ludlow et al 2008	
PreXion (Terarecon)	189–388		Ludlow et al 2008	
CB MercuRay (Hitachi)	407	283–1,073	Ludlow et al 2008	Ludlow et al 2006 Okano et al 2009 Ludlow et al 2008
Iluma (Imtec Imaging)		98–498		Ludlow et al 2008

*The studies have been divided into dentoalveolar (using a smaller FOV) and craniofacial (with the FOV covering the whole face).[3]

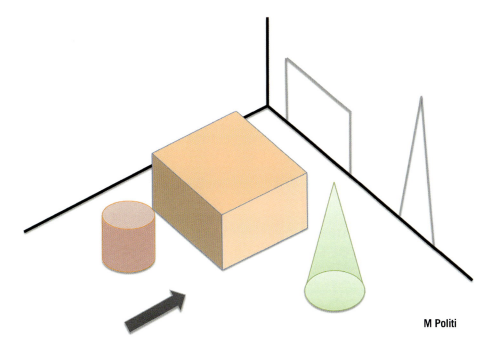

Fig 1-1 The information provided by one projection is not sufficient to get a sense of the 3D structure under investigation.

M Politi

Computed Tomography

The invention of computed tomography by Sir Godfrey Hounsfield in the early 1970s has been considered by many as the greatest step forward in the field of radiology after the discovery of x-rays. Using this new technique, he could obtain a cross-axial image of the head using a beam of strictly collimated x-rays in motion.

The first computed tomography units used allowed only the study of cranial structures. It was installed at Atkinson Morley Hospital of London in 1971, and it was only used to investigate and study brain conditions.

CT is an x-ray tomographic method based on the attenuation of a radiating beam crossing thin axial sections of the patient in many angles. The basic principle of CT lies in the possibility of reconstructing a 3D image by combining a great number of 2D axial images.

In its simplest form, a CT scanner is composed of two parts: sensors and a gantry containing a tube that emits rays.

The gantry turns around the bed where the patient lies, and the beam of emitted x-rays is strictly collimated and aimed at a series of scintillation detectors or ionization chambers. After each rotation of the gantry, the bed is advanced a few millimeters until the volume under investigation has been completely exposed (Fig 1-2).

Depending on the mechanical layout of the scanner, we can distinguish four generations of CT scanners. The first two generations of CT scanners were replaced at the end of the 1970s by third- and fourth-generation scanners, which are still in use. In third- and fourth-generation CT units, the ray-emitting tube and the array of detectors rotate synchronously around the patient. The row of detectors covers the whole width of the rotating beam.

In fourth-generation units, the crown of detectors covers the circumference of the gantry and does not move during scanning; only the gantry rotates around the patient. Attenuation occurs partly due to energy absorption by the structures crossed by x-rays and partly by x-ray scattering.

Attenuation can be expressed by the following equation:

$$I = I0e^{-md}$$

where I is the intensity of the rays transmitted (ie, radiation exiting the tissues), $I0$ is the intensity of incident rays (entering the tissues), m is the so-called total linear factor of tissue attenuation, and d is the distance

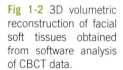

Fig 1-2 3D volumetric reconstruction of facial soft tissues obtained from software analysis of CBCT data.

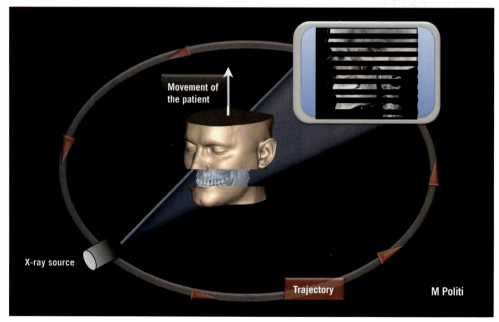

covered by rays crossing tissues (tissue thickness).

The factor of attenuation m is determined by the atomic number and the density of electrons in tissues. The higher the density, the atomic number, and the quantity of electrons, the higher the factor of attenuation. The atomic number and the density of electrons are therefore two parameters determining the radiographic attenuation property of tissues. It should be considered that the factor of attenuation also depends on the energy of the x-rays.

The gantry, ie, the structure containing the scanning device, can be tilted by ± 30 degrees to make oblique scans, and this angle is most often used to investigate head, neck, and spinal marrow.

The beam collimation settings drive the thickness of the CT section, but the gantry emits a cone beam of diverging rather than parallel rays. To obtain slices of a reasonably even thickness, it is necessary to use collimators inside the gantry; in some CT units there are additional postpatient collimators to optimize the section profile.

The ideal section profile is a rectangle whose height perfectly corresponds to the desired slice thickness so that all points outside of it do not contribute to the attenuation measured while the points inside it contribute to CT 5 numbers.

The section profiles actually have round edges, which means that adjacent regions contribute to generating an image.

The detectors measure attenuation values of the rays emerging from the examined body. In conventional CTs, the detector was single-layered and voxels were anisotropic, while nowadays systems with double or split detectors are based on an array of detectors, which are twice as wide as a conventional CT detector and split in the middle. Real multidetector or multilayer systems can acquire at least four sections simultaneously.[14]

During image processing, a CT number is assigned to each voxel depending on the degree of x-ray attenuation of that specific voxel.

The CT number is defined as:

$$1{,}000 \times (\mu - \mu_{water})/\mu_{water}$$

The unit of measurement for CT attenuation is called the Hounsfield unit (HU). The values are arranged according to a scale where −1,000 represents air attenuation and 0 is water attenuation. The scale maximum value is not predefined, and the range of CT numbers varies depending on the number of bits per pixel in the tomograph (eg, from −1,024 to 3,071 HU with 12 bits or up to 64,500 HU for 16 bits).

Reconstruction algorithms or convolution filters, called kernels, are used to reconstruct images starting from raw data and determine the ratio between spatial resolution and image background noise. Background noise limits contrast resolution and hence the capability of differentiating objects showing minimal attenuation differences from surrounding objects.

Kernels can be hard or soft: high-definition hard ones enhance spatial resolution but also disproportionately increase image background noise; soft or smooth ones reduce background noise but also spatial resolution.

Spiral CT

Spiral CT consists of a gantry capable of rotating continuously. The patient is not scanned plane by plane but instead is advanced along the scanning plane, with the bed being pushed forward at an even speed while raw data are acquired.

The advantages of spiral CT are continuous acquisition of data and short scanning time. Most of the drawbacks of spiral CT depend on the use of old tomographs requiring a reduced x-ray dose at each rotation, which can induce an increase in the background noise of the image.

The space between the reconstructed sections is called the interval, increment, or reconstruction index. It is worth remembering that the reconstruction interval has nothing to do with the collimation of the beam and the thickness of the layer; rather, it defines how much the axial sections overlap.

While in conventional CT the patient's bed is moved between one scan and the other, in spiral CT the table is advanced at each gantry rotation; this is known as the table increment (Fig 1-3). The ratio between collimation and table advancement is called the pitch, and two rules have to be considered:

1. If the pitch is slightly < 1: the dose of rays absorbed by the patient increases, but the quality of images improves.
2. If the pitch is > 2, the target volume will be undersampled with inevitable creation of artifacts.

Depending on circumstances, either of these two may be preferred.

The maximum scanning time in spiral CT depends on the gantry: the higher the required dose, the shorter the available scanning time.

Cone Beam Computed Tomography

Although CBCT has existed for about 25 years, only in the last 10 years have these machines experienced great technical advancements, with structural changes promoting their growth in the clinical dental and maxillofacial fields. Current tomographs are characterized by several features:

- Development of a compact, relatively cheap, and high-quality detector system

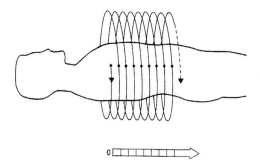

Fig 1-3 Patient scanning: the horizontal arrow shows the advancement of the patient's bed during data acquisition.

- Enough processing power to reconstruct cone beam images
- Manufacturing of highly efficient gantries capable of multiple exposures
- Limited scanning volumes (eg, head and neck), thus eliminating the need for a portal with rotation speed below 1 second

The first CBCT system marketed for oral and maxillofacial imaging in 1998[10] was the NewTom (Quantitative Radiology). It was also the first approved by the Food and Drug Administration (FDA) in April 2001.

Cone beam tomographs can have different layouts: some look like conventional CT units such as the NewTom DVT 9000 (Quantitative Radiology), while others look like panoramic radiograph units where the patient sits (i-CAT, Imaging Sciences; Accuitomo, Morita; Scanora, Soredex) or stands (ProMax, PlanMeca; Galileos, Sirona).

These machines are very different from conventional computed tomographs in terms of the way that images are acquired. The whole volume is not reconstructed from a progressive scan along the z-axis using a collimated beam, but instead through a single 360-degree pendular movement of a cone beam, hence the name *cone beam tomography* (Fig 1-4).

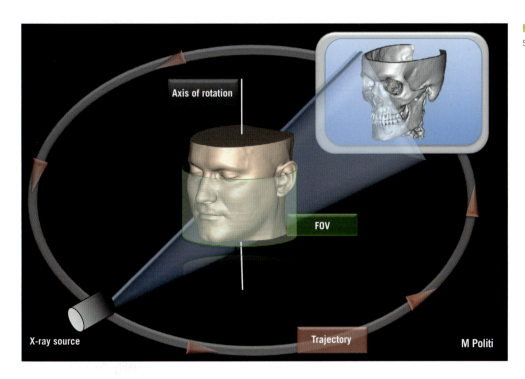

Fig 1-4 Cone beam scanning layout.[15]

The cone beam covers the whole target area with the possibility of selecting different FOVs.
The size of the FOV can vary according to the region under investigation (Fig 1-5):

- Small: often used for examining single teeth, for instance impacted teeth, root morphology, supernumerary teeth, etc, or potential recipient sites for implants or temporary anchorage devices (TADs).
- Medium: includes the mandible, superior maxilla, or both; commonly used to obtain information about occlusion relationships or facial asymmetries, when bilateral temporomandibular joint (TMJ) assessment is needed, or, in general, when the overall status of basal bone in the maxilla needs to be assessed.
- Large: includes the entire head. This FOV helps clinicians to visualize the relationships among skeletal frameworks and between teeth and skeletal frameworks and to assess patients with severe face dysmorphism requiring orthognathic surgery or patients needing maxillofacial surgery in general.[16]

It is therefore important when prescribing this exam to select the proper FOV, as an error could expose the patient to an ineffective radiation load for the diagnostic goals.
If the entire maxillofacial structure including TMJs must be examined, the use of a caliper can help clinicians in selecting the proper FOV.
In patients who have completed their growth, a 15-cm area is often inadequate to include the TMJ area.

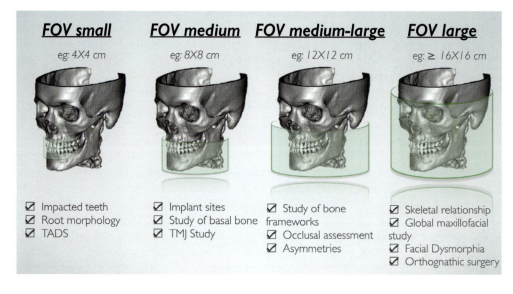

Fig 1-5 Representation of the main FOV required.

The scanning time is variable depending on the type of equipment used and the desired CT resolution. Radiologic acquisition allows visualization of a cylindric volume, which can have different sizes according to the FOV selected: 4 to 24 cm in height and 4 to 21 cm in diameter.

The detection system used can be of two essential types:

1. Flat detector panels (FDPs): allow direct x-ray conversion into a high spatial-resolution digital signal. It consists of a crystal panel with scintillators immersed in a photodiode matrix incorporated in a layer of amorphous solid silicon (aSi:H) or a layer of selenium. Incident x-rays are photochemically converted into light by the scintillating film. The light is directly transmitted to the photodiodes, where the charge intensity signal has been saved. Transistors in the aSi:H layers transmit a signal of intensity proportional to the charge saved in the photodiodes, which is in turn proportional for incident photons on the scintillator layer.
2. Charge coupling sensors (brilliancy intensifiers): the system detects the x-ray image and converts it into a visible-light image, which is then transferred to a charge-coupled device (CCD) camera to be displayed on a monitor.

The FPD detector potentially offers higher space resolution with comparable intensity of background noise as opposed to its intensifier/charge coupler predecessors.[17]

These sensors are directly connected to a computer. Their use is very similar to that of video cameras. Their property is to convert x-rays or light into an electrical signal, which is transferred by cable and analyzed by the electronic processor.

The origin of each signal from the surface sensor is known and codified. The computer easily reconstructs the radiographic matrix received from the sensor and, therefore, also the image of the object crossed by x-rays.

The image is thus visualized on the display of the processor almost in real time, with an evident benefit from a diagnostic and clinical point of view (eg, monitoring during surgical procedures), and it can be later printed out or stored in digital format. Reconstruction algorithms in tomographic imaging allow the clinician to obtain multidimensional images by inverting one-dimensional projection data. The most commonly used reconstruction formula for CBCT is the modified Feldkamp algorithm.[18]

The Feldkamp algorithm is essentially a 3D adaptation of the filtered retroprojection method used in 2D fan-beam reconstructions.[11,19]

The filtering or convolution process entails application of a kernel or mathematical filter to the projection of data before they are retroprojected. Filtering reduces blurring, which is otherwise present in the retroprojection process.

Raw data as acquired by scanning are processed by the computer and quantified in small cubes called voxels, which consist of elementary information (Fig 1-6). The computer software is capable of selecting any sequence of voxels and changing their spatial arrangement with a simple cursor to produce sections on three orthogonal planes, axial, coronal, and sagittal, which are called secondary or multiplanar reconstructions.

Multiplanar reconstructions in turn allow the redistribution of voxels on many other planes, bending them until panoramic-like images of the mandible and other target structures are obtained together with actual 3D reconstructions.

2D images are basically represented on three planes (axial, sagittal, and coronal), but the various software systems can process images on panoramic-like and radial planes, as seen with the Dentalscan program, or on oblique planes, as for a TMJ study.

In many of these software systems there are preinstalled algorithms to manipulate images, and from these we can obtain various reconstructions starting from a DICOM file.

- Panoramic-like image: this is similar to a panoramic radiograph, but it is much sharper as there is no overlapping of the spinal column and no projection artifacts like the "burnout" areas that are often observed in the anterior region.[20]
- Multiplanar reconstruction (MPR): multiplanar reconstructions are 2D images reconstructed from a series of axial image data. Coronal and sagittal reconstructions are generated by extracting and visualizing from the mass of data only the voxels that are placed one upon the other within the coronal or sagittal planes.
- Ray-sum: the mean value of CT numbers in one direction is calculated, or these numbers are added. The result simulates a conventional radiograph of the sectioned volume.
- Maximum intensity projection (MIP): see DICOM File Synthesis later in this chapter.
- Volume rendering techniques (3DVRT): these assign a range of density values to CT numbers, thus providing a better definition of objects or a semitransparent visualization of structures. This creates a realistic visualization of 3D volumetric data, therefore allowing the detection of conditions and assessment of anatomical relations.

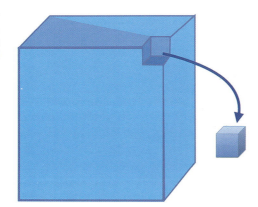

Fig 1-6 Representation of isotropic voxels, which are the same size in all three spatial dimensions.

Image Postprocessing

DICOM

At the beginning of the 1980s, the American College of Radiology and the National Electrical Manufacturers Association joined their efforts to standardize the encoding of images obtained with CT and magnetic resonance imaging (MRI).
After some improvements, in 1993 the term Digital Imaging and Communications in Medicine (DICOM) was coined.[21]
DICOM data consist of:

- A DICOMDIR (DICOM directory) file, including information on a patient, information on the specifications for acquiring images, and a list of images corresponding to the axial slices comprising the 3D images
- A number of sequentially codified images corresponding to the axial slices

After scanning, the radiologic unit allows, through its software, the data to be converted from its own format into a DICOM file that can be exported; this is the first step in managing 3D data.[22]
The DICOM file is then uploaded into dedicated software systems that have tracing, viewing, and many other tools, allowing clinicians to obtain all the information necessary to plan an ideal treatment.

Management of DICOM Files

The data produced by CT, whether standard or volumetric, are sets of images representing axial slices.
These images are usually printed out on large films and then viewed like conventional 2D images; even if these images make it easier to visualize the various anatomical structures, we need to get back to 3D data in raw format to do a quantitative analysis.
A digital radiograph is composed of pixels, or small square elements distributed in rows and columns (Fig 1-7).

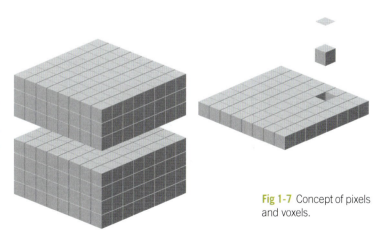

Fig 1-7 Concept of pixels and voxels.

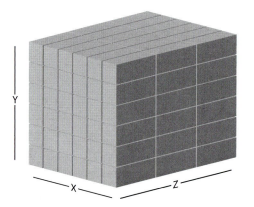

Fig 1-8 Graphic representation of anisotropic voxels.

Each pixel has a brightness or color value in the scale of gray representing the density of x-rays of the corresponding structure. If one includes the third dimension, a volume is obtained, and when this is acquired, it can be broken down into many primary structures called voxels. Each voxel, like a pixel, represents a certain level of x-ray absorption.

The size of voxels influences image resolution: the smaller they are, the higher the image resolution. In conventional CT, voxels are anisotropic, ie, unequal in the three dimensions, as the greatest dimension is given by the slice thickness on the axial plane (Fig 1-8). Even if the voxel surface can be reduced to 0.625 mm^2, the depth usually ranges between 1 and 2 mm.

With the advent of MSCT, CT voxels are isotropic, ie, equal in the three x, y, and z dimensions, as with CBCT. Cone beam tomography produces isotropic voxels whose dimensions can vary between 75 and 300 μm, allowing for resolution in the 0.4- to 0.07-mm range.

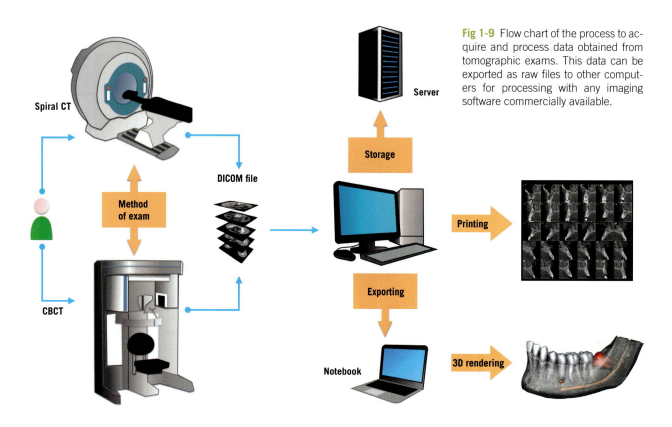

Fig 1-9 Flow chart of the process to acquire and process data obtained from tomographic exams. This data can be exported as raw files to other computers for processing with any imaging software commercially available.

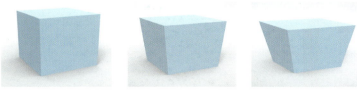

Figure 1-9 summarizes the postprocessing of images.

It therefore can be concluded that the quality of images in CBCT is not superior to that of spiral CT, but it is nevertheless more than satisfactory, most of all in the assessment of hard tissues.[23,24]

3D Volume Reconstruction

Numeric reconstruction algorithms in volumetric radiologic equipment and dedicated software systems receive raw data produced by the radiologic instrument and process the data appropriately, producing a density or radiopacity associated with each voxel comprising the irradiated volume.

First, we know that a 3D object needs a 3D space.

It is therefore as if we were to take a photo of the object and draw it. This task is performed by the software, which projects the object on the monitor in two different ways (Fig 1-10):

1. Perspective mode: similar to what we would see with our own eyes
2. Orthogonal mode: maintains the dimensions of the parts of the object, irrespective of their distance from the monitor, so that parallel lines remain parallel

The latter mode is used by software systems to prevent changes in the shape and size of structures according to the visual angle.

Perspective projections (Fig 1-11) can be generated by changing the parallel lines used to generate orthogonal projections with voxel lines that diverge from a visible point behind the apparent volume at such a distance that, on the display, the observer

Fig 1-10 Orthogonal, perspective, and highly perspective object projections (left to right).

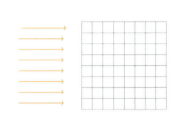

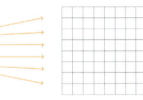

Fig 1-11 Parallel and perspective projections, with visualization of the lateral view of voxels and the observing eye in front of the display.

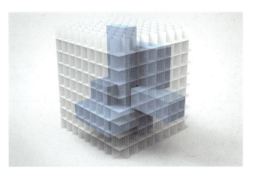

Fig 1-12 Volume composed of voxels. Some voxels are transparent so as to show the object inside.

can see the smallest characteristics the object is taking on, depending on its position. For instance, it can be deeper or shallower in some parts than in others.

The volumetric data acquired by CT or MRI does not contain only the target structures; they also represent the space enclosing an object (Fig 1-12). They are composed of external voxels that have absorbed a small dose of rays (the air around the patient's head); therefore, they are black.

To reach the target structures, external voxels are eliminated, but unfortunately their value is not a good indicator of the corresponding histologic tissues because a voxel can contain more than one type of tissue (eg, mucosae, bone, and muscle).

The relationship between transparence of a voxel and its value is specified by the transfer function, which is a mathematical formula coupling the value of a voxel and its transparence value. It can be simple or complex.

The transfer functions not only can use the value of single voxels, but they can also be combined with other data such as the values of adjacent voxels, in an attempt to improve the segmentation of an object. An example is the selection of voxels lying on the surface between two different structures (skin surface).

The visualization of the 3D object is based on a threshold filter identifying the critical value dividing voxels into visible and invisible ones. After selecting the filter, the software will create the 3D image accordingly.

More filters can be applied to the same image to distinguish tissues with different densities. Transparence is an option that allows visualization of hard tissues through soft tissues (which are made transparent).

The visualization of an object can be influenced by several factors:

- The image contrast
- The image background noise caused by collimation of the ray beam and the voxel thickness
- The threshold filter applied by the operator

There are two methods for reconstructing an object so that it can be viewed: *(1)* 3D surface rendering (shaded surface display) and *(2)* volume rendering technique.

3D Surface Rendering (Shaded Surface Display)

This method represents the superficial reconstruction of our target object/subject, giving a realistic 3D visualization of the surface structure within the mass of acquired data. This method allows separation of the target object from its background. It is called *segmentation*, and it can be simple or very complex depending on the contrast of the object, which can vary according to two factors:

- The CT number of the target structure
- The difference between the CT number of the object and the background density (Fig 1-13)

Both the shaded surface display and the volume rendering technique require segmentation to define the target volume and to separate it from the structures that must not be displayed on the 3D image (Fig 1-14).

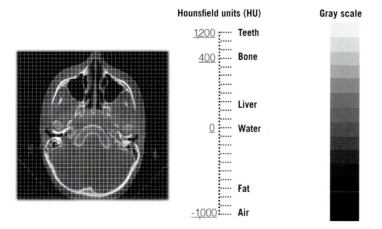

Fig 1-13 Hounsfield scale.

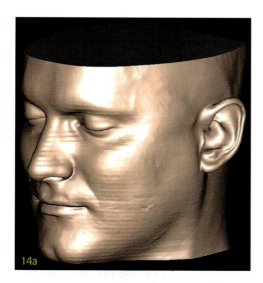

Fig 1-14a Soft tissue segmentation of the patient.

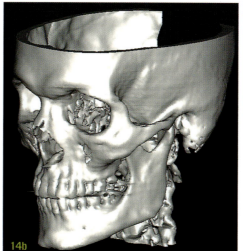

Fig 1-14b Hard tissue segmentation of the patient.

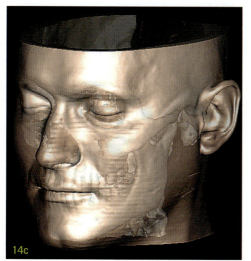
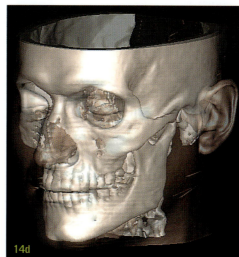

Figs 1-14c and 1-14d Two kinds of transparence filters have been used: a low one *(c)* and a medium one *(d)* to obtain a global view of the object acquired, including both soft and hard tissues.

There are several factors influencing segmentation:

- Bone thickness and mineralization
- Space resolution and image contrast
- Software reconstruction algorithm
- Scattering (a phenomenon whereby some rays exit the absorbing body, after having crossed it, in directions different from the incident beam; this is called scattered radiation and can be caused by implants, crowns, and amalgam fillings)
- Dexterity and experience of the operator

Figure 1-15 shows examples of the scattering phenomenon.

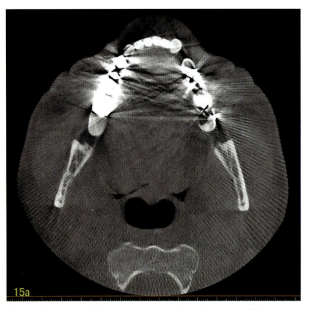
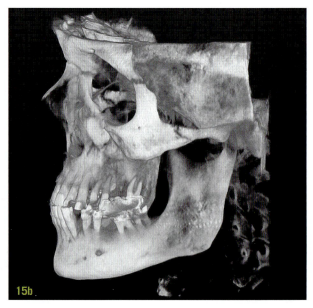

Figs 1-15a and 1-15b Both the axial slice *(a)* and the 3D rendering *(b)* show how the presence of metallic elements causes background noise, potentially leading to severe loss of information.

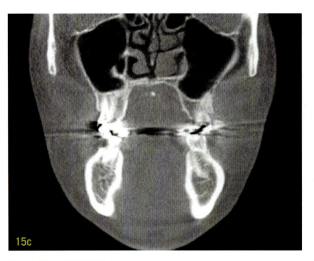
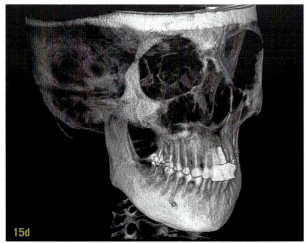

Figs 1-15c and 1-15d Another example of metallic elements causing "noise" in the image: *(c)* coronal section; *(d)* 3D rendering.

One of the segmentation methods entails the use of a threshold filter that identifies the critical value, or the range where voxels are visible while the mass of external data are made invisible.

The ideal threshold value for segmentation is the value showing a structure in its real size. In theory, the optimal value is nothing else but the mean value between that of the target object and that of surrounding structures.

The thickness of the CT section plays a fundamental role because it is strictly correlated to the accuracy in the 3D reconstruction of a surface; as the section thickness increases, a greater number of elements in the structure will be displayed incorrectly. Threshold-setting errors can be due to several factors:

- Poor process accuracy
- Excessively long time required to perform object segmentation correctly
- Lack of experience of the operator

When the threshold is lowered, more voxels contribute to the image of the structure, thus increasing the apparent diameter and volume of the structure. This offsets partial-volume effects and allows the smallest structures to be displayed realistically (Figs 1-16 and 1-17).

If on the contrary the threshold value is too low, and the CT number of the single pixels exceeds the threshold in relation to the background noise of the image, so-called flying pixels will be displayed (Fig 1-18a).

When the threshold is raised, a smaller number of pixels contributes to recon-

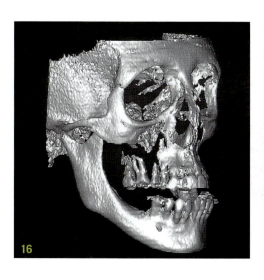

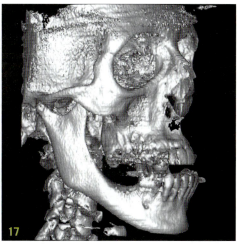

Fig 1-16 An example of error in segmentation: because of the low density in the maxilla, the maxillary molars are suspended in space.

Fig 1-17 Modifying the threshold value during segmentation, ie, using a correct value, makes it possible to obtain a realistic object reconstruction without molars that are suspended in space.

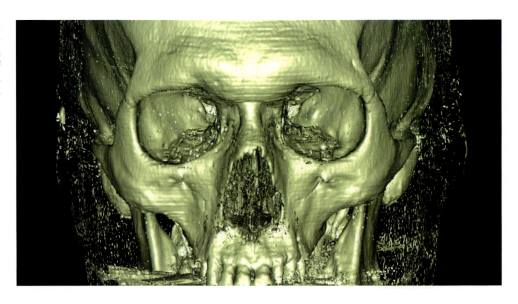

Fig 1-18a 3D image in which excessive lowering of the threshold has caused the presence of so-called flying pixels, impairing clear segmentation.

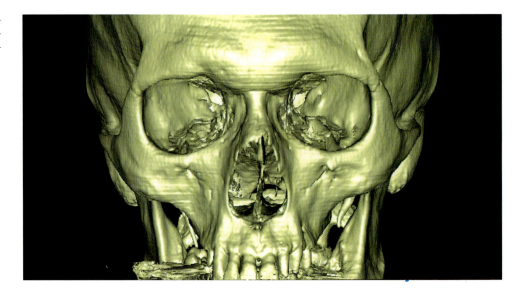

Fig 1-18b The same image using a higher segmentation threshold, resulting in no flying pixels.

structing the structure, thus reducing its apparent diameter and volume (Fig 1-18b). Low-density structures and flying pixels are eliminated, but artifacts like pseudodefects, bone dehiscences, or fenestrations can appear in the 3D rendering.

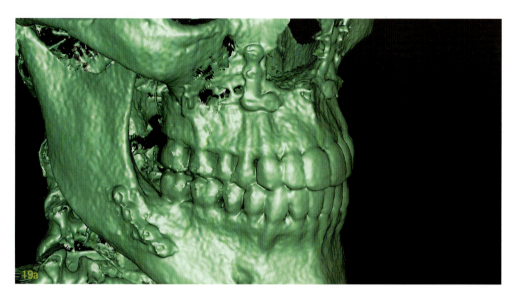

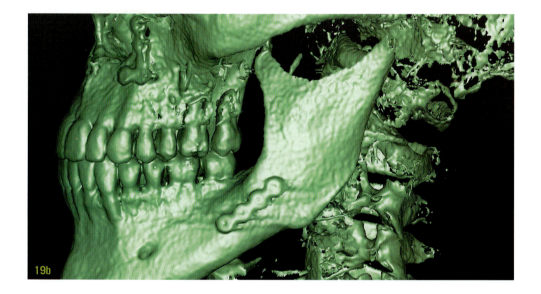

Figs 1-19a and 1-19b Right (a) and left (b) lateral views showing that, with the same threshold, there can be different densities at the level of the tuberosity.

The two structures that are most at risk are the the maxilla and the mandibular condyle (Fig 1-19).
In the maxilla, variation in density of the bone, especially in the palate and tuberosity, can create severe artifacts like fenestrations or bone defects (Fig 1-20).

The mandibular condyle is very difficult to display because of its anatomical structure, which consists primarily of trabecular bone covered with a very thin layer of cortical bone. It is also difficult to separate the articular disk from the surrounding structures (Fig 1-21).

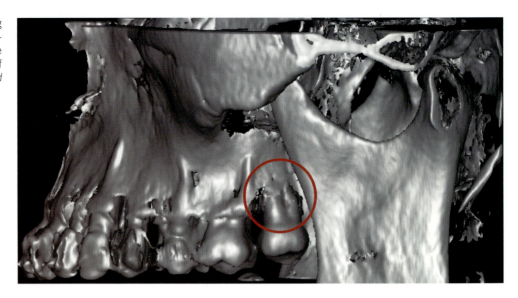

Fig 1-20a 3D rendering in which a periodontal defect seems to be present at the level of the second molar *(red circle)*.

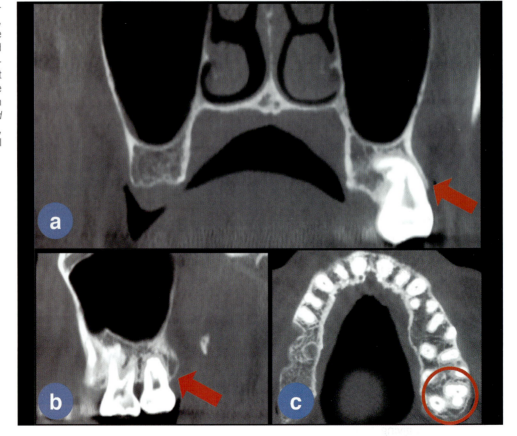

Fig 1-20b Another image of the same patient, showing in detail the bone level in the second molar region; this confirms the use of incorrect segmentation because there is no defect in this image *(arrows and circle)*: a, coronal slice, b, sagittal slice, c, axial slice.

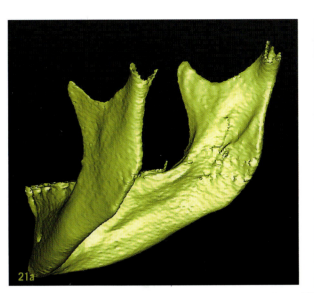 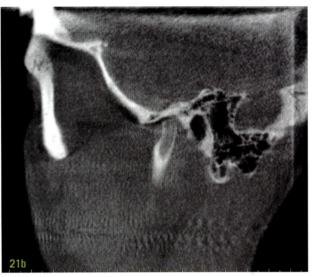

Figs 1-21a and 1-21b The (a) condyle and (b) articular disk are difficult to display.

Volume Rendering Technique

The volume rendering technique (VRT) aims to reproduce the whole volume rather than just surfaces. Potentially, all voxels are visible, but transparence is applied selectively so that we can observe the volume inside.

There are different techniques used to obtain a reconstruction of a 3D object through direct rendering; one of them is called *ray casting*, which takes light rays in the opposite direction, ie, from the computer monitor towards the volume.

For each pixel on the monitor we have a light ray moving towards the volume. As each ray crosses the object, the computer calculates how light is absorbed by the voxels along the way and infers the color of the corresponding pixel on its monitor.

VRTs assign a range of density values to CT numbers, thus giving a better definition of object contours or a semitransparent view of structures.

The quality of the images is high, and the user has a complete range of image effects at his or her disposal.

Shaded surface display techniques are a binary process, ie, only the voxels below the threshold value are displayed, while the rest are assigned a density of zero. In VRT the density values of voxels are continuous, ie, they range from 0% to 100%. The way in which VRT images appear depends on the density curve, which can be manual (more time-consuming) or preselected.

It should always be kept in mind that the actual rendering capabilities depend greatly on the selection of the transfer function, as the voxel value is not sufficient for the separation of different anatomical structures.

DICOM File Synthesis

2D cephalometric radiographs have been used for over a century to evaluate skeletal and dental relations in orthodontics.

A fundamental requisite for this kind of analysis is its reproducibility, which mainly depends on projection and errors in identifying landmarks.[25,26]

With the ongoing development of CT scanners, 3D craniofacial imaging techniques have opened up new opportunities in orthodontic assessment, treatment, and follow-up, allowing very realistic visualization of the morphology in cranial skeletal structures.

Two algorithms are used for synthesizing lateral and posteroanterior radiographs starting from a CBCT/MSCT scan (Fig 1-22).

Ray-sum technique: The 3D data are visualized by the sum of all the values of the voxels encountered from the point of view to the projection plane, dividing this number by the number of voxels (Fig 1-23).

Maximum intensity projection (MIP): The images are obtained by projecting the target volume on a viewing plane and selecting the highest CT numbers in the direction of the projection, or angle of view. Viewing is impaired as this technique conceals less dense structures along the way from the point of view to the projection plane (Fig 1-24).[27]

In studies by Kumar et al both in vivo[28] and on dry skulls[29] it has been shown that cephalometric measurements obtained from synthesized cephalometric radiographs are not different from those of conventional cephalometry.

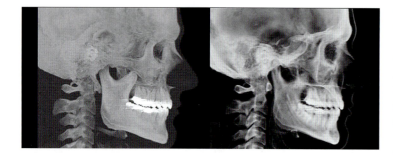

Fig 1-22 CBCT reconstruction of lateral cephalometric radiographs using the MIP *(left)* and ray-sum *(right)* techniques.

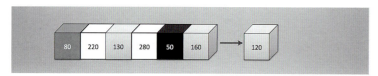

Fig 1-23 Diagram of the ray-sum process of image reconstruction.

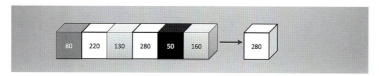

Fig 1-24 Diagram of the MIP process of image reconstruction.

Also, Cattaneo et al[27] showed that there are no statistically significant differences between the results obtained using these two types of cephalometric radiographs.
Cephalometric analysis obtained using the ray-sum method is more reproducible than conventional analysis because of the absence of projection mistakes and errors in landmark identification of similar structures, thus improving the accuracy[22]; moreoever, it is more reliable than MIP, in which less dense structures along the same line of view are concealed.

Furthermore, it is possible to evaluate separately the right and left sections of the skull, thus overcoming the inevitable overlapping of bilateral structures.
In 2D cephalometric radiographs, many landmarks are defined as the highest or lowest point in a structure, and the third dimension in landmark location is not defined. Therefore, it is worth underlining that landmarks should be indicated following strict definitions relating to visualization on three separate slices (Fig 1-25).

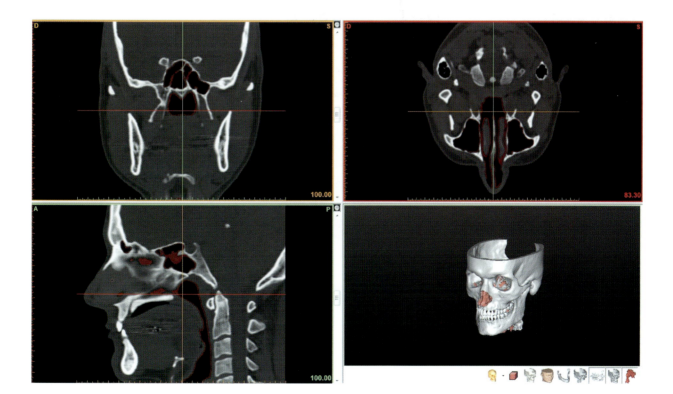

Fig 1-25 MPR software window. The location of a landmark occurs using simultaneous viewing of the axial, coronal, and sagittal slices and surface rendering.

References

1. Broadbent BH. A new x-ray technique and its application to orthodontia. Angle Orthod 1981;51:93–114.
2. Digital Imaging and Communications in Medicine (DICOM). Rosslyn, Virginia: National Electrical Manufacturers Association (NEMA), 2008.
3. SEDENTEXCT Project. Radiation Protection: Cone Beam CT for Dental and Maxillofacial Radiology. Provisional Guidelines (version 1.1 May 2009). http://www.sedentexct.eu/system/files/sedentexct_project_provisional_guidelines.pdf. Accessed 16 December 2009.
4. Zonca G, Pignoli E, Benetti C, Paglia L. La radioprotezione del paziente: Dosi a confronto. Dent Mod 2008;3:62–78.
5. Siewerdsen JH, Jaffray DA. Cone-beam computed tomography with a flat-panel imager. Med Phys 1999;26:2635–2647.
6. Tam KC, Samarasekeva S, Somer F. Exact cone beam CT with a spiral scan. Phys Med Biol 1998;43:1015–1024.
7. Farman AG. ALARA still applies. Oral Surg Oral Med Oral Pathol Oral Radiol Endod 2005;100:395–397.
8. Compagnone G, Angelini P, Pagan L. Monitoring of the medical radiological exposures of the population of the Emilia-Romagna Region. Radiol Med 2006;111:469–480.
9. Loubele M, Bogaerts R, Van Dijck A, et al. Comparison between effective radiation dose of CBCT and MSCT scanners for dentomaxillofacial applications. Eur J Radiol 2009;71:461–468.
10. Mozzo P, Procacci C, Tacconi A, Martini PT, Andreis IA. A new volumetric CT machine for dental imaging based on the cone-beam technique: Preliminary results. Eur Radiol 1998;8:1558–1564.
11. Katsumata A, Fujishita M, Maeda M, Ariji Y, Ariji E, Langlais RP. 3D-CT evaluation of facial asymmetry. Oral Surg Oral Med Oral Pathol Oral Radiol Endod 2005;99:212–220.
12. Hoelberg C, Steinehäuser S, Geis P, Rudzki-Jason I. Cone beam computed tomography in orthodontics: Benefits and limitations. J Oral Orthop 2005;66:434–444.
13. Ludlow JB, Laster WS, See M, Bailey LJ, Hershey HG. Accuracy of measurements of mandibular anatomy in cone-beam computed images. Oral Surg Oral Med Oral Pathol Oral Radiol Endod 2007;103:534–542.
14. Park IC, Bowman D, Klapper L. A cephalometric study of Korean adults. Am J Orthod Dentofacial Orthop 1989;96:54–59.
15. Farman GA, Scarfe WC. The basics of maxillofacial cone beam computed tomography. Semin Orthod 2009;15:2–13.
16. Kapila S, Conley RS, Harrell WE Jr. The current status of cone beam computed tomography imaging in orthodontics. Dentomaxillofac Radiol 2011;40:24–34.
17. Siewerdesen JH, Moseley DJ, Burch S, et al. Volume CT with a flat-panel detector on a mobile, isocentric C-arm: Pre-clinical investigation in guidance of minimally invasive surgery. Med Phys 2005;32:241–254.
18. Proffit WR, Fields HW, Sarver DM. Ortodonzia Moderna. Milan: Elsevier Masson, 2008.
19. Khoury A, Siewerdsen JH, Whyne CM, et al. Intraoperative cone beam CT for image-guided tibial plateau fracture reduction. Comput Aided Surg 2007;12:195–207.
20. Lascala CA, Panella J, Marques MM. Analysis of the accuracy of linear measurements obtained by cone beam computed tomography (CBCT-NewTom). Dentomaxillofac Radiol 2004;33;291–294.
21. Halazonetis DJ. From 2-dimensional cephalograms to 3-dimensional computed tomography scans. Am J Orthod Dentofacial Orthop 2005;127:627–637.
22. Grauer D, Cevidanes LSH, Proffit WR. Working with DICOM craniofacial images. Am J Orthod Dentofac Orthop 2009;136:460–470.
23. Harvold EP. The Activator in Orthodontics. St Louis: Mosby, 1974.
24. Hashimoto K, Kawashima S, Kameoka S, et al. Comparison of image validity between cone beam computed tomography for dental use and multidetector row helical computed tomography. Dentomaxillofac Radiol 2007;36:465–471.
25. Ahqvist J, Eliasson S, Welander U. The cephalometric projection. Part II. Principles of image distortion in cephalometry. Dentomaxillofac Radiol 1983;12:101–108.

26. Baumgaertel S, Palomo JM, Palomo L, Hans MG. Reliability and accuracy of cone-beam computed tomography dental measurements. Am J Orthod Dentofac Orthop 2009;136:19–25.
27. Cattaneo PM, Bloch CB, Calmar D, Hjortshøj M, Birte M. Comparison between conventional and cone-beam computed tomography-generated cephalograms. Am J Orthod Dentofac Orthop 2008;134:798–802.
28. Kumar V, Ludlow J, Soares Cevidanes LH, Mol A. In vivo comparison of conventional and cone beam CT synthesized cephalograms. Angle Orthod 2008;78:873–879.
29. Kumar V, Ludlow J, Mol A, Cevidanes L. Comparison of conventional and cone beam CT synthesized cephalograms. Dentomaxillofac Radiol 2007;36:263–269.

G Perrotti
M Politi
G Lorè

2

Changes in Basal Bones from Infancy to Senescence

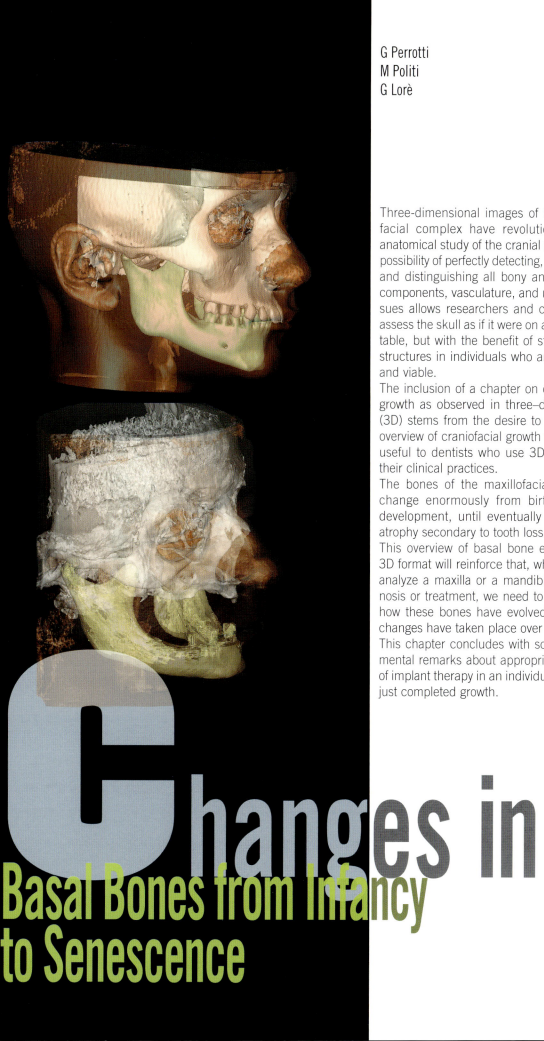

Three-dimensional images of the craniofacial complex have revolutionized the anatomical study of the cranial region. The possibility of perfectly detecting, separating, and distinguishing all bony and nonbony components, vasculature, and nervous tissues allows researchers and clinicians to assess the skull as if it were on a dissection table, but with the benefit of studying the structures in individuals who are still alive and viable.

The inclusion of a chapter on craniofacial growth as observed in three–dimensional (3D) stems from the desire to provide an overview of craniofacial growth that will be useful to dentists who use 3D images in their clinical practices.

The bones of the maxillofacial complex change enormously from birth through development, until eventually the bones atrophy secondary to tooth loss.

This overview of basal bone evolution in 3D format will reinforce that, whenever we analyze a maxilla or a mandible for diagnosis or treatment, we need to remember how these bones have evolved and what changes have taken place over time.

This chapter concludes with some fundamental remarks about appropriate staging of implant therapy in an individual who has just completed growth.

Growth and Development of Facial Bones in 3D Images

According to Moyers, growth is the sum of normal changes in the quantity of living matter. It represents the quantitative aspect of development, and it is measured in units of increase per units of time. Moreover, differentiation (transformation of cells into specialized entities) and translocation (change in position) are part of this development process.[1]

In bones, several types of cells are involved:

- *Osteoblasts:* cells responsible for new bone formation by secreting fundamental components of the extracellular organic matrix and controlling its mineralization. They form a sort of fence on bony surfaces and perform active deposition.
- *Bone-lining cells:* inactive, elongated cells deriving from osteoblasts that cover the bone surface.
- *Osteocytes:* star-shaped cells trapped in the bone surface, derived from osteoblasts and involved in maintaining the viability of the bone matrix.
- *Osteoclasts:* multinucleated cells responsible for resorption of mineralized bone tissue.

There are three patterns of cell growth:

- *Hypertrophy:* increase in cell volume
- *Hyperplasia:* increase in cell number
- Secretion of extracellular material: growth in tissue volume not coupled with an increase in the number or size of cells

These processes drive the development of all tissues.[2]

Skeletal growth derives from three distinct processes: chondrogenesis (cartilage formation); endochondral ossification (process of transformation of cartilage into bone in sites exposed to pressure); and intramembranous ossification (process of bone formation from undifferentiated mesenchymal tissue in sites exposed to tension).

The peak of development of the cartilaginous skeleton occurs in the third month of intrauterine life; in the fourth month, vascular-haematic elements start penetrating into various locations. These regions become ossification centers, where cartilage is transformed into calcified tissue whose rate of growth increases to match that of cartilage. On the contrary, the bones that do not derive from the chondroskeleton are formed by direct secretion of the bone matrix inside connective tissues; this intramembranous bone formation is typical of the cranial vault and of the maxilla and mandible.[3]

The stomatognathic system is a multifunctional complex. From an anatomical-topographic point of view, it occupies the medium and lower thirds of the face. Its functions are related to swallowing, phonation, mimics, esthetics, chewing, and breathing.

The growth of this complex is a differential process in which there are different times for the maturation of the various components, and it involves a set of various organs and tissues that are functionally interdependent.[1]

Growth control is regulated by three classes of factors:

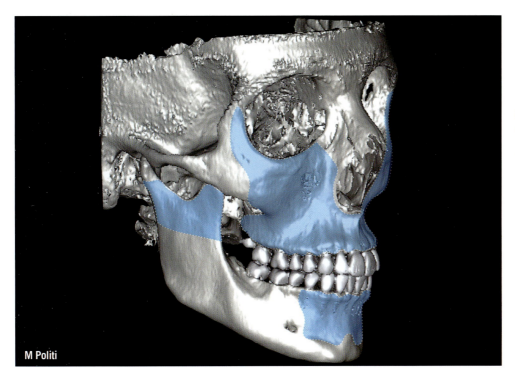

Fig 2-1 Areas of bone resorption in the middle and lower thirds of the face.

- *Genetic factors:* intrinsic in the individual
- *Epigenetic factors:* local (eg, encephalon) and general (eg, hormones)
- *Environmental factors:* can be local (eg, muscular strength and functions of the stomatognathic system) or general (eg, nutrition and oxygen tension)[4]

Three fundamental phases can be recognized in growth: ossification, starting in the prenatal period and continuing after birth; organization, allowing structures to grow harmoniously even if in different ways and at different paces; and adaptation, determining the architecture of the stomatognathic system.[5]

Several local-regional changes occur in the proportions among the various craniofacial structures, and endless structural adaptations occur so as to optimize the skeletal structure.

The mechanisms of bone growth result from two processes: apposition, formation of new bone on the cortical surface in the direction of growth, and resorption, bone loss from the surface opposing that on which apposition occurs (Fig 2-1).[2]

The external (periosteal) and internal (endosteal) surfaces of a bone are completely covered in "fields of growth" arranged as a mosaic: each area of apposition corresponds to an area of resorption on the opposing surface. The result is defined as translocation, and it is associated with an increase in volume due to the prevalence of apposition over resorption.[3]

Bone growth in general is characterized by the presence, inside or outside the surface, of an uneven series of "areas of growth" consisting of different soft or cartilaginous structures with osteogenic activity.

The growth "program" for bones is not contained inside the tissues themselves but rather in the soft tissues covering them: in muscles, mucosa, and vascular and nervous structures. The irregularity in the shape of bones is therefore a consequence of different functional demands coming from muscle insertions.[1,3]

Some "areas of growth" are further defined as "centers of growth," as they are very active, important sites. The different rate and level of growth of some parts as opposed to others causes the morphologic variation known as *remodeling*,[1] which reaches its maximum rate during infancy and adolescence and decreases markedly in adulthood, thus allowing normal relationships among the various bones to be maintained while growth processes tend to pull them away from one another.

The remodeling process[1] associated with translation, which is in turn due to bone deposition and absorption, causes two movements:

- Cortical drift, defined as a movement of repositioning or displacement of a growing bone, induces a movement towards the bone apposition surface.
- Dislocation or displacement, defined as a movement of the whole bone undergoing remodeling, causes formation of a space between bones where further bone will then grow. It can be due to intrinsic growth of bone (primary displacement) (Fig 2-2) or to the growth of other bones (secondary displacement) (Fig 2-3).

The maxillofacial complex of a child is not just a miniature version of an adult one; it has different proportions that change during development.[1,3]

The craniofacial complex can be divided into four areas that develop in quite different ways:

- Cranial vault: the bones covering the superior and outer surface of the brain
- Base of skull: the bone floor under the brain, which is also the dividing line between the skull and the face
- Nasomaxillary complex: consists of nose, maxilla, and small associated bones
- Mandible

The cranial vault consists of a series of flat bones that form with an intramembranous growth mechanism. Growth occurs mainly at the level of the skeletal sutures, while remodeling of internal and external surfaces occurs via periosteal activity, allowing the morphologic changes that take place during growth.

The neurocranium is the model on which the maxillofacial complex models itself. At birth it is about 10 times larger than the face. This proportion decreases by up to three times in adults. The cranial vault grows extensively and rapidly in the first year of life, reaching 80% of its adult size at the end of the second year and completing its growth at 8 to 10 years of age. Because the encephalon at 10 years has completed 95% of its development, it needs a container with enough volumetric capacity to contain it.

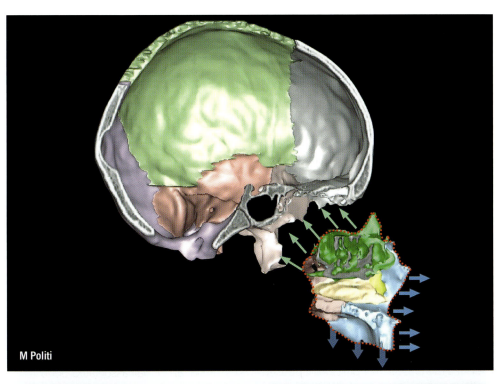

Fig 2-2 Primary dislocation or displacement of the maxilla. The maxilla is pushed inferiorly and anteriorly by the growth of soft tissues, causing the opening of the superior and posterior suture spaces. This phenomenon induces apposition of new bone tissue on both sides of the sutures.

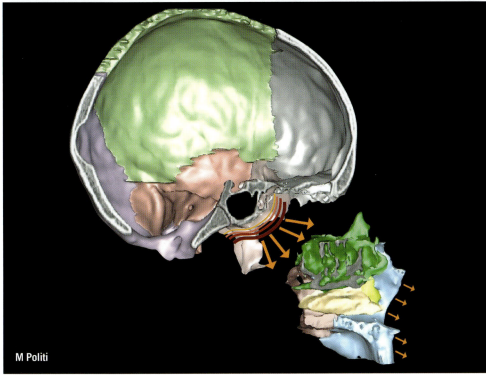

Fig 2-3 Secondary dislocation or displacement of the maxilla caused by the growth of the base of the skull, middle cranial fossa, and temporal lobe.

The growth of the cranial vault is sutural; the circumference of individual bones increases while their curvature decreases at the same time. This growth is also appositional because the cortical layer gets thicker.[6,7]

At about 10 years of age, the facial bones have completed only 75% of their growth. The base of the skull, which is the junction between the neurocranium and the facial complex, has an endocranial part that contains the brain mass and an exocranial part that supports the whole structure. Because of their different development patterns, the various components require different amounts of time to achieve complete maturation at the same point in time. The base of the skull presents both endochondral (bone apposition along the axial zone at level of the sutures) and appositional patterns of growth.

The base of the skull originates from a cartilaginous skeleton in which some ossification centers are already present in the embryonic phase; these centers establish the basal, occipital, sphenoid, and ethmoid bones. The skull base can be considered as an autonomous unit of growth developing at the same time as the encephalon but independently from it.[7]

The nasomaxillary area develops, on the contrary, through intramembranous ossification with two mechanisms:

- Active growth of the maxillary and nasal structures, or primary displacement
- Passive growth, or secondary displacement, induced by the growth of the base of the skull pushing the maxilla forward (see Fig 2-3)[8]

The passive movement of the maxilla is an important growth mechanism at the time of the primary dentition; with completion of the encephalic development at about 7 or 8 years of age, growth at the level of the synchondroses slows noticeably, and this mechanism gradually becomes less important.

In the period from 7 to 15 years, about one-third of the total maxillary movement is due to secondary displacement driven by growth of the middle cranial fossa and the temporal lobe (see Fig 2-3), while the remaining part is the result of active growth in maxillary structures in response to stimuli coming from the development of soft tissues.

In eumorphic individuals, the nasomaxillary complex grows as a vector pointing downward and forward with anterior rotation along three directions: posteroanteriorly at the level of the tuberosity (Fig 2-4), laterally at the level of the external surface, and vertically and downwards at the level of the sutures (Fig 2-5). The superior and posterior sutures are arranged ideally to allow this kind of repositioning, and the space that develops is then filled by active bone proliferation. The sutures therefore maintain the same width while the various maxillary processes get longer; bone apposition occurs on both sides of the suture so that the bones that articulate with the maxilla will also become larger (see Figs 2-2 and 2-3).[3]

It is important to note that as the maxilla grows downward and forward, its anterior surface undergoes remodeling, and much of the bone tissue is resorbed from this surface. The whole anterior surface of the maxilla presents an area of bone resorption but not of apposition, as bone is removed from the entire anterior surface except for a small area at the level of the anterior nasal spine.

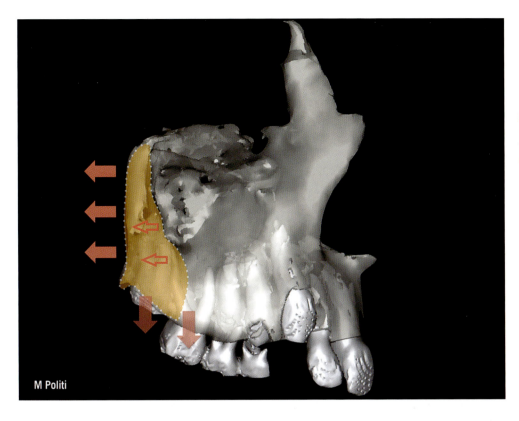

Fig 2-4 Growth of the maxillary tuberosity: the vector of growth is posterior, lateral, and downward.

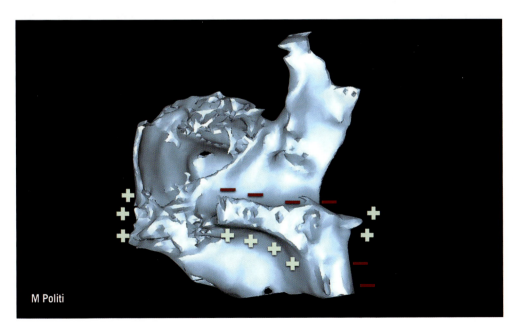

Fig 2-5 Areas of apposition and resorption with the growth vector of the maxilla pointing downward and forward. Notice the presence of a major resorption center at the level of the nasal floor as opposed to an area of apposition on the palatal side. This causes downward and forward movement of the nasal floor and of the palatal vault.

Another very important resorption area is located at the level of the nasal floor in association with a center of bone apposition on the oral side (see Fig 2-5). This process induces a downward and forward movement of the palatal vault. On the anterior surface, as already mentioned, the bone is reabsorbed, thus partially nullifying the translation forward. The transversal development of the palate, on the contrary, occurs due to growth at the level of the middle palatal suture.

It is worth underlining that alveolar development, dental eruption, and migration of dental elements in association with alveolar movement play a very important role in the vertical growth of the maxilla. These processes, together with the downward movement of the maxilla, determine the final vertical height of the maxilla.[1,3]

The mandible is the most mobile bone in the skull, and it is of vital importance as it is involved in chewing, facial expressions, and preservation of the airway. It grows in a relatively constant way until puberty: the mandibular ramus increases by 1 or 2 mm per year, the length of the mandible by 2 or 3 mm per year.

The mandible is a macroskeletal unit comprised of four microskeletal units: body (basal unit) and condyle, coronoid process, angle, and alveolar process. Most of its growth is associated with remodeling due to muscle insertions (coronoid and angular units) and with tooth eruption (alveolar unit). Only a small percentage is due to intrinsic factors (basal unit) (Fig 2-6).[6]

The condylar cartilage, which was considered in the past as an autonomous center of growth, is in fact an important zone of adaptation to articular forces. It grows in a direction driven by regional functional adaptation in response to peristaltic factors and, only secondarily, in response to genetic factors.[9,10] Conversely, compensation growth of the condyle is of paramount importance to maintain functional relations between the mandible and the skull base.[11]

Many authors, particularly in the past, have stated that the condyle is the main force driving the downward and forward movement of the mandible. Several studies have nevertheless demonstrated that it is possible to have adequate function and a normal position of the mandible without condyles. According to this theory, the soft tissues drive the anteroposterior movement of the mandible, while the condyle performs the task of maintaining contact with the skull base.[3]

The growth vector of the mandible in eumorphic individuals is downward and forward with an anterior rotation of about 2 mm in relation to the maxilla. The body of the mandible moves forward, thus offsetting the growth of the maxilla in the sagittal plane.[1,3,6]

Lavergne and Grasson[12] have stated that mandibular rotation is influenced by the intrinsic growth of the mandible, by the position of the maxilla in space, and by its rotation. The mandible undergoes remodeling all along its surface, and this increases its size. Vertical growth of the ramus promotes vertical growth of the nasal region and tooth eruption, and it is also correlated with the direction of condylar growth: backward and downward in the case of anterior rotation; forward and upward in the case of posterior rotation.[13] New bone apposition usually occurs on the posterior edge of the ramus, while resorption occurs on the anterior edge. These processes induce a drift, causing a posterosuperior displacement and a consequent increase in intercondylar distance, if one considers the mandible as a single unit (Fig 2-7). The mandible becomes longer as the ramus grows in the direction opposite to the chin, and what once was the posterior surface of the ramus now becomes its center and, later, its anterior surface through remodeling. During infancy the ramus is located approximately where the primary first molar erupts. The progressive posterior rearrangement creates space for the second primary molars and, later, for the permanent molars (Fig 2-8). Often this growth ends before enough space has been created to allow for the eruption of the permanent third molars, which, as a consequence, will remain unerupted.[1,3]

Similar to that of the maxilla, the development of the mandible is characterized by the concomitant action of primary and secondary dislocation: the former allows elongation of the mandible due to posterosuperior remodeling of the ramus, while the latter occurs due to the expansion of the middle cranial fossa causing anteroinferior displacement. Nevertheless, because the growth of the middle cranial fossa mainly occurs anterior to the condyles, secondary dislocation of the mandible is not as great as maxillary dislocation.[3]

Displacements due to growth are related to maxillary movements. The primary purpose of the displacement of the mandible is to maintain continuous juxtaposition of the maxillary and mandibular dentoalveolar arches. The growth of the sphenoid-occipital complex is an equivalent of the growth in the nasopharynx and in the mandibular ramus. The ramus grows dorsally, and the mandible is dislocated anteriorly. Thus the sagittal relation between the mandibular arch and the nasomaxillary complex is restored after the latter has advanced. Moreover, vertical growth is correlated with the development of the skull base and of the nasomaxillary complex.

A further feature of mandibular growth is that chin prominence becomes more marked, not so much through apposition of new bone tissue in this area but rather through resorption in the area between it and the alveolar process.[3]

The alveolar bone is a portion of the maxilla and mandible that forms and supports the bony sockets of teeth; the alveolus constitutes the functional matrix for bone growth. Alveolar bone develops together with the formation and eruption of dental elements.[2,3]

Apposition/remodeling processes occur simultaneously, although on opposing surfaces, under a precise functional stimulus.[14] As already seen, vertical mandibular growth depends on the development of the ramus in a posterosuperior direction and on the alveolar processes, which will be in turn influenced by the type (hypo- or hyperdivergent) of face. The importance of the normal development of the alveolar processes for vertical maxillary growth is proven by the effects of ankylosis of primary teeth.

Fig 2-6 The growth of the mandible and of the other bones results from a process of remodeling with resorption *(blue arrows pointing at surface)* and apposition areas *(red arrows pointing away from surface)*.

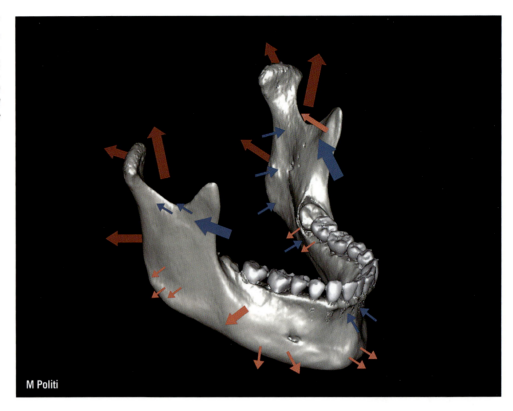

Fig 2-7 Vertical growth of the ramus.

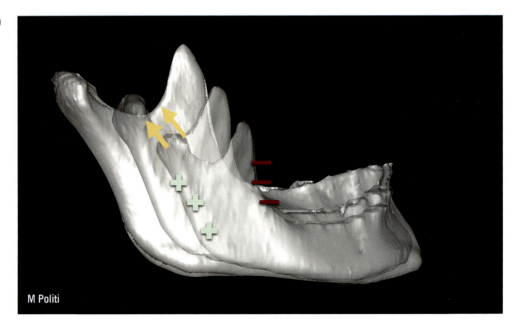

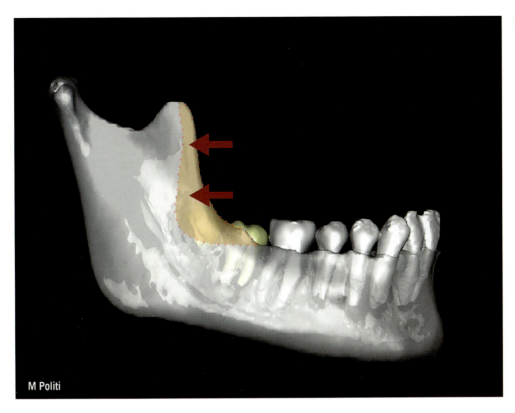

Fig 2-8 Resorption of the anterior edge of the mandibular ramus occurs simultaneously with the eruption of the mandibular molars.

Growth in width, on the contrary, is partly due to the natural divergence of the rami and hence to their growth and partly to the extent of apposition on the outer surface of the ramus. The intercondylar and gonial distance therefore increase, while the width of the dental arch does not change significantly (Fig 2-9).[3]

At birth the mandible is relatively small and has a cartilage structure at the symphysis, which allows rapid transversal growth. At 12 months, the anterior part supports the erupted primary incisors and has already reached an almost-adult size. Molar eruption is possible because by about 10 years of age, the mandible has grown sufficiently to accommodate them. It is therefore dorsal growth of the mandible that allows complete eruption of all teeth. When analyzing the length of the mandible during cephalometric analysis, one should bear in mind that it is correlated with the length of the maxilla (condylion-point A [Co-A]) and with the facial height (anterior nasal spine-menton [ANS-Me]).[15]

In the sagittal plane the face, beginning in the fourth year of growth, grows by 7 mm at the level of the nasion (N), by 14 mm at the level of the ANS, and by 21 mm at the level of the pogonion (Pog). In the vertical plane, at 4 years of age, the growth ratio between the upper anterior facial height (N-ANS) and the lower anterior facial height (ANS-Me) is 1:3.

Later, until 12 years of age, this ratio changes because of differential growth in favor of the lower (+ 0.7 mm) as opposed to the upper.

Fig 2-9

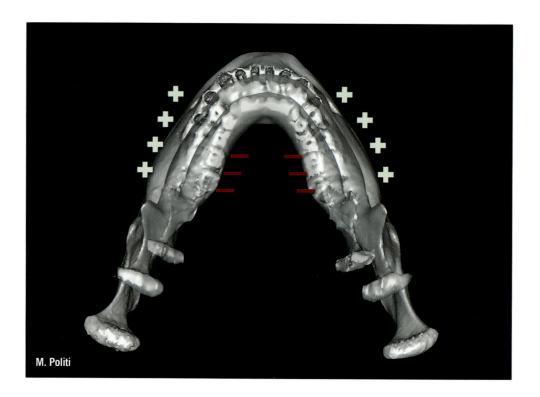

Therefore, at age 12, N-ANS = ANS-Me + 5.6 mm.

After this age, the growth ratio varies depending on gender; in boys differential growth continues until 20 years, while in girls the ratio of N-ANS to ANS-Me returns to 1:1. At the end of growth, the following values are typical:

- In males with a normal vertical growth ratio, N-ANS = ANS-Me + 11.2 mm
- In females with a normal growth ratio, N-ANS = ANS-Me + 5.6 mm

These cases are classified as normal skeletal vertical occlusion; if the ratio is higher, there is a skeletal open bite, which, if it is not compensated for, leads to growth of the mandible in posterior rotation. If, on the contrary, this ratio decreases, there is skeletal deep bite with horizontal growth of the mandible in anterior rotation.[6]

According to Fränkel and Fränkel,[16,17] for orofacial development to occur physiologically, it is necessary to meet several biophysical and biomechanical requirements:

- There must be physiologic space in the oral and nasopharyngeal cavities.
- The posture of the orofacial muscles during infancy must be correct.
- The valves in the orofacial region must function properly.

Any abnormality in these biomechanical and biophysical parameters can lead to altered craniofacial development and therefore to dysgnathia.[18]

Theories on Control of Craniofacial Growth

As outlined above, there are genetic, epigenetic, and environmental factors regulating and controlling bone growth.
Many theories have tried to explain the determinants of bone development.[14,19] The prevailing idea is now that there is a close association between the epigenetic control of cartilage tissue on bone and a bone/cartilage response to signals from surrounding tissues outside the skeletal system. There are three theories that try to identify the determinants of craniofacial growth:

- Bone tissue contains the information necessary for its development.
- Cartilage drives craniofacial growth while the bone responds secondarily and passively (epigenetic control).
- The matrix of soft tissues enveloping skeletal tissues is the main factor in skeletal growth, with bone and cartilage being consequential elements.

The main difference among these theories lies in the site where genetic control is exerted. According to the first theory, genetic control occurs directly at the bone level through differentiation of growth sites and centers; the former are places where growth occurs, and the latter are areas where growth takes place independently because it is controlled genetically. All growth centers are also growth sites but not the other way around, and growth represents the genetic expression of all growth centers. According to this theory, sutures between membranous bones of the skull and ossification centers of basal bones are considered to be growth centers. It has nevertheless been demonstrated that sutures and periosteal tissues are not determinants of craniofacial development as they do not have an intrinsic growth capability; on the contrary, structural growth seems to respond to external influences under various circumstances. Sutures therefore need to be considered as areas of reaction rather than primary drivers.[19]

According to the second theory, it is cartilage that drives craniofacial growth. This is supported by the fact that cartilage grows at level of the jaws while bone tissue simply replaces it. Several studies have nevertheless demonstrated that an adequate function and normal mandibular position are possible even without condyles. According to this theory, it is therefore soft tissue that drives the anteroposterior movement of the maxilla, while the condyle has the task of maintaining contact with the skull base.[3]

The third theory attributes control of growth in the craniofacial skeleton to adjacent soft tissues. In an article titled "The Primary Role of Functional Matrices in Facial Growth,"[20] Moss and Salentijn state that facial growth occurs in response to functional needs and that it is mediated by soft tissues containing the maxilla. In this perspective, it is the soft tissues that grow, while cartilage and bone react to that growth. Growth in the craniomaxillofacial complex proves this hypothesis; for instance, development of the cranial vault is a direct response to brain growth.

The pressure exerted by the growing encephalon mass separates skull bones at the sutural level, and the skull progressively adapts itself to the brain. The mechanism whereby functional needs are trans-

ferred is still unknown, but it seems to be fundamental for bone growth in general.
A synthesis between the theory of epigenetic control through cartilage and the theory of the functional matrix driving craniofacial growth seems to be the most plausible; the first theory, which was prevalent until 1960, has now been largely abandoned.[3]

Bone Resorption and Atrophy of the Basal Bone

Maxillary and mandibular bone resorption means a loss of bone at the cortical level (or, in extreme cases, at the basal level), which can occur transversally or vertically or both.

Early loss of teeth and of the function associated with them progresses to a condition of bone atrophy of alveolar and basal bones, with deficits in the vertical and sagittal dimensions impacting vertical height and facial esthetics.

One of the most commonly adopted classifications nowadays was developed by Cawood and Howell in 1988.[21] The authors highlighted the differences between alveolar and basal bone; the former reabsorbs according to fairly consistent patterns that are specific for the affected site, while the latter seldom undergoes resorption unless it is exposed to irritative or incongruous stimuli.

Their classification differs for the maxilla and mandible; in the anterior mandible, in the interforaminal region, bone resorption is almost completely vestibular with horizontal progression. On the contrary, in the posterior region there is more vertical resorption. In the maxilla, resorption is horizontal in both the anterior and posterior regions.

Bone atrophy therefore has been classified into five classes for the maxilla and six classes for the mandible, and each class is associated with a specific bone morphology. Different regions of the same arch can simultaneously present different classes.

A summarizing classification has been proposed by Testori et al[22] in which areas of bone atrophy are subdivided into regional, multiarea or total, and extreme resorption. The following pages contain examples of this classification system using images obtained through processing of Digital Imaging and Communications in Medicine (DICOM) data from cone beam computed tomography scans prescribed prior to implant placement.

1

Maxillary Posterior Bone Resorption
Type A: Hyperpneumatization of the sinuses

Normal interarch distance
Ridge height ≤ 5 to 8 mm
Crestal ridge width ≥ 6 mm

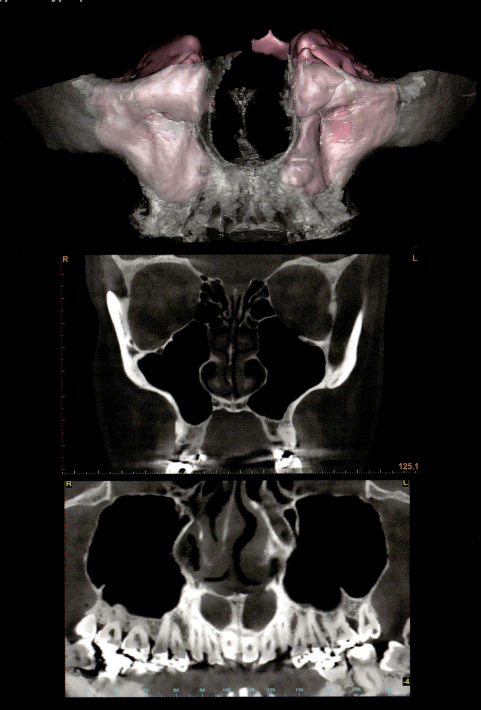

2
Maxillary Posterior Bone Resorption
Type B: Transverse deficiency

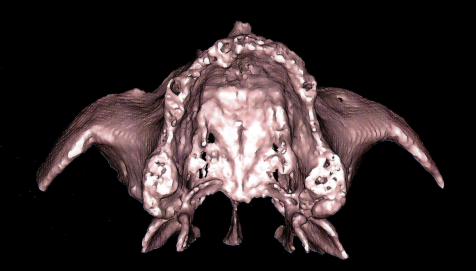

Normal interarch distance
Ridge height between 5 and 8 mm
Crestal ridge width ≤ 6 mm

3

Maxillary Posterior Bone Resorption
Type C: Vertical deficiency

Increased
interarch distance
Ridge height
≤ 5 mm
Crestal ridge width
≥ 6 mm

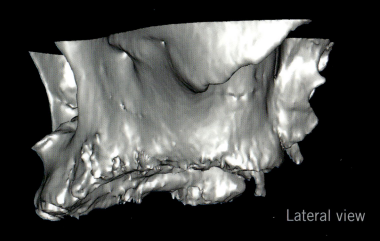

Lateral view

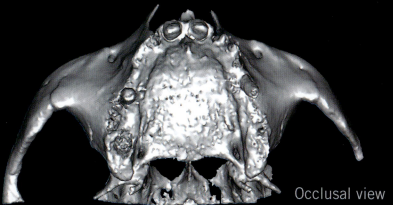

Occlusal view

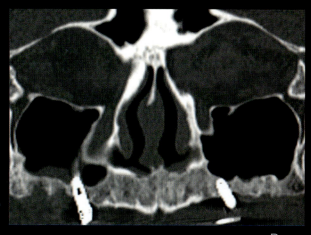

Panoramic view

Type D: Combined deficiency

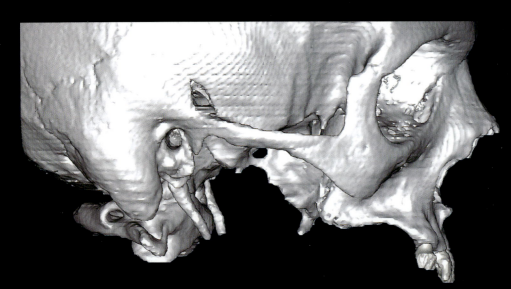

Increased interarch distance
Ridge height
≤ 5 mm
Crestal ridge width
≤ 6 mm

Lateral view

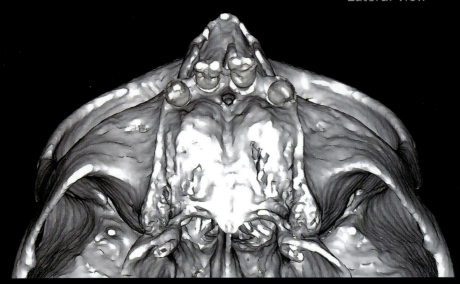

Occlusal view

Maxillary Anterior Bone Resorption

Type A: Transverse deficiency

Normal interarch distance
Ridge height
> 10 mm
Crestal ridge width
< 6 mm

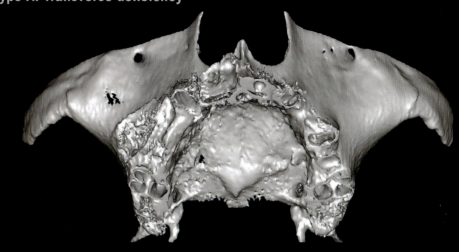

Type B: Vertical deficiency

Increased interarch distance
Ridge height
≤ 10 mm
Crestal ridge width
≥ 6 mm

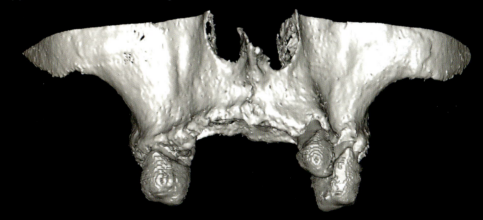

Type C: Combined deficiency

Normal interarch distance
Ridge height
< 10 mm
Crestal ridge width
< 6 mm

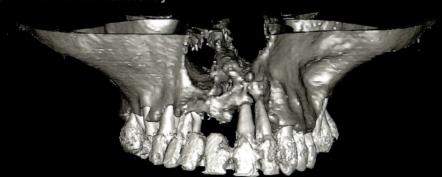

6

Multiarea/Total Resorption with Normal Maxillomandibular Relationship

Type A: Transverse deficiency

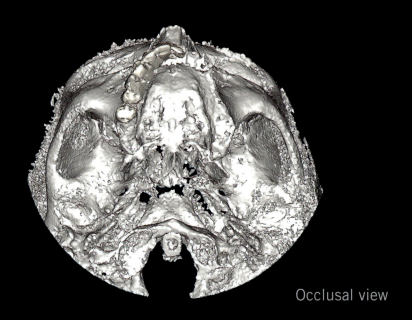

Occlusal view

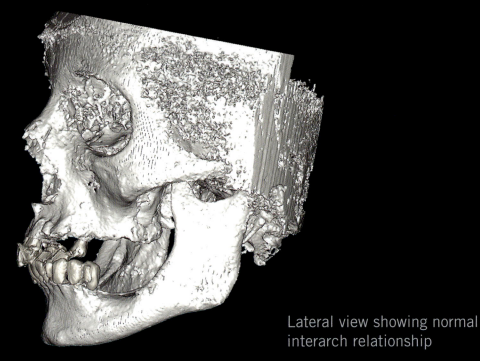

Lateral view showing normal interarch relationship

7

Multiarea/Total Resorption with Normal Maxillomandibular Relationship

Type B: Vertical deficiency

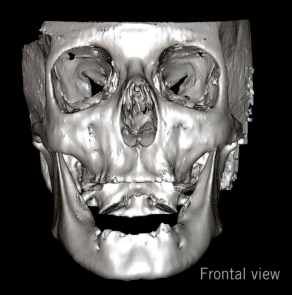
Frontal view

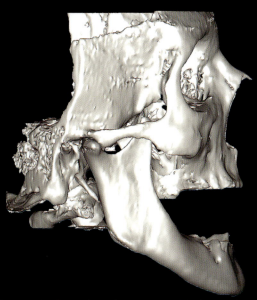
Lateral view showing normal interarch relationship

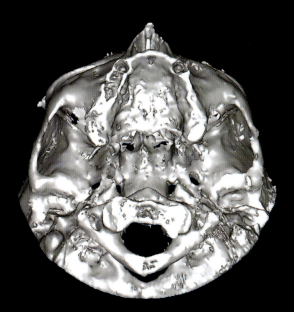
Occlusal view

Type C: Combined deficiency

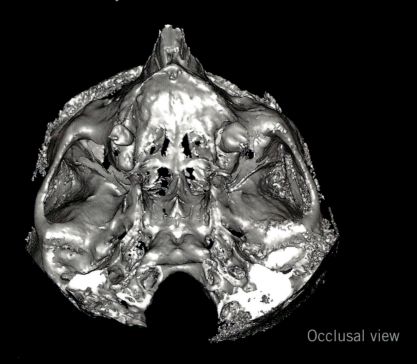

Occlusal view

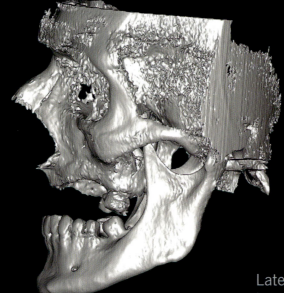

Lateral view showing altered interarch relationship

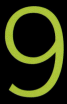

Edentulous Mandible Without Resorption in Vertical or Transverse Dimensions

Altered 3D maxillomandibular relationship
Increased interarch distance
Variable crestal ridge thickness

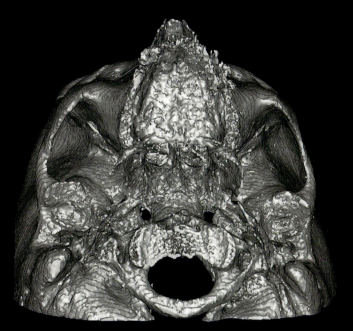

Occlusal view

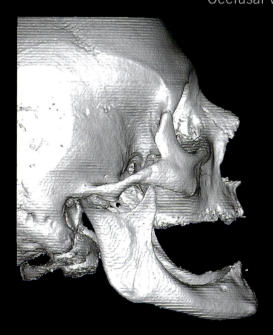

Lateral view

10
Posterior Atrophy Without Involvement of the Anterior Areas

Advanced atrophy with severe resorption, including basal bone
Increased interarch distance

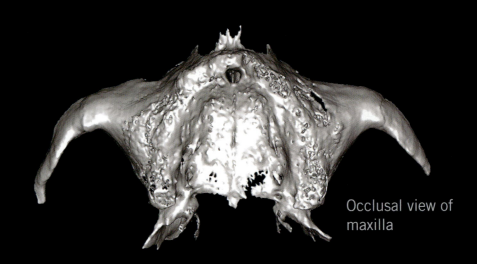

Occlusal view of maxilla

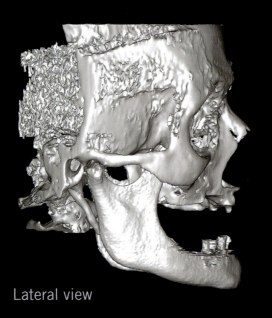

Lateral view

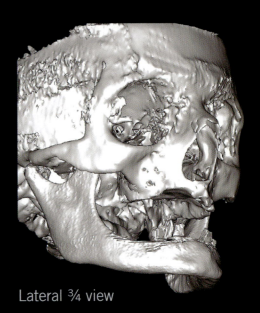

Lateral ¾ view

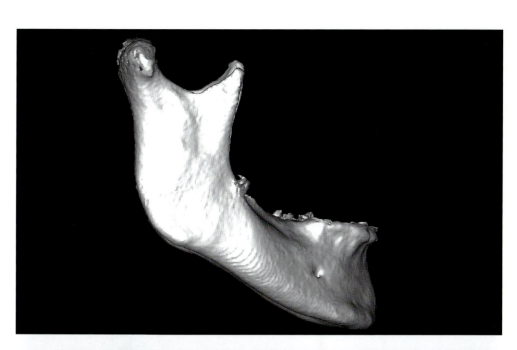

Fig 2-9 Edentulous mandible without resorption in vertical or transverse dimension.

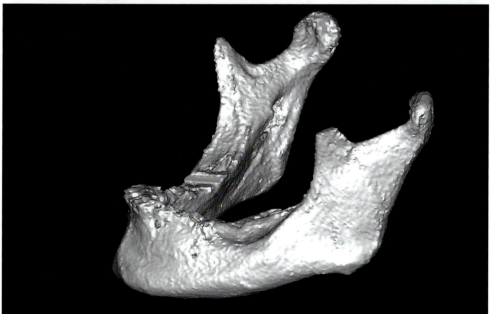

Fig 2-10 Posterior regional atrophy with no involvement of the anterior areas.

For the mandible, on the contrary, Gerber's classification is used, in which the gonial angle and the sigmoid notch progressively tend to widen (Figs 2-9 to 2-12). The muscle process elongates, and the condyle and the fontal process dorsalize. Correct staging of bone atrophy severity and hence classification of patients into the above categories allows the clinician to address potential treatment options and to develop a suitable treatment plan.

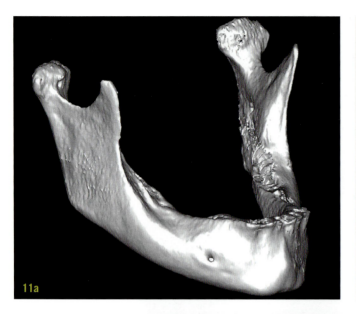
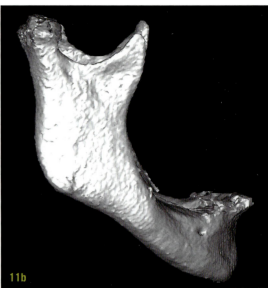
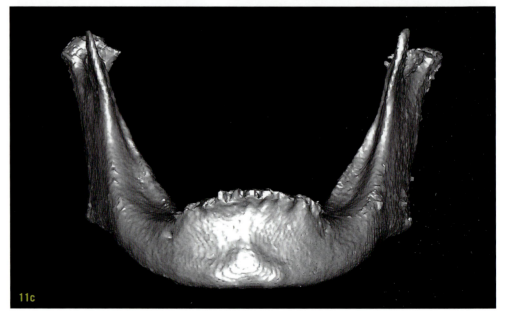

Figs 2-11a to 2-11c Mandibular growth. Diffuse atrophy with greater involvement of the posterior regions: *(a)* lateral ¾ view; *(b)* lateral view; *(c)* frontal view.

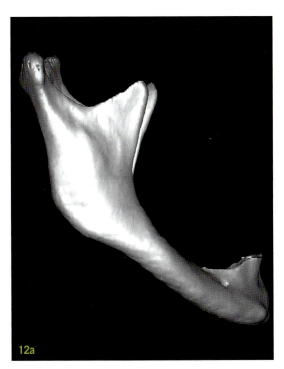 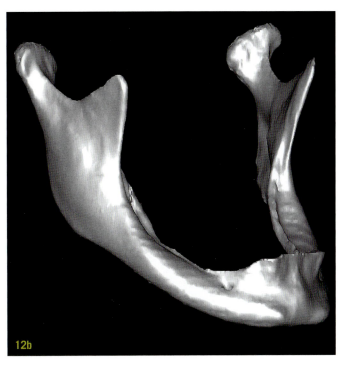

Figs 2-12a and 2-12b Total atrophy of the mandible with an increase in transverse distance from ridge crest to ridge crest: *(a)* lateral view; *(b)* lateral ¾ view.

Implant Therapy and Craniofacial Growth

In patients with a normal facial profile (Fig 2-13), the placement of an implant must be postponed until growth has been completed. In brachycephalic or dolichocephalic patients (Figs 2-14 and 2-15), further growth and the continuous eruption of adjacent teeth can jeopardize a successful outcome if implant placement occurs before the age of 20 years because the result may be a prosthetic crown in infraocclusion to natural teeth, which are spontaneously extruded.

In implant planning, the age and gender of patients must be considered; the critical period of growth in girls is 9 to 15 years, and in boys it ranges from 9 to 11 years (primary growth). If one adds the variability associated with facial biotype (brachycephalic and dolichocephalic individuals show significant changes until 25 years), the critical period becomes longer. It is therefore clear that chronologic age is not sufficient to determine the end of growth.

The clinician must assess actual growth, based on the following:

- Overlapping cephalometric tracings of radiographs taken at intervals of 6 to 12 months
- A period of 1 year with no growth-associated changes
- Height monitoring over 2 years, ensuring that annual growth is less than 0.5 cm/year
- Observation of dental changes within the arches, eg, eruption of the second molars

The population can be classified in normal, brachycephalic, and dolichocephalic individuals. Each of these facial types presents particular features in the development of the maxillary bones.

The studies carried out by Kokich[23] indicate that growth of the craniofacial complex continues after puberty. The marked growth difference between the genders is evident mostly until the age of 15 years.

In the second decade of life, residual growth is similar in boys and girls but is nevertheless present until 20 to 25 years of age, more noticeably in individuals with dysgnathic long faces rather than in normodivergent or short-faced individuals.

Another aspect to be considered is the potential residual eruption of the maxillary incisors after 15 years of age; this is more evident in females, with a vertical increase of about 1 mm, and it is also correlated to anterior occlusion and overjet. Mandibular incisors often show residual eruption of at least 1 mm after age 18 years.

The teeth in the lateroposterior areas express their greatest eruption potential until 15 years, after which eruption becomes less than 0.5 mm, correlated to the vertical skeletal dimension and the intercuspation pattern of teeth.

In light of these remarks about craniofacial growth, it should therefore be considered that, even if there are no primary contraindications to the placement of implants in individuals during secondary growth, there

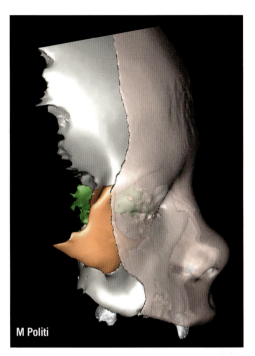

Fig 2-13 3D rendering of a 12-year-old patient with a transparent overlay of soft tissues using a kernel.

is a potential risk of infraocclusion of the implant-supported crown 4 to 5 years after the restoration of an implant, most frequently in the anterior region (Fig 2-16).

Therefore, the above diagnostic parameters for growth completion have to be considered. After deciding to proceed with an implant-supported prosthetic treatment, it is necessary to assess occlusal relationships very carefully to avoid passive eruption because of improper intercuspation.

In patients with anodontia or marked oligodontia, it is possible to place implants in the anterior maxilla or mandible before the pubertal growth spurt; only limited changes occur in this area after 5 or 6 years of age, especially when teeth are absent.

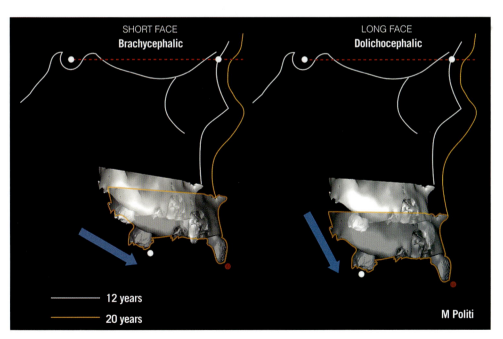

Fig 2-14 These images show the growth direction of the maxilla and the eruption of the maxillary incisors and first molars in brachycephalic and dolichocephalic individuals. In dolichocephalic patients, vertical growth is greater both in terms of growth quantity and of secondary growth potential, which expresses itself after 15 years, than in brachycephalic individuals.

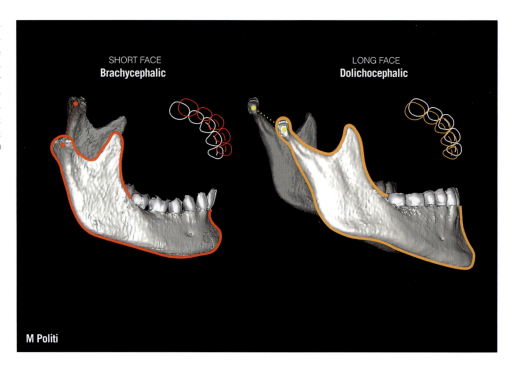

Fig 2-15 Image showing the pattern of mandibular growth (bone resorption and apposition along the inferior border, the dentoalveolar edge, and the condyle) in brachycephalic and dolichocephalic individuals between 10 and 19 years of age.

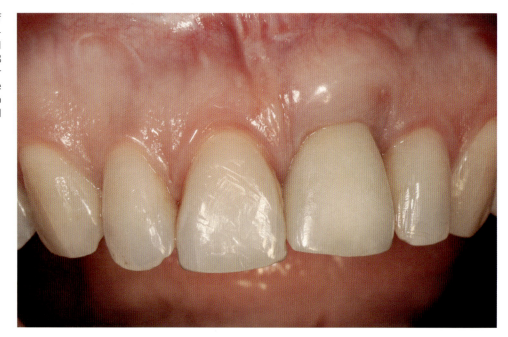

Fig 2-16 Example of an incisor in infraocclusion: the implant had been placed at age 18 years, and 6 years later the incisal edge of the prosthetic crown was no longer at the same level as the natural teeth.

References

1. Enlow DH. Facial Growth, ed 3. Philadelphia: Saunders, 1990.
2. Lindhe J, Lang NP, Karring T. Parodontologia clinica e implantologia orale, ed 5. Milano: Ermes, 2009.
3. Proffit WR, Fields HW Jr, Sarver DM. Contemporary Orthodontics, ed 4. St Louis: Mosby/Elsevier, 2007.
4. van Limborg J. A new view of the control of the morphogenesis of the skull. Acta Morph Neerl Scand 1970;8:143–160.
5. Darwis WE, Messer LB, Thomas CD. Assessing growth and development of the facial profile. Pediatr Dent 2003;25:103–188.
6. Giannì E. La nuova ortognatodonzia. Padova: Piccin-Nuova Libraria, 1980.
7. Ranly DM. Craniofacial growth. Dent Clin North Am 2000;44:457–470.
8. Crago C, Proffit WR. Distraction osteogenesis. In: Proffit WR, White RP Jr, Sarver DM (eds). Contemporary Treatment of Dentofacial Deformity. St Louis: Mosby, 2003.
9. Moss ML. A functional analysis of human condylar growth. J Prosthet Dent 1960;10:1149–1160.
10. Moss ML. Genetics, epigenetics, and causation. Am J Orthod 1981;80:366–375.
11. Roald KL, Wisth PJ, Bøe OE. Changes in craniofacial morphology of individuals with hypodontia between the ages of 9 and 16. Acta Odontol Scand 1982,40:65–74.
12. Lavergne J, Gasson N. A metal implant study of mandibular rotation. Angle Orthod 1976;46:144–150.
13. Björk A. Prediction of mandibular growth rotation. Am J Orthod 1969;55:585–599.
14. Moss ML, Salentijn L. The capsular matrix. Am J Orthod 1969;56:474–490.
15. McNamara JA Jr. A method of cephalometric analysis. In: Clinical Alteration of the Growing Face, Monograph 12, Craniofacial Growth Series. Ann Arbor: Center for Human Growth and Development, University of Michigan, 1983.
16. Fränkel R, Fränkel C. Functional approach to treatment of skeletal open bite. Am J Orthod 1983;84:54–68.
17. Fränkel R, Fränkel C. Ortopedia orofacciale con il regolatore di funzione. Milano: Masson, 1991.
18. Poggesi MP, Iannarilli G, Fidanza F, Rossi F. Ortodonzia funzionale: Effetti terapeutici ed indicazioni dell'attivatore e del regolatore di funzione di Frankel. Attualità Odontostomatologiche 1999;3:5–16.
19. Enlow DH, Hans MG. Essentials of Facial Growth. Philadelphia: Saunders, 1996.
20. Moss ML, Salentijn L. The primary role of functional matrices in facial growth. Am J Orthod 1969;55:566–577.
21. Cawood JI, Howell RA. A classification of the edentulous jaws. Int J Oral Maxillofac Surg 1988;17:232–236.
22. Testori T, Weinstein RL, Wallace S. La chirurgia del seno mascellare e le alternative terapeutiche. Viterbo, Italy: ACME, 2005:125–127.
23. Kokich VG. Maxillary lateral incisor implants: Planning with the aid of orthodontics. J Oral Maxillofac Surg 2004;62(9, suppl 2):48–56.

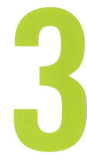

T Testori
L Fumagalli
A Parenti
F Grecchi
M Mantovani
L Pignataro
G Pozzi
A Zerbi

3

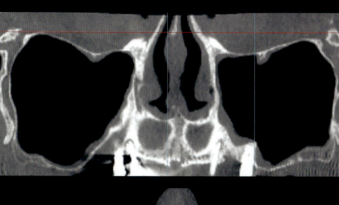

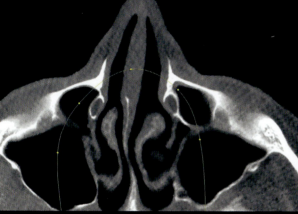

Radiologic investigations using images acquired with the latest-generation cone beam computed tomography (CBCT) scanners have reached a high degree of accuracy, allowing integration of three–dimension (3D) analysis of anatomical structures with the clinical examination.

This recent integration translates into more accurate treatment plans and better-planned surgical procedures that are less dependent on the clinician's experience.

Although modern imaging allows one to operate with more confidence, a good knowledge of physiologic anatomy and the learning curve of the clinician are still the mainstays in preventing, or at least minimizing, the risks connected with any surgical procedure.

The aim of this chapter is to illustrate 3D radiologic images of the anatomical areas relevant for oral and maxillofacial surgeons, combined with interesting pathologic presentations that can be difficult to interpret by using conventional two–dimensional (2D) radiology alone.

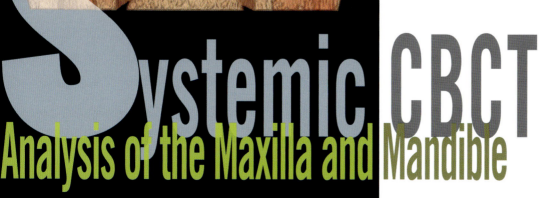

Systemic CBCT
Analysis of the Maxilla and Mandible

Radiologic and Clinical Anatomy of the Maxilla

A 3D analysis of the maxillofacial area is fundamental to assess the exact spatial arrangement of anatomical structures, which will allow the clinician to more accurately diagnose and plan any surgical (oral, maxillofacial, implant) procedure.

There is great individual variability in the anatomy of the maxillary and mandibular area, and this can influence surgical procedures. Through careful 3D multiplanar assessment, it is possible to gain a clearer picture of treatment options, which would be difficult to identify using only 2D images. The dose of rays absorbed by the patient raises controversy about the actual indications for performing this kind of test. Nevertheless, as outlined in the literature, a 3D exam is warranted if the information obtained will extend a real benefit to the patient in terms of diagnosis and treatment.[1]

The quantity of rays absorbed by a patient during a CT is definitely higher than that absorbed during CBCT.[2-4] Conversely, the dose reduction when using CBCT instead of CT results in images of lower quality.[5-7] Nevertheless, in choosing the ideal type of 3D examination, the diagnostic value of the test itself shall be considered while limiting the field of view of image acquisition to the area that is clinically relevant in line with the as low as reasonably achievable (ALARA) principle.

Knowledge of physiologic anatomy is of paramount importance in assessing radiologic anatomy.

With CBCT, it is possible to analyze landmarks in hard and soft tissues and in dental structures. The great quantity of information obliges the clinician to a systematic approach in the analysis of radiographic examinations in order to deliver an accurate diagnosis.

The aim of this chapter is to illustrate the physiologic anatomy and anatomical variations of the maxilla and mandible while highlighting the most frequent pathologies in these two areas.

The analysis starts from a 2D image such as a panoramic radiograph, which is used in a rational evaluation process that allows the clinician to assess the various anatomical areas rationally and systematically.

To this purpose, it is useful to divide the maxilla into three regions (Table 3-1):

- Anterior region: incisive bone and adjacent structures
- Lateroposterior region: maxillary sinus
- Posterior region: maxillary tuberosity area

The anatomical structures of these areas must be assessed in the three planes of space, as they cannot be fully viewed on a 2D image.

The use of panoramic images provides clinicians with a systematic and rational mental process.

It is possible to label the anatomical structures starting from the region of the nasal septum, proceeding towards the posterior region of maxillary tuberosity (Fig 3-1).

Table 3-1 Relevant anatomical structures: Maxilla
Region A: Anterior maxilla
Nasal septum
Anterior nasal spine
Nasopalatal canal
Nasolacrimal duct
Lateral nasal wall
Nasal turbinates
Region B: Lateroposterior maxilla
Orbit
Maxillary sinus
Infraorbital foramen
Zygomatic process
Region C: Maxillary tuberosity area
Greater palatine foramen
Maxillary tuberosity
Pterygoid process of the sphenoid
Articular fossa

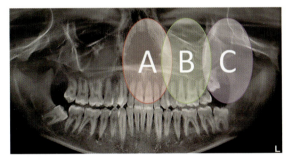 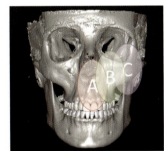 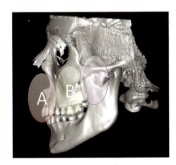

Figs 3-1a to 3-1c The three regions of the maxilla: *(a)* panoramic radiograph; *(b)* frontal 3D view; *(c)* lateral 3D view.

Anatomy of the Maxilla

The maxilla consists of two main bones: the maxillary and the palatal bones. The maxillary bone comprises most of its volume, and this bone consists of a central body and four processes: the alveolar, the zygomatic, the palatal, and the nasal processes (Fig 3-2).

Region A: Anterior Maxilla

In the medial maxillary region, there is the piriform aperture into the nasal cavity (Fig 3-3).
Inside the nasal cavity are the convolutions of the three turbinates, which, from the lateral wall of the nose, develop vertically in a caudal direction with a medial course and divide the nasal cavity into three chambers called meati (inferior, middle, and superior). The meati are

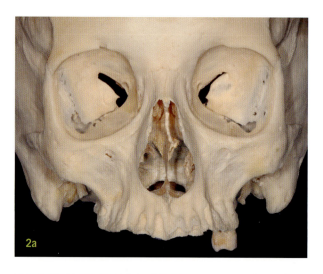
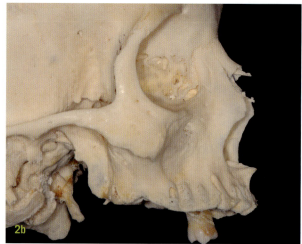
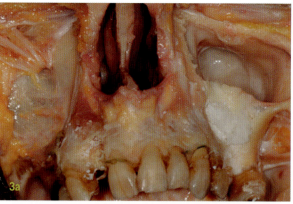
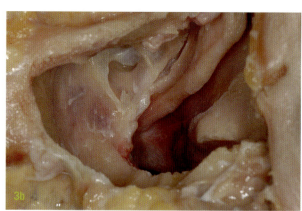
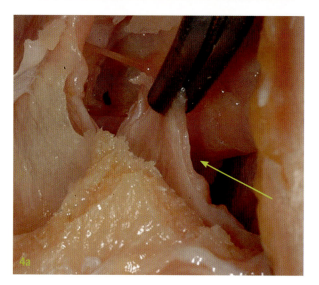

Figs 3-2a and 3-2b Osteology of the maxilla, showing its relationship with the adjacent palatal, sphenoid, zygomatic, and nasal bones.

Figs 3-3a and 3-3b Relationship between the maxilla and the nasal cavity. It is possible to very clearly see the area of the maxillary sinus, the relationship with the nasal cavity, and the emergence of the infraorbital bundle. In the left maxillary sinus, a sinus elevation has been performed. For teaching purposes, the vestibular bony table has been removed to show the graft volume in relation to the sinus width.

Figs 3-4a and 3-4b Detail of the mucosal coating of the nasal cavity. Its thickness is greater than the membrane enveloping the maxillary sinus.

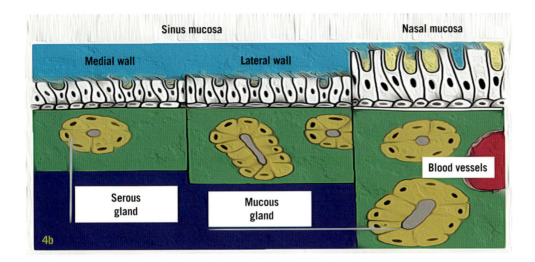

coated by ciliated pseudostratified respiratory epithelium (Fig 3-4).

Patency and ventilation of the nasal fossae can be impaired by pathologic processes of the nasal mucosa and/or congenital or acquired structural alterations.

The nasal cavity is separated from the maxillary sinus by a thin bony wall. In some cases, the dorsal part of this nasal-sinus wall in the middle meatus can be void of bone or dehiscent (accessory ostium).

The nasopalatine (incisive) canal is an anatomical structure located in the anterior part of the maxilla that originates from the base of the nose, emerging at the retroincisal level and containing the neurovascular bundle. The retroincisal part of the mucosa is innervated by the nasopalatine nerve and vascularized by the nasopalatine artery (Fig 3-5).

The nasolacrimal duct connecting the orbit and the nasal cavity is enclosed between

Figs 3-5a to 3-5e Nasopalatine canal. It is possible to see the two foramina on the nasal side joining as they emerge at the palate. In some cases, the foramen has a larger diameter, and the canal is very wide.

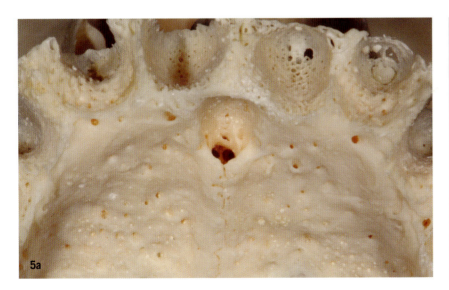
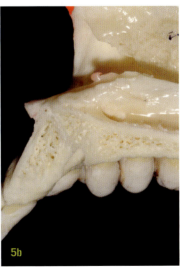

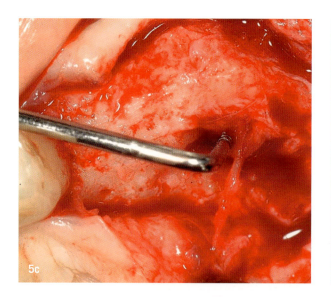

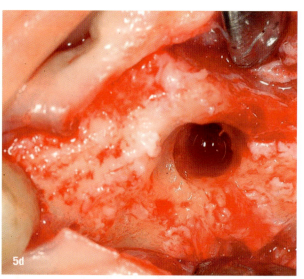

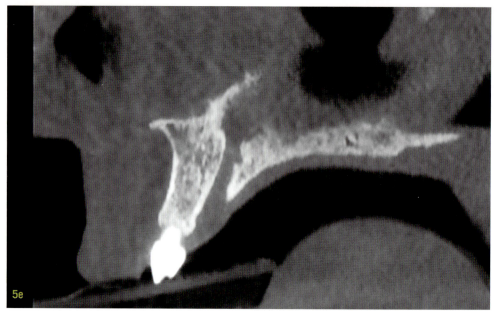

the medial wall of the maxillary sinus and the lateral wall of the nose.

The duct terminates in the inferior meatus and has the function of draining the lacrimal fluid (Fig 3-6).

Lateral to the piriform aperture, below the infraorbital notch, is the infraorbital foramen. The canal of the same name contains the infraorbital bundle, consisting of nervous and vascular components. The infraorbital nerve provides sensory innervation to the suborbital, perialar, and upper perilabial regions (Fig 3-7).

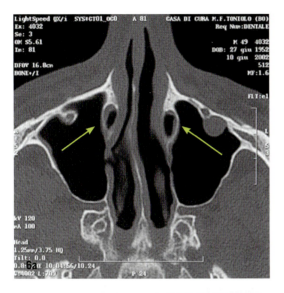
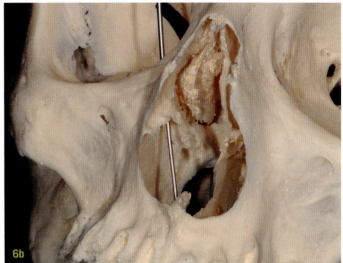
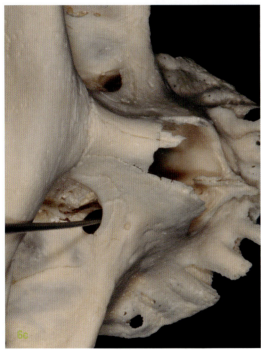

Figs 3-6a to 3-6c Radiologic and anatomical depictions of the nasolacrimal duct. Its course can be traced with a probe.

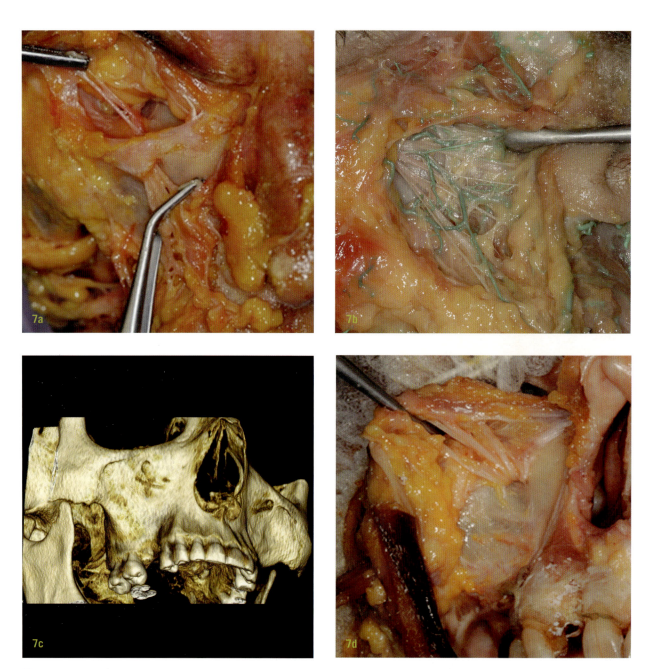

Figs 3-7a to 3-7d Infraorbital bundle. The cadaver was dissected to show the course of the bundle, originating in the region of the canine fossa.

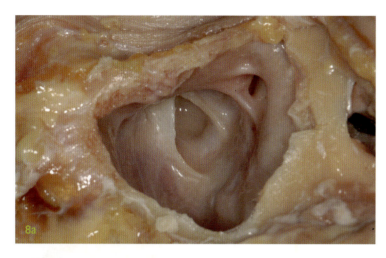
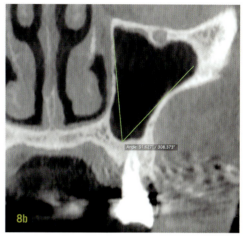
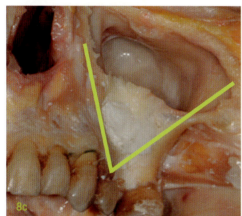

Figs 3-8a to 3-8c Relations of the maxillary sinus and anatomical variability of the angle between its mesial and lateral walls are shown *(yellow lines)*.

Region B: Lateroposterior Maxilla

Inside the body of the maxillary bone there is an airway cavity in communication with the nasal cavities called the maxillary sinus or antrum of Highmore (Fig 3-8a).

The volume of the maxillary sinus varies, but in most cases, it extends from the region of the first premolar to the second molar. Its lateromedial width is equally variable. A sinus can be wide, with a very open angle between the lateral and medial walls, or it can be very narrow, with a more acute angle (Figs 3-8b and 3-8c).

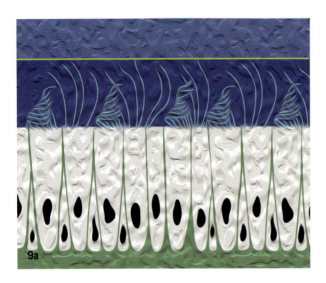
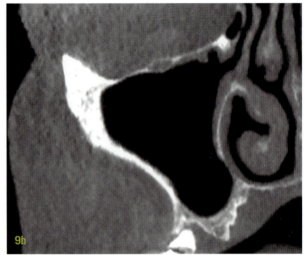
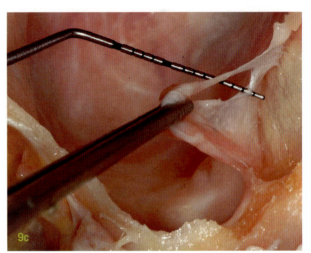

Figs 3-9a to 3-9c Epithelium of the sinus membrane. The cilia have the function of pushing the mucus secreted by muciparous cells towards the drainage ostium.

It is very important to consider this variability in planning preimplant surgical procedures such as a maxillary sinus elevation because the width of the sinus can influence the perforation rate of the sinus membrane.[8]

The internal surface of the maxillary sinus is coated by ciliated pluristratified epithelium (Fig 3-9a), and it has a physiologic thickness of 100 to 500 μm. This epithelium cannot be detected on CBCT images (Figs 3-9b and 3-9c).

Secondary to inflammatory processes, its thickness can increase to several millimeters, becoming radiographically visible (Figs 3-9d and 3-9e).

These inflammatory reactions can be local or systemic and can induce complete obliteration of the maxillary sinus, with severe effects on its homeostasis.

Some cases of sinus membrane thickening can be treated surgically by removing the cystic formation (Figs 3-9f to 3-9i).

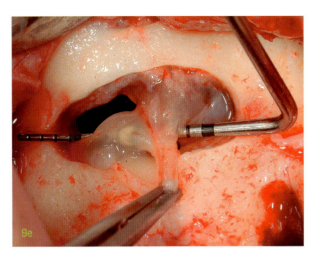

Figs 3-9d and 3-9e Clinical and radiologic evidence of sinus membrane thickening.

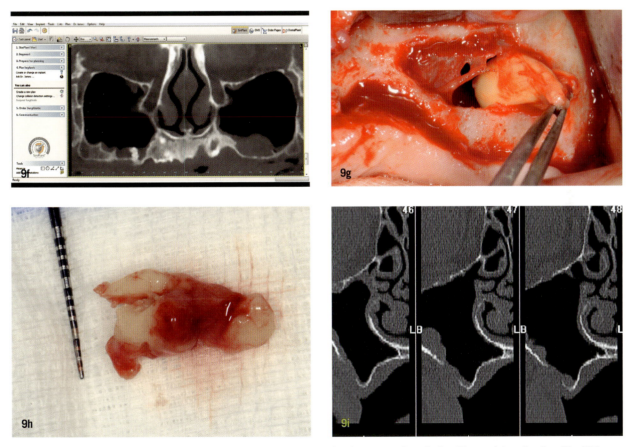

Figs 3-9f to 3-9i Localized thickening of the mucosa. The cystic formation has been treated surgically with complete extirpation. The 3D image at 2 months shows complete healing of the maxillary sinus.

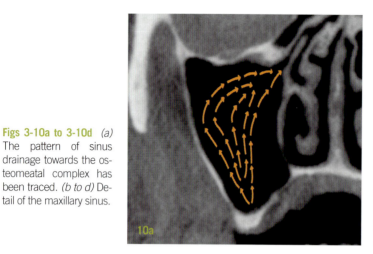
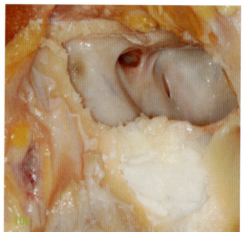

Figs 3-10a to 3-10d *(a)* The pattern of sinus drainage towards the osteomeatal complex has been traced. *(b to d)* Detail of the maxillary sinus.

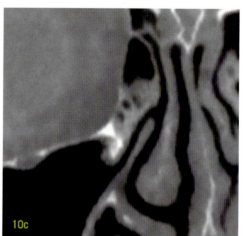

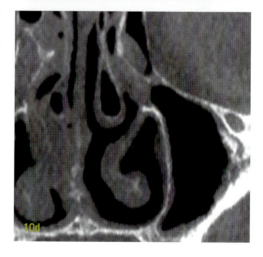

The function of the sinus membrane is to maintain the homeostasis of the maxillary sinus, draining the secreted mucus towards the osteomeatal complex (Fig 3-10a). This anatomical structure is located in the superior and posterior part of the medial wall of the maxillary sinus, and it consists of a canal that terminates at the level of the middle turbinate (Fig 3-10b). Anatomical variations or pathologic alterations of the osteomeatal complex or of adjacent structures can impair the physiologic drainage of the maxillary sinus and promote the development of pathologic processes. According to the Otorhinolaryngology School of Milan, Italy, potential anatomical abnormalities (eg, maxillary sinus septa, conchae bullosae, Haller cells) that are considered as contraindications to maxillary sinus elevation must be treated surgically (preliminary to and not simultaneous with the sinus elevation procedure) only when they interfere with the antrum drainage and ventilation, ie, when the patient's history is indicative of previous sinus pathologies and imaging shows mucosal alterations in the osteomeatal complex and in the maxillary sinus (Figs 3-10c and 3-10d).

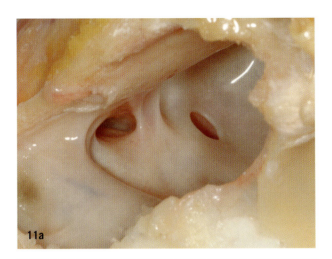

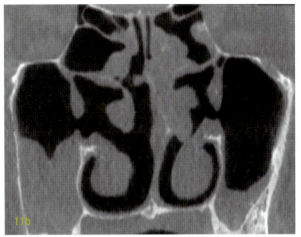

Figs 3-11a to 3-11c *(a and c)* Visual and *(b)* radiographic evidence of accessory foramina.

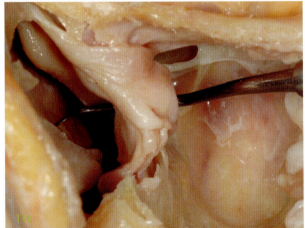

On the contrary, mucosal cysts, which can be large enough that they can obstruct the physiological maxillary ostium after a sinus elevation, can be treated by transantral window evacuation puncture simultaneous with a maxillary sinus elevation.[9,10]

Along the medial wall of the maxillary sinus, accessory ostia can sometimes be found. They open into the middle meatus in the area of nasal fontanels that are posterior to the osteomeatal complex. In the fontanel area, coalescence may occur between the mucosa of the nasal fossa and that of the maxillary sinus. The two mucosae are separated by a thin fibrous reticulum without a bony wall in between (Fig 3-11).[11]

The maxillary sinus can be a single large cavity, or it can be divided into bony septa called Underwood septa that subdivide the maxillary sinus volume into various chambers (Fig 3-12).

Figs 3-12a to 3-12c Underwood septa. These fins of bone typically have a lateromedial course, but it is also possible to find septa with a mediodistal or more convoluted course.

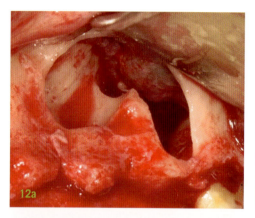
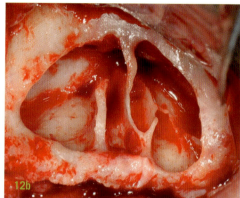
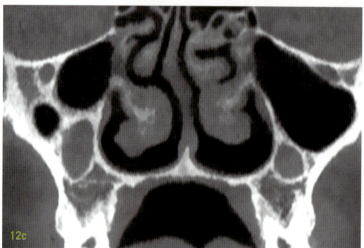

Usually these bony formations have a lateromedial course, but sometimes they can be more convoluted and develop in multiple directions. It is important to underline how these chambers are never completely closed; they are always in communication with the antrum so as to guarantee its ventilation.

An anatomical peculiarity of this region is the presence of a vessel, the alveolar antral artery, along the lateral wall of the maxillary sinus (Figs 3-13a to 3-13c). This vessel is a vascular anastomosis between the infraorbital artery and the posterior superior alveolar artery that runs in an anteroposterior direction at the level of the most caudal portion of the maxillary sinus (Fig 3-13d).[12,13]

The vessel is not always visible radiographically because in some cases it does not flow intraosseously (Fig 3-13e) but rather within the mucosa of the maxillary sinus.

The presence of this vessel can increase the risk of intraoperative complications during maxillary sinus elevation procedures because of potential bleeding (Fig 3-13f).

Figs 3-13a to 3-13f Alveolar antral artery. The vessel can have an intra- or extraosseous course. When the vessel is intraosseous, it is visible radiographically and must be studied to plan the most appropriate antrostomy.

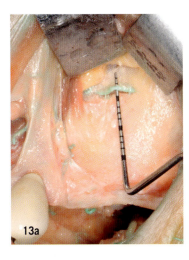

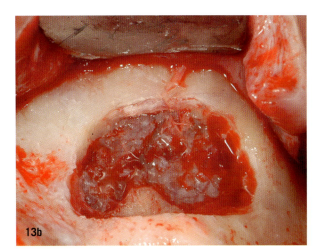

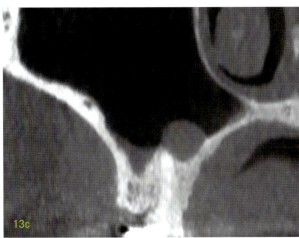

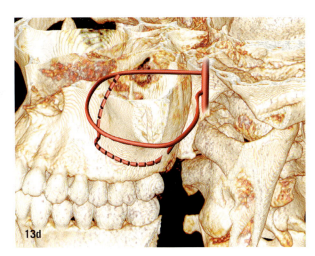

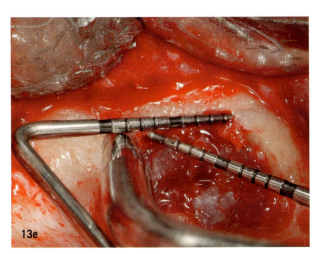

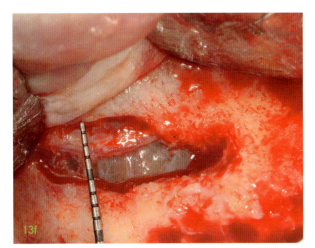

Region C: Maxillary Tuberosity Area

Greater Palatine Foramen

Posterior to the palate between the horizontal plane of the palatal process and the alveolar process is the location of the palatine foramen, the opening of the canal containing the greater palatine artery. Its landmark is placed between the maxillary second and third molars (Fig 3-14).

The vessel is located between the alveolar process and the palatal process of the maxillary bone. During harvesting of palatal

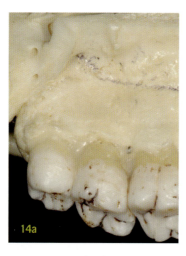
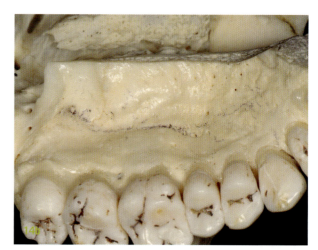
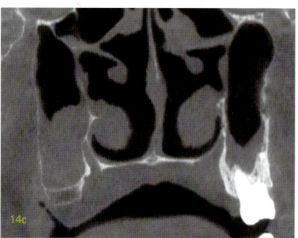

Figs 3-14a to 3-14c Course and emergence of the palatal bundle. Its emergence in the posterior area of the maxilla must be studied prior to palatal harvesting procedures.

connective tissue, it is uncommon to cut this vessel, as it flows very deep inside a protective bony sheath. It is nevertheless possible to damage the more superficial secondary branches, but this inconvenience can be easily managed surgically due to the small diameter of these vessels. The pterygoid processes of the sphenoid can be of surgical interest. They are an anatomical area where dental implants may be stabilized (Fig 3-15).

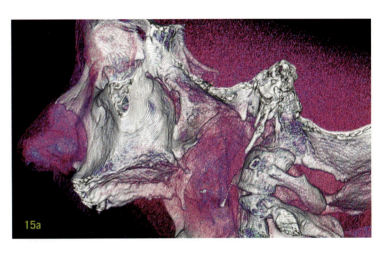

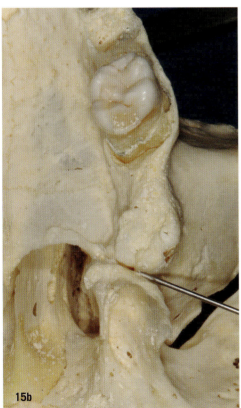

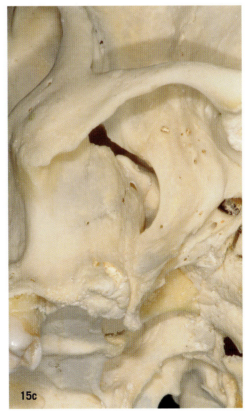

Figs 3-15a to 3-15c Pterygoid processes of the sphenoid and their relationship with the posterior maxilla are shown in (a) 3D reconstruction and (b and c) a dry skull.

Radiologic and Clinical Anatomy of the Mandible

The mandible is an unpaired median bone consisting of a main body and two ascending rami; the temporomandibular joint is the anatomical unit that connects the mandible to the temporal bones.

The mandibular body has a horseshoe form. It can be more or less square or triangular shaped (U- or V-shaped) (Fig 3-16). The mandible has two surfaces, external and internal.

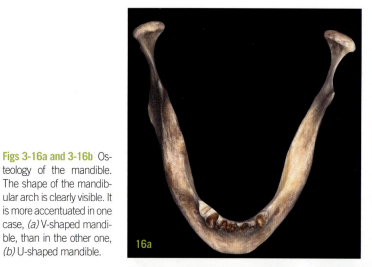
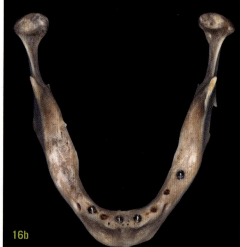

Figs 3-16a and 3-16b Osteology of the mandible. The shape of the mandibular arch is clearly visible. It is more accentuated in one case, *(a)* V-shaped mandible, than in the other one, *(b)* U-shaped mandible.

Figs 3-17a and 3-17b Area of the symphysis menti, or mandibular symphysis. These views show the typical position of the dental axis with reference to the mandibular body.

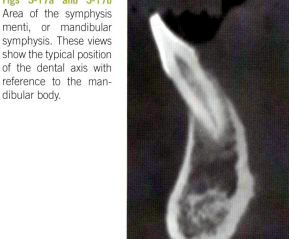
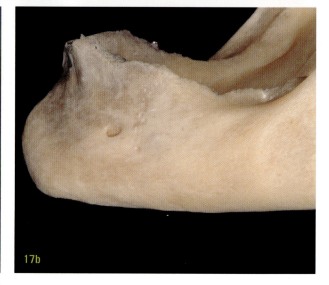

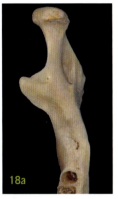 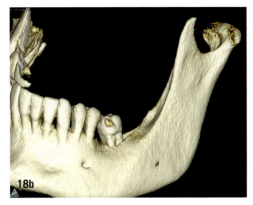 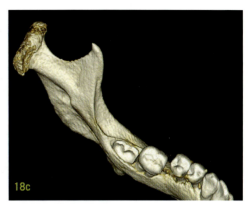

Figs 3-18a to 3-18c Region of the mandibular ramus. The articular condyle and the coronoid process, where the temporalis muscle inserts, are shown. The internal surface is the location of the mandibular foramen.

On the external surface in the premolar region, there is the mental foramen; on the internal surface, the mandibular foramen is in a more posterior position.

In the anterior region of the mandible there is the symphysis, the area where the two hemiarches unite (Fig 3-17). The mandibular rami consist of two processes; the coronoid process is anterior, and the posterior process ends in the articular condyle (Fig 3-18).

The mandibular body and the ramus join together at the mandibular angle. Anterior to the angle, on the lateral surface, the masseter muscle inserts; on the medial surface, the medial pterygoid muscle inserts of the mandibular angle. The external pterygoid muscle (also called the lateral pterygoid) inserts on the condyle.

Anterior to the masseter insertion, along the mandibular edge, is the antegonial notch, where the facial artery is located (Fig 3-19). Similar to the maxilla, it is possible to outline a systematic, rational approach to the analysis of the mandibular anatomical structures. This rational assessment starts in the area of the symphysis, continues with the mandibular body, and ends with the area of the ascending ramus (Fig 3-20).

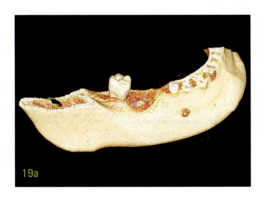 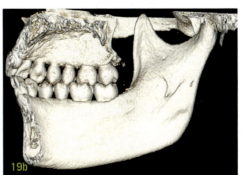

Figs 3-19a and 3-19b The antegonial notch on the mandibular edge can be more or less marked. Behind it, the masseter muscle and, on the internal side, the external pterygoid muscle insert.

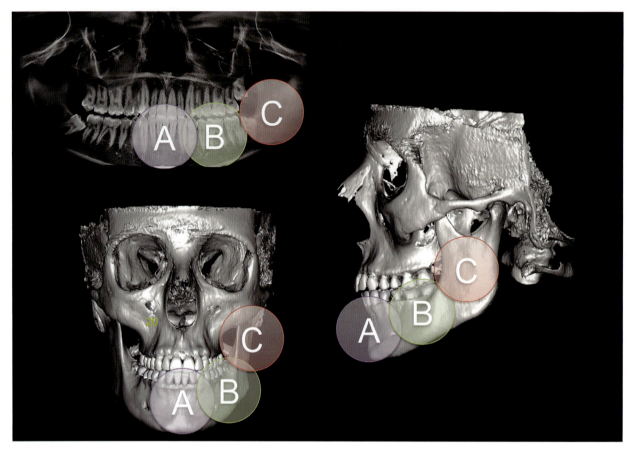

Fig 3-20 The three regions of the mandible are shown in a panoramic radiograph and in frontal and lateral 3D views.

Table 3-2 Relevant anatomical structures: Mandible
Region A: Symphysis
Mylohyoid line
Incisive nerve
Perforating branches of the sublingual artery
Genial tubercles
Region B: Lateroposterior mandibular body
Mandibular canal
Mental foramen
Submandibular fossa
Region C: Mandibular ramus
Mandibular canal
Third molar
External oblique line
Gonial angle

Region A: Mandibular Symphysis

The region anterior to the mental foramen, the symphysis area, region A in this systemic analysis, is characterized in the sagittal plane by an anterior concavity between the inferior border of the mandible and the alveolar process (Fig 3-21).

Physiologic anatomy may be altered in some patients, in whom the anteroposterior thickness of the symphysis area is greatly reduced. Cases of "hourglass" symphysis are not infrequent. These patients present with thin cortical bone apical to the alveolar process.[14] This constriction leads to major problems in implant-prosthetic rehabilitation in the frontal mandibular region, especially in the absence of an accurate 3D case assessment (Fig 3-22).

Another structure in this region is the incisive branch of the mandibular nerve. This anatomical structure is not located inside a proper canal but instead is a neuroplexus; anatomical sections and radiologic findings do not show it surrounded by cortical bone (Fig 3-23).

The genial tubercles are important landmarks (Fig 3-24). These bony processes are located along the median line of the lingual side of the symphysis and are the insertion area for the genioglossal muscle and, more inferiorly, for the geniohyoid muscle.

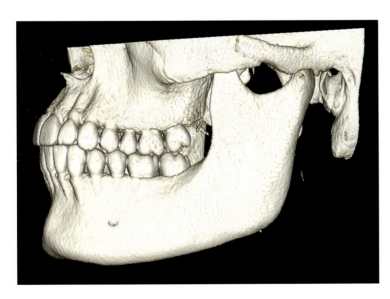

Fig 3-21 Concavity of the alveolar process in the mandible, where the symphysis is located. This area must be carefully assessed in anterior implant rehabilitation cases because the prosthesis axis and the residual alveolar crest axis may differ.

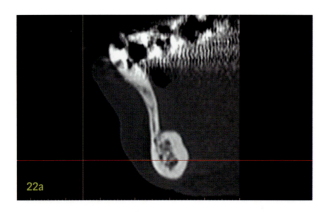
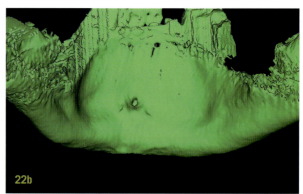

Figs 3-22a to 3-22c Anatomical variations of the symphysis area. These cases are difficult to treat surgically due to the presence of a thin layer of bone between the inferior mandibular border and the teeth.

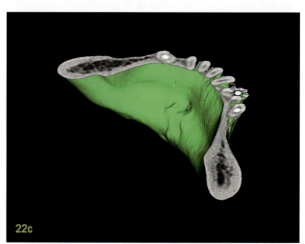

Figs 3-23a and 3-23b Course of the incisive branch. The neurovascular bundle does not traverse the mandible inside hollow cortical bone but instead within the trabecular bone.

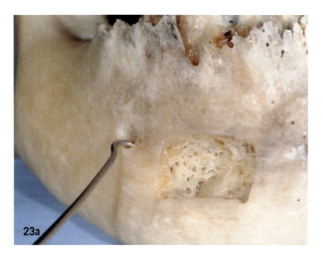
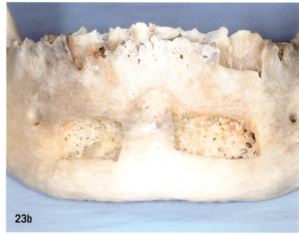

These bone projections are an important indicator of resorption in the residual alveolar crest—especially in totally edentulous patients—because they seldom undergo bone resorption. In edentulous patients with severe atrophy, the genial tubercles may be located at the level of the residual ridge, creating a lingual prominence that can greatly limit oral hygiene measures in patients with a fixed implant rehabilitation. Another anatomical peculiarity of the symphysis is the presence of arterial branches that perforate the lingual cortex (Fig 3-25). These vessels connect the sublingual artery with the intraosseous vascular network of the mandibular artery.[15]
Foramina on the lingual side of the mandible. Through these foramina a vascular anastomosis is formed between the incisive branch of the mandibular artery and the lingual artery.

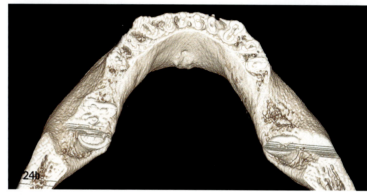

Figs 3-24a and 3-24b Genial tubercles; area of insertion of the genioglossal and geniohyoid muscles. These bone formations do not undergo atrophy in patients with extreme mandibular resorption because of continuous stimulation from the muscles.
Figs 3-25a and 3-25b Foramina on the lingual side of the mandible. Through these foramina a vascular anastomosis is formed between the incisal ramus of the mandible and the lingual artery.

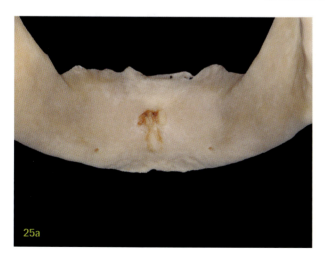
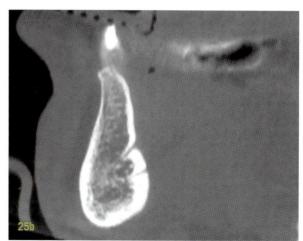

Region B: Lateroposterior Mandibular Body

In region B the most relevant anatomical structure is the mental foramen, which is usually located in the premolar region. Its size and shape are variable. There are round or oval-shaped foramina. Close to the main foramen, it is not infrequent to find accessory foramina containing sensory fibers (Fig 3-26).

The course of the mandibular canal is variable in proximity to the mandibular foramen. In some patients there is a loop that departs from the canal and runs superiorly and inferiorly. In other patients, the neurovascular bundle proceeds anteriorly without any loop.[16]

On the lingual side, the mylohyoid line (the insertion of the mylohyoid muscle) is an important landmark dividing the oral cavity and the submandibular fossa (Fig 3-27). The mylohyoid muscle is the floor of the

Figs 3-26a to 3-26e Anatomical variants of the mental foramen. There are a variety of mental foramina shapes, and it is not infrequent to find accessory foramina close to the main foramen.

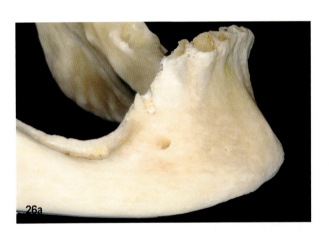
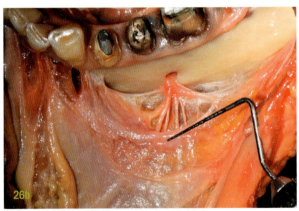
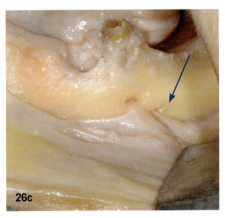
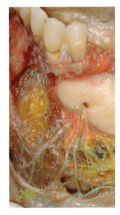
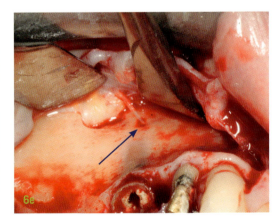

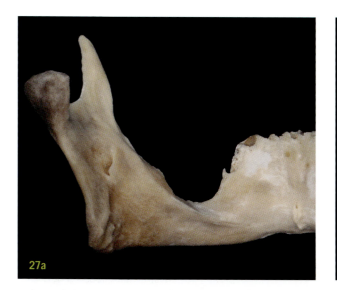
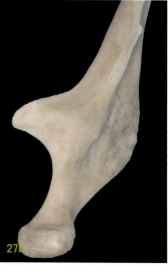

Figs 3-27a to 3-27c The mylohyoid line is the area of insertion of the mylohyoid muscle that separates the oral cavity from the structures of the neck.

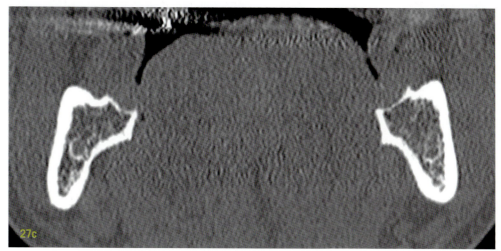

oral cavity. Caudal to the mylohyoid line, there is a fossa containing the submandibular gland. This concavity can be more or less accentuated; when the fossa is more pronounced, the residual crestal space for implant placement is reduced (Fig 3-28).

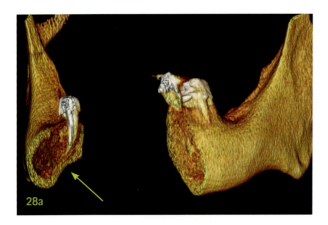
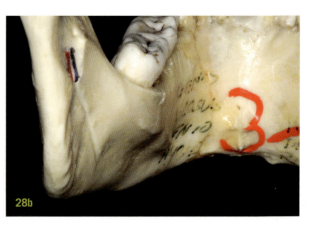

Figs 3-28a and 3-28b In the posterior mandibular region, on the lingual side, the submandibular fossa accommodates the gland of the same name *(arrow)*. The undercut thus formed can reduce the volume of bone available for implant placement.

Region C: Mandibular Ramus

The most important anatomical structure in the mandible is the neurovascular bundle consisting of an artery, a vein, and a nerve, which is located inside the mandibular canal (Fig 3-29). The entrance to the canal may sometimes be protected by an anatomical structure called the spine of Spix, or the canal may open directly on the internal surface of the ascending ramus (Figs 3-30a to 3-30d). The canal progresses cranio-caudally towards the mental foramen in a direction that is from the lingual to the buccal; its height in relation to the mandibular border varies, and it has a more or less close relationship with the third molars. In cases of partial or total third molar impaction, the relationship between the neurovascular bundle and the roots of the tooth must be carefully assessed (Fig 3-30e). In some clinical cases, the neurovascular bundle runs between two roots fused at the apex. This anatomical peculiarity needs to be carefully considered preoperatively because it will determine the surgical proce-

Figs 3-29a and 3-29b Course of the mandibular canal along the mandibular body.

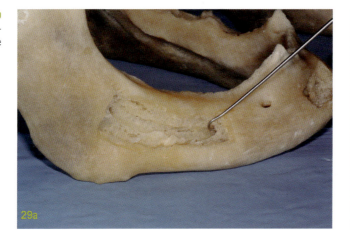
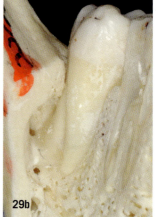

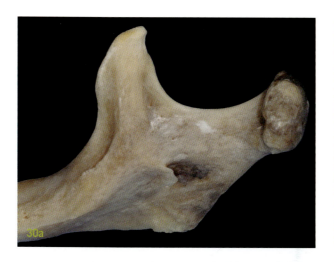
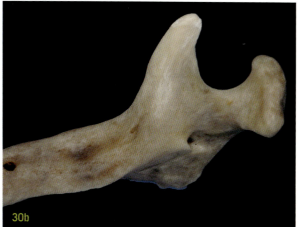
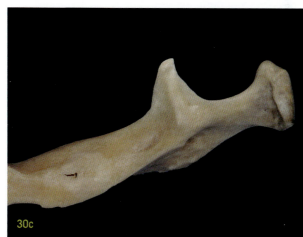
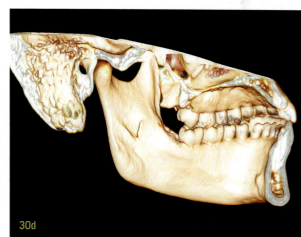
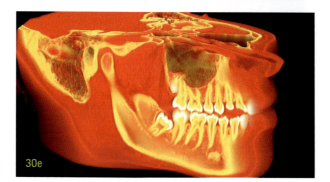

Figs 3-30a to 3-30d Mandibular canal and anatomical variability of the spine of Spix, which is a bone formation covering the access to the mandibular canal in some patients.

Fig 3-30e Relationship between the mandibular canal and the third molar.

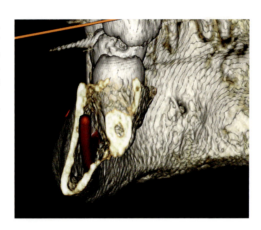

Fig 3-31 Anatomical variation of the mandibular canal. Usually the mandibular canal is positioned lingual to the roots of the third molar. Here, however, it is located buccal to the tooth.

Figs 3-32a to 3-32d Anatomical variations of the mandibular canal. *(a to c)* A bifurcation is evident with imaging. *(d)* The mandibular canal is not surrounded by cortical bone but, as in the symphysis region, the neurovascular bundle runs through trabecular bone. This explains why it is difficult to detect its course in patients in whom the bone trabeculae are not clearly visible.

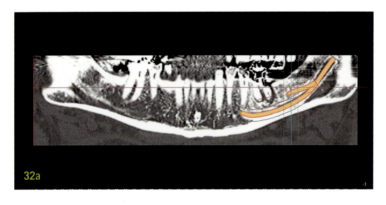

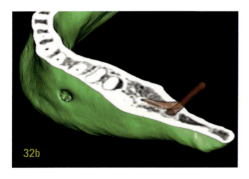

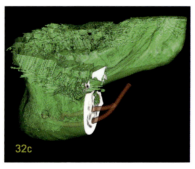

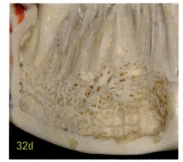

dure to avoid potential neurologic lesions (axonotmesis or neurotmesis).

Direct contact between the mandibular canal and the root of a tooth on either the lingual or buccal side is not infrequent. Moreover, the position of the tooth may vary. Usually the mandibular third molar is located buccal to the mandibular canal. There are nevertheless cases of the inverse relationship in which the tooth is positioned lingually (Fig 3-31). Extraction of this tooth without first analyzing this anatomical variant can result in a high risk of paresthesia.[17]

In the literature, there have been case reports of a double course of mandibular canal containing an accessory neurovascular bundle (Figs 3-32a to 3-32c).[18] The mandibular canal is not always delimited by cortical bone. This characteristic explains why it is not always possible to detect the course of the canal on CBCT images (Fig 3-32d). Distal to the third molar, one may frequently find a bone formation called the retromolar or Robinson canal (Fig 3-33).[19]

On the external surface of the mandibular body, there is a linear bone prominence, the external oblique line, which starts from the anterior edge of the mandibular ramus and develops caudally and anteriorly towards the mental tubercles. Its position must be carefully considered when harvesting bone from the mandibular ramus (Fig 3-34).

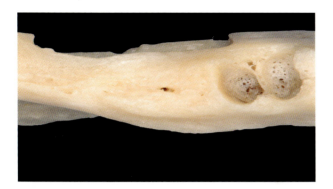

Fig 3-33 Retromolar or Robinson canal. This canal emerges near the third molar.

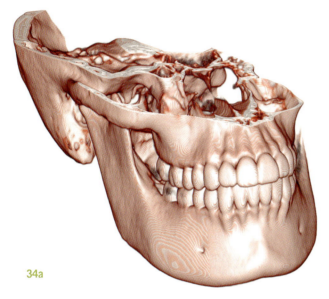

Figs 3-34a to 3-34d Mandibular ramus: the external oblique line is an important landmark when harvesting bone from the mandibular ramus.

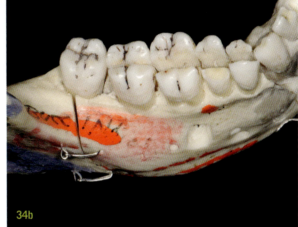

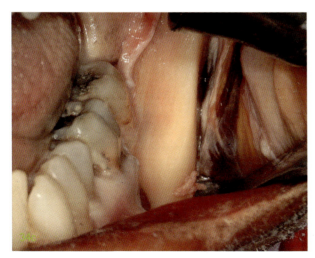

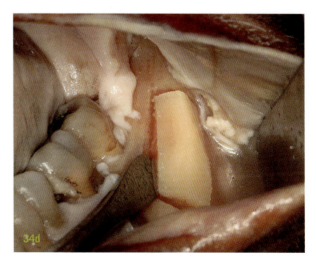

Conclusion

In-depth knowledge of the anatomical structures in the orofacial region is fundamental for the dentist operating in this region. This knowledge allows the dentist to use the correct technical and surgical procedures and to plan the best, most up-to-date, and most ethical approaches to achieve an ideal clinical outcome.

In this perspective, anatomy is no longer interpreted as a theoretical, partly forgotten subject matter but as a vital 3D reality—the field where dentistry operates.

Inadequate anatomical preparation is often the cause of iatrogenic vascular or neurologic complications after surgical procedures that are not intrinsically complex.

In the mandible, for instance, the mandibular nerve and its branches, a sensory and a motor nerve, have many anatomical variations, particularly at the level of the mental foramen and the incisive canal.

Iatrogenic neurologic lesions of the sensorineural component in this nerve, such as transient or permanent paresthesia after surgical procedures (eg, extraction of the mandibular third molar or implant placement), can be major complications with medicolegal consequences.

The authors therefore recommend proper radiologic assessment and comparison with actual anatomy, including two-finger palpation of the alveolar crest. Further investigation with specific 3D examinations like CT is fundamental to detect anatomical variations. Considering the quantity of data that modern radiologic examinations can provide, it is extremely important to have a rational assessment process so that no important information is omitted.

The extension of the CBCT acquisition plane allows the clinician to view structures that are not specifically in the domain of dentistry, and this must prompt dentists to gather knowledge of ear, nose, throat, and maxillofacial anatomy so as to be able to refer their patients to the appropriate specialist in case of visible pathology in the CBCT image.

Clinical Examples

The images displayed in the following pages have been acquired with the following systems: NewTom VGi, Quantitative Radiology; Galileos, Sirona; i-CAT Cone Beam 3D Imaging, Imaging Sciences.

Relevant anatomical structures: Maxilla

Region A: Anterior maxilla
Nasal septum
Anterior nasal spine
Nasopalatal canal
Nasolacrimal duct
Lateral nasal wall
Nasal turbinates

Region B: Lateroposterior maxilla
Orbit
Maxillary sinus
Infraorbital foramen
Zygomatic process

Region C: Maxillary tuberosity area
Greater palatine foramen
Maxillary tuberosity
Pterygoid process of the sphenoid
Articular fossa

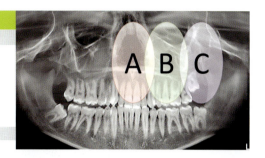

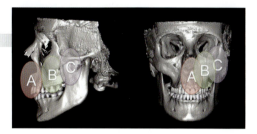

Relevant anatomical structures: Mandible

Region A: Symphysis
Mylohyoid line
Incisive nerve
Perforating branches of the sublingual artery
Genial tubercles

Region B: Lateroposterior mandibular body
Mandibular canal
Mental foramen
Submandibular fossa

Region C: Mandibular ramus
Mandibular canal
Third molar
External oblique line
Gonial angle

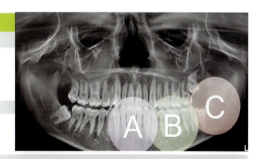

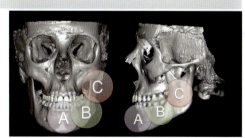

Normal Anatomy

Maxillary sinus elevation in healthy conditions

The presurgical image shows the absence of reactive phenomena of the sinus mucosa and the patency of the osteomeatal complex.
The postsurgical image shows the ideal retention of the grafting material and the absence of inflammatory processes of the sinus mucosa.

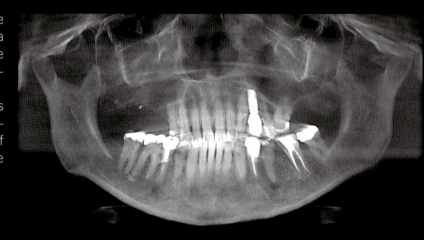

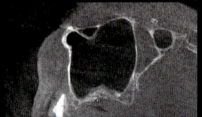
Sagittal section

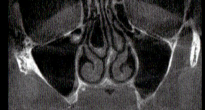
Coronal section

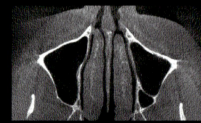
Axial section

The three-dimensional reconstruction makes it easy to visualize the bone volume created in respect to total air volume of the maxillary sinus.
The implant is surrounded along its circumference by the bone grafting material.

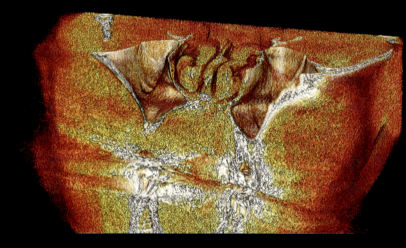

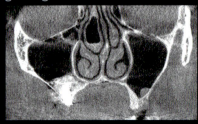

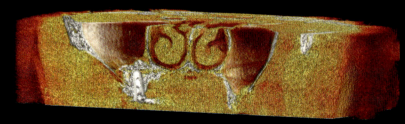

2 Normal Anatomy

Maxillary sinus

Image of the maxillary sinus is shown in a CBCT panoramic image and horizontal section.

The sinus appears well ventilated, with a patent osteomeatal complex. The anatomical structures, such as the nasolacrimal duct and the nasal cavity with the turbinates and their relationship with the maxillary sinus, are well visible.

The maxillary sinus has no radiopacity, and the sinus mucosa does not exhibit inflammatory processes.

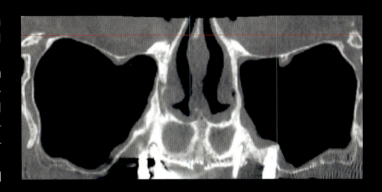

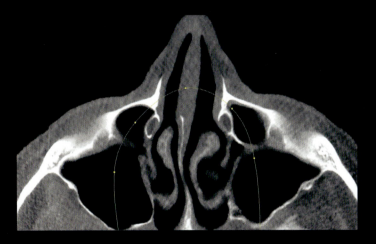

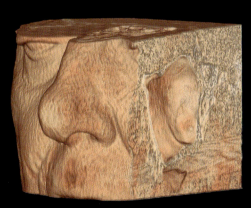

Sagittal section

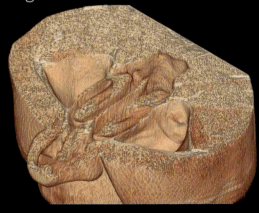

Axial section

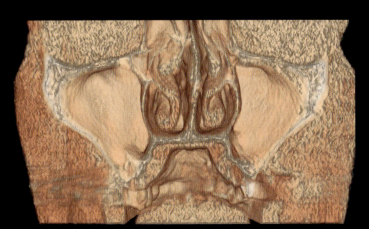

Coronal section

Maxillary sinus septum (Underwood septum) with an oblique course is visible. The septum delimits an anterior and medial cavity.
Laterally, the sinus mucosa appears slightly thickened.
Along the lateral wall of the maxillary sinus the bone groove housing the anastomosis between the superior posterior alveolar and infraorbital arteries is visible.

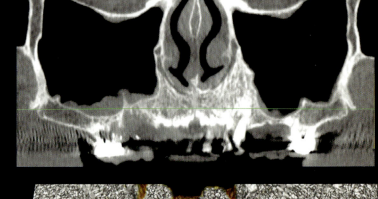

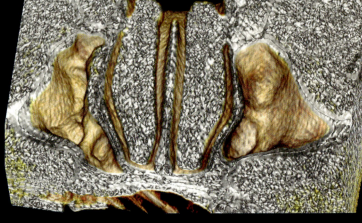

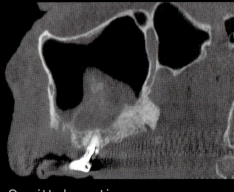

Sagittal section

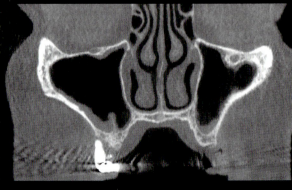

Coronal section

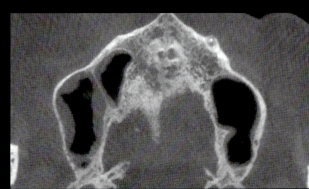

Axial section

Normal Anatomy

Maxillary sinus: Circumflex artery

Pronounced radiologic evidence of the circumflex artery course along the maxillary sinus lateral wall. The groove created along the bony table is clearly visible. The course appears normal, starting from the tuberosity region and continuing horizontally towards the piriform aperture.

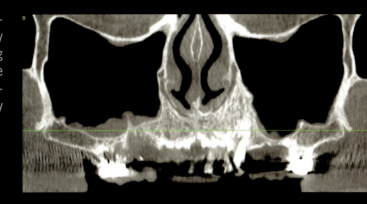

Sagittal section

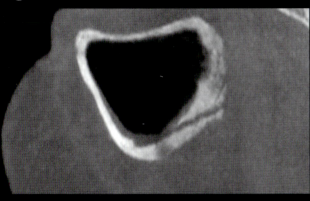

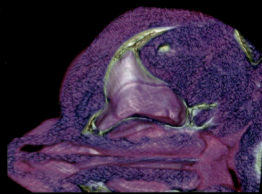

Three-dimensional reconstruction, with a horizontal section passing through the maxillary sinus. It is possible to see the vessel's course on the vertical plane.

Coronal section

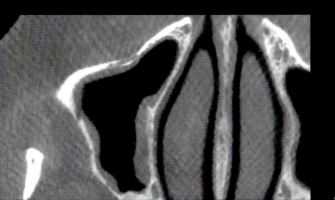

Axial section

5 Normal Anatomy
Vascular network

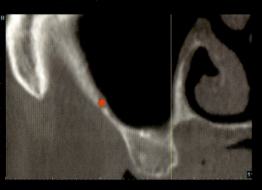

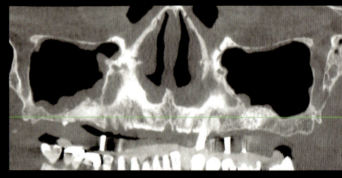

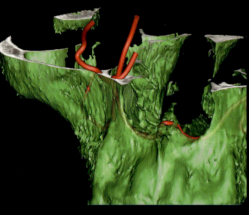

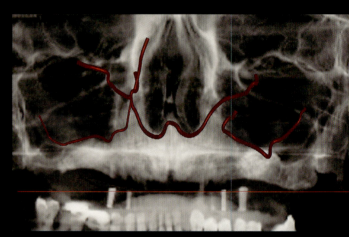

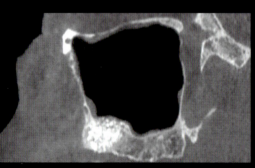

Reconstruction of the vessel's course in the incisive bone region.
The course has been traced following the foramina within the bone component, where possible. The extraosseous branches, not visible, are not traced.
It is possible to note the complex network vascularizing the nasal and incisive bone regions.

Sagittal section

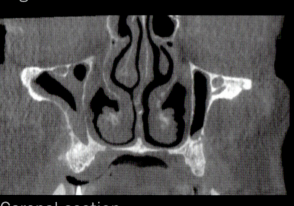

Coronal section		Axial section

6 Normal Anatomy

Nasopalatine canal

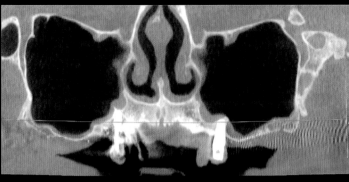

Sections through the nasopalatine canal. It is possible to see the relationship between the central incisors and the retroincisal area.

The course of the nasopalatine canal can be variable. In some patients, the canal appears as a single canal up to the nasal portion. In other patients, it appears as two distinct canals merging in the middle.

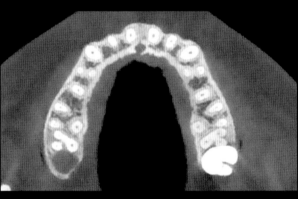

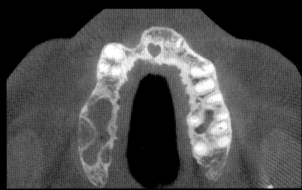

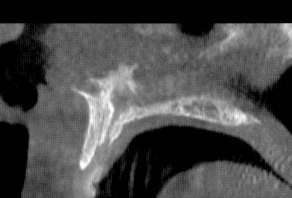

Sagittal section

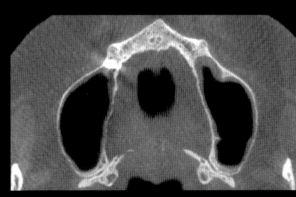

Axial section

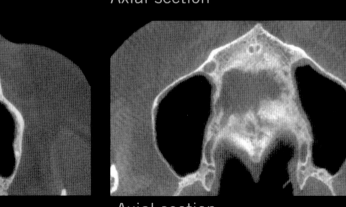

Axial section

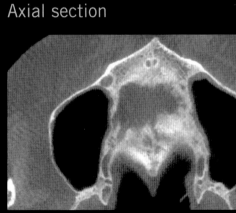

Axial section

Normal Anatomy

Maxillary sinus septa (Underwood septa)

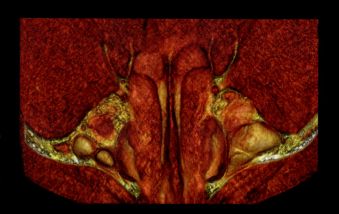

Right maxillary sinus with multiple chambers due to the presence of the Underwood septa.
The posterior recess appears almost completely closed by bone walls and is radiopaque because of the stagnation of secretions.

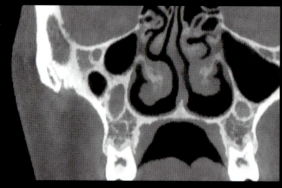

Coronal section

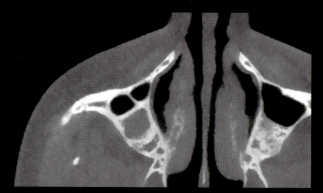

Axial section

8 Normal Anatomy

Maxillary sinus: Reactive thickening due to sinus elevation procedure

Maxillary sinus mucosa reacts to the sinus elevation intervention with a traumatic ciliostasis, which reduces the secretion drainage towards the osteomeatal complex. Moreover, an edema establishes in the mucous layer, reducing the free residual volume within the maxillary sinus.

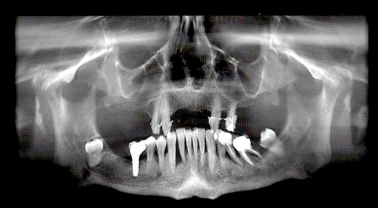

Axial section	Coronal section	Sagittal section

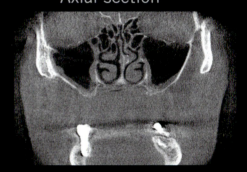 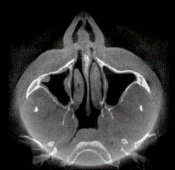 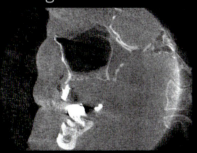

Preoperative

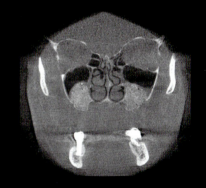

Postoperative

This phenomenon is normal and must not be considered pathologic; on the contrary, it must be considered in relation to the extent of the sinus elevation procedure.

An excessive elevation of the maxillary sinus mucosa may lead to an iatrogenic closure of the osteomeatal complex with sinus ventilation arrest.

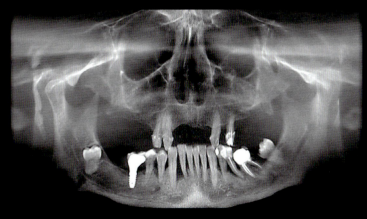

9 Normal Anatomy

Maxillary sinus septa (Underwood septa)

Maxillary sinus chambers are shown. The septum has an oblique course in an anteroposterior direction. It is important to visualize the sections in the different reference planes in order to understand their direction.

During an antrostomy procedure or membrane elevation, the clinician must take particular care with the sinus membrane to avoid lacerations.

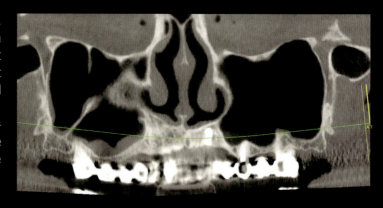

Axial section

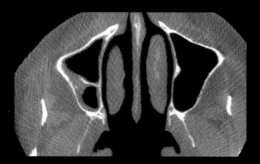

Coronal section

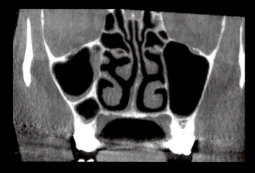

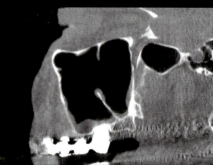

Sagittal section

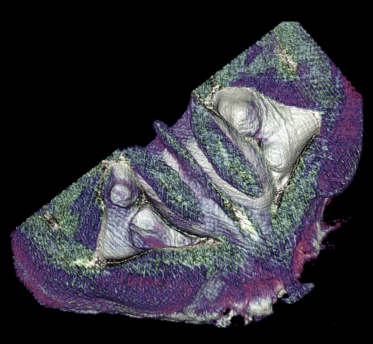

10 Normal Anatomy
Palatine arteries

It is possible to see the neurovascular bundle emerge in the posterior section of the maxilla.
The course of the canal has been marked in the 3D reconstructions. During the surgical intervention, the neurovascular bundle has been isolated along its course.
The bundle measures approximately 3 mm tranversely.

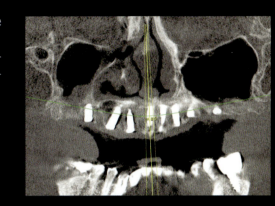

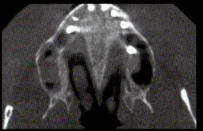
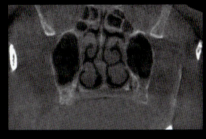
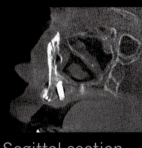

Axial section   Coronal section   Sagittal section

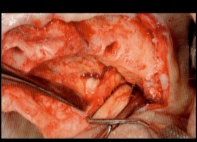
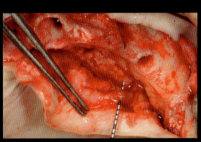
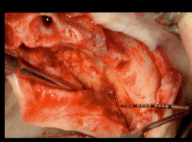

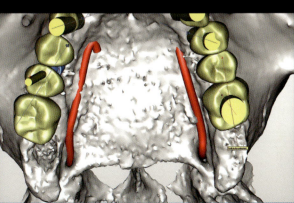
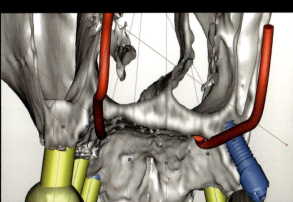

The accessory ostium is located more caudally and posteriorly than the main ostium. This accessory foramen is a not-infrequent anatomical finding, and it is in communication with the nasal cavity superior to the inferior turbinate.

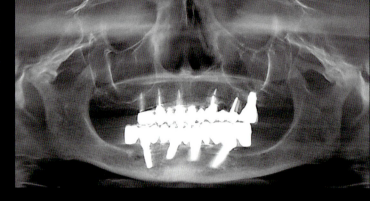

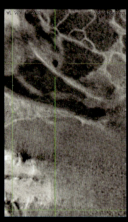

Sagittal section

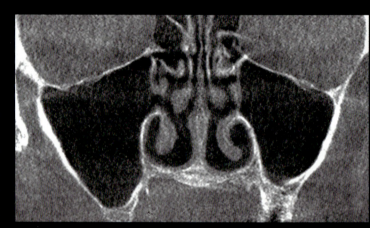

Coronal section

In the 3D reconstruction it is possible to highlight the accessory ostium's location, posterior to the nasolacrimal canal.

During a classic maxillary sinus elevation procedure, it is difficult to see this formation, because it is located cranial to the antrostomy (approximately in the middle of the canal cavity width in a craniocaudal direction).

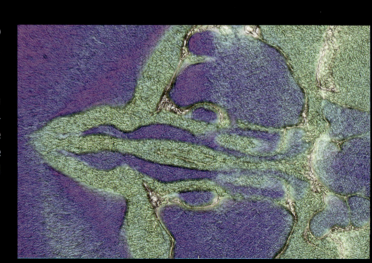

Axial 3D image

12 Anatomical Variations
Maxillary sinus

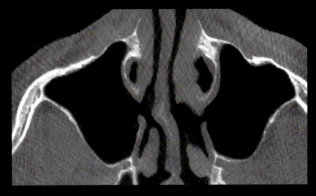
Axial section

Maxillary accessory ostia in the presence of a septum deviation with medialmeatal spurs are visible.
The ostia are located in the middle meatus, superior to the inferior turbinate. The accessory ostium measures approximately 5 mm and has an elongated shape in the anteroposterior direction, as shown in the 3D reconstruction. In the 3D reconstruction it is possible to see the middle turbinate through the accessory ostium.

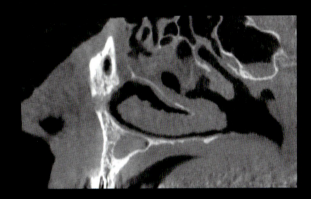
Sagittal section

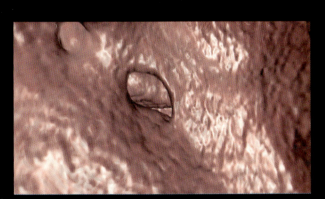

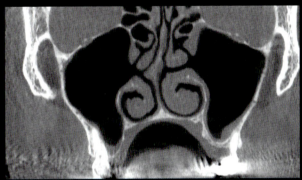
Coronal section

13 Anatomical Variations
Maxillary sinus

Presence of an accessory ostium along the lateral sinus wall.
This formation is located more caudally and posteriorly than in the osteomeatal complex that is patent.

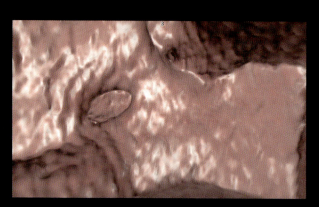

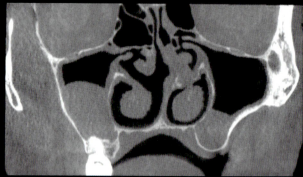
Coronal section

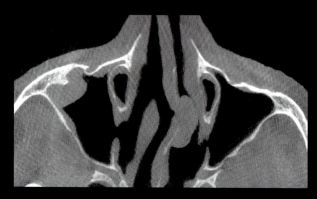
Axial section

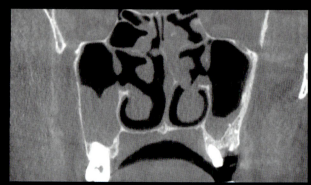
Coronal section

14 Anatomical Variations
Maxillary sinus

Anatomical variation of the maxillary sinus.
In the CBCT panoramic image, the sinus appears to have a normal shape, with radiopacities located in the sinus mucosa.
In the coronal and axial reconstructions it is possible to see an irregular anatomy of the anterior recess of the maxillary sinus, which is characterized by sinus extensions in the medial direction at the landmark between the palatal lamina and the nasal floor. The recess is found to be very deep, almost to the median line.
A sinus elevation that results in accidental closing of this extension of the anterior recess would block the sinus drainage, leading to a severe iatrogenic sinusitis.

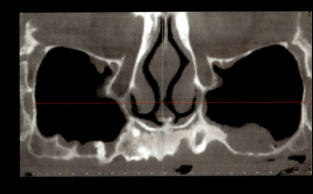

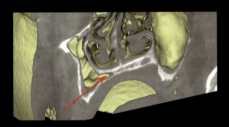

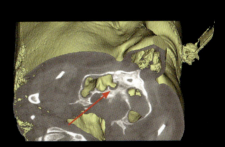

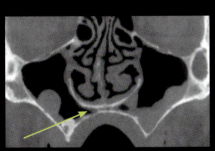

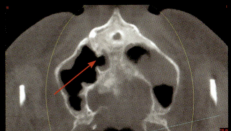

Coronal section   Axial section

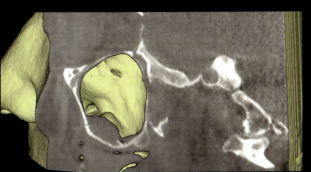

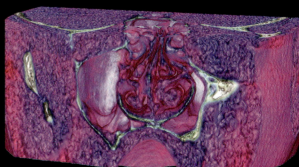

15 Anatomical Variations

Maxillary sinus: Ectopic third molar in the maxillary sinus

No other pathology is visible in this sinus. In the absence of symptoms, it is not necessary to intervene surgically to remove the ectopic tooth that is in balance with the sinus homeostasis.

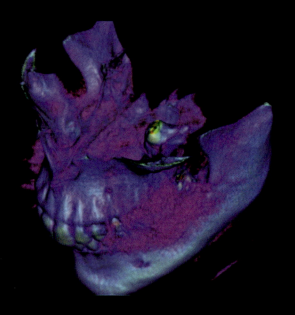

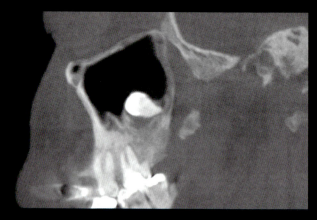

Sagittal section

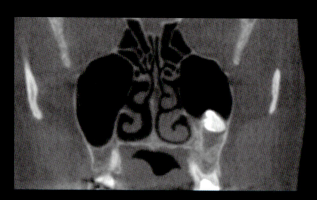

Coronal section

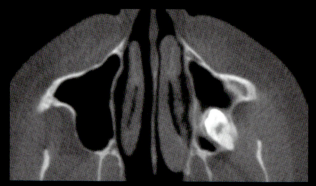

Axial section

16 Anatomical Variations

Maxillary sinus: Thickened vestibular wall of maxillary sinus

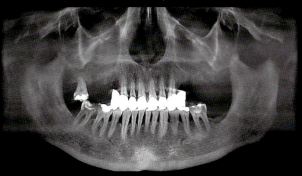

The cortical bone delimiting the maxillary sinus appears heavily thickened as compared to normal anatomy, and, moreover, it appears very corticalized. If a sinus elevation is planned, it is advisable to perform the antrostomy by erosion.

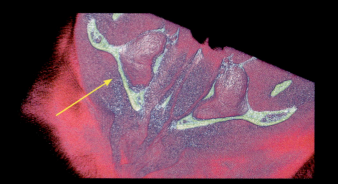

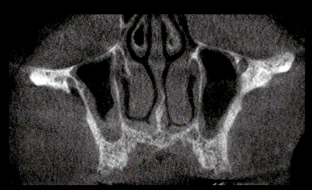

Coronal section

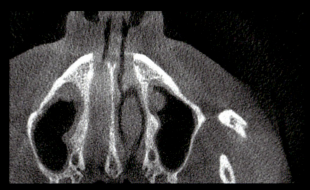

Axial section

17 Anatomical variations

Maxillary sinus: Bilateral "silent sinus syndrome"

The patient has a reduced maxillary sinus volume with expansion of the nasal cavities and depression of the orbital floor.

It is possible to see the typical alteration of the alveolar crest with an increase of the quantity of the alveolar bone and marked depression of the canine fossa.

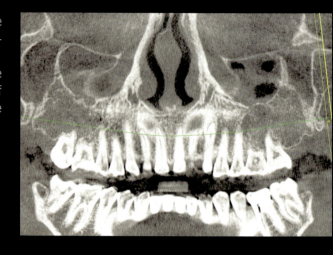

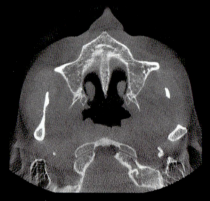

Axial section

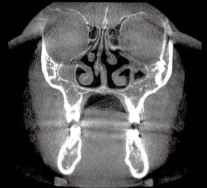

Coronal section

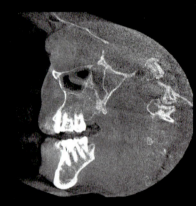

Sagittal section

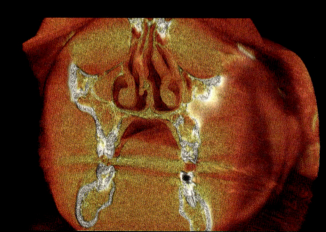

18 Anatomical Variations
Infraorbital canal

Abnormal course of the infraorbital canal. In normal anatomy, its course is located more cranially, between the orbital floor and the maxillary sinus roof, and it proceeds in the anterior direction before opening onto the maxilla at the infraorbital foramen, below the orbit. On the contrary, in this patient the canal detaches more posteriorly and proceeds forward, passing through the maxillary sinus.
Laterally, the canal is linked to the maxillary sinus lateral wall by a thin, layer of bone.
In the view of the coronal plane, it is possible to highlight the diameter of the canal, which is completely ossified, and its direction.
In the 3D reconstructions it is possible to see the anterolateral recess created by the infraorbital canal with the maxillary sinus wall.
This event must be carefully investigated, as the location of the infraorbital foramen is, as a result, more caudal. In case of a surgical intervention in the maxilla (for example, a sinus elevation), the periosteal releasing incisions must be superficial and not involve the submucosal plane.

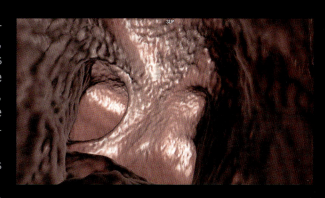

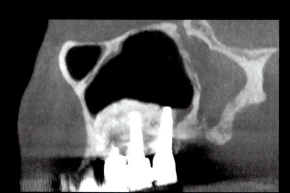

Sagittal section

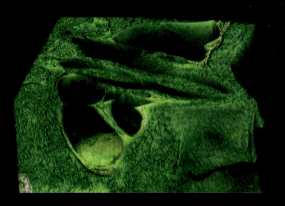

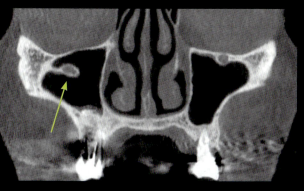

Coronal section

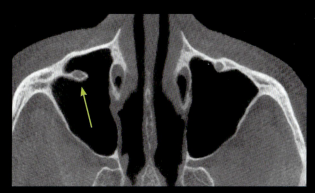

Axial section

19 Anatomical Variations

Canalis sinuosus: Anastomosis between vascular structures

Along the anterior margin of the maxillary sinus, on the boundary of the piriform aperture, the radiographic assessment highlights the course of a vessel that, starting from the infraorbital foramen, proceeds to the base of the nose, merging at the level of the nasopalatine foramen.

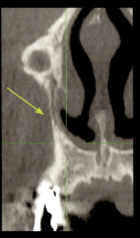
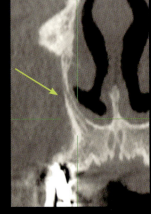

Coronal section

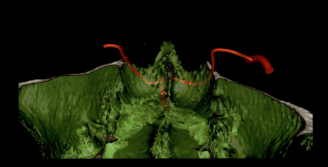
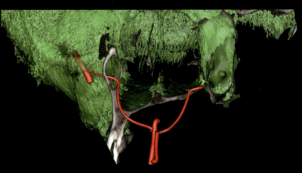

20 Anatomical Variations
Canalis sinuosus: Vascular anastomosis

Radiologic evidence of vascular anastomosis between a branch coming from the maxillary sinus lateral wall, the infraorbital artery, and the nasopalatine canal. In the section shown, the anatomical area of the convergence of the vascular canals located in correspondence to the apex of the anterior recess of the maxillary sinus can be seen. Such a formation is called canalis sinuosus and runs in a craniocaudal direction, emerging at the level of the anterior palatal area between the canine and the central incisor.[20-22]

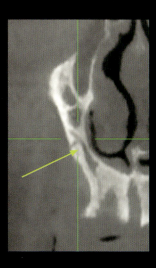
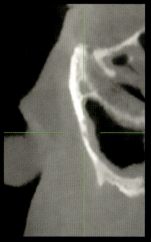
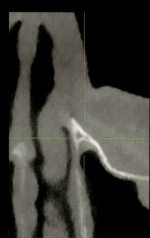

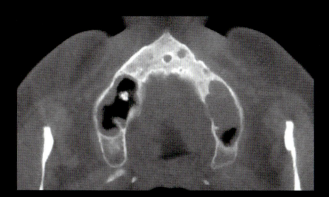

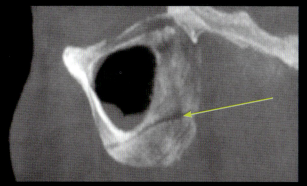

Sagittal section

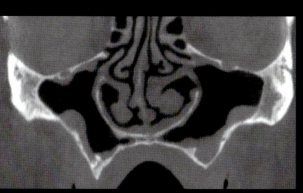

Coronal section

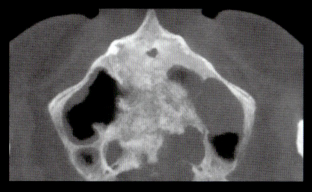

Axial section

21 Anatomical Variations

Canalis sinuosus

This anatomical variation is clearly visible in this patient. The alveoloantral artery has an intrabony diameter of 3 mm in the anterior area, merging with the vessels coming from the infraorbital artery.
In the 3D image its course is particularly evident.[20-22]

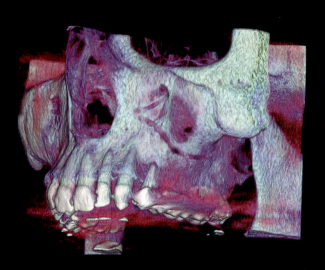

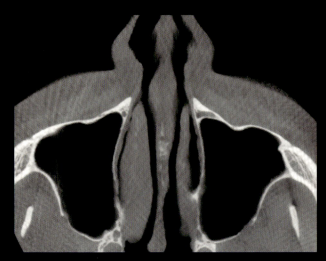

Axial section

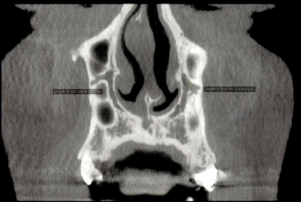

Coronal section

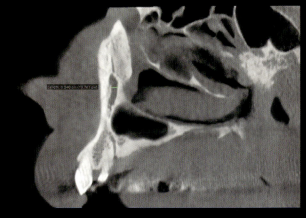

Sagittal section

22 Anatomical Variations

Nasal septum: Nasal septum deviation with two accessory ostia

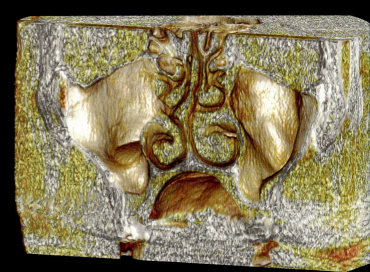

If the patient must undergo a sinus elevation, this anatomical variation must be investigated by a specialist (otorhinolaryngologist or ear, nose, and throat [ENT] specialist). The nasal septum deviation can involve an alteration of the sinus ventilation, with an increased risk of sinusitis.

Coronal section

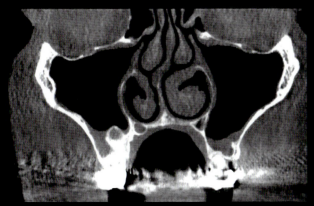

Axial section

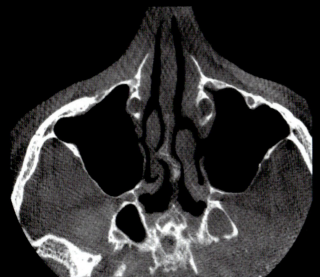

23 Anatomical Variations
Maxillary sinus: Septum with oblique course

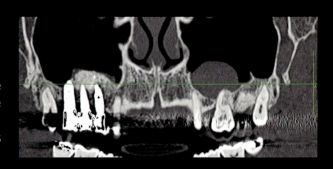

The septum starts from the lateral wall of the nose and runs toward the lateral wall of the sinus. In the 3D reconstruction it is possible to better see its course. Moreover, a domed thickening of the sinus mucosa is present, clearly visible in the 3D view.

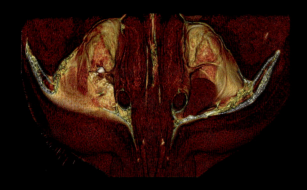
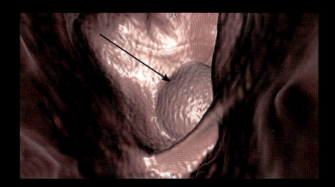

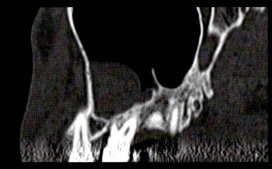

Sagittal section

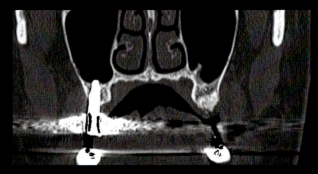

Coronal section

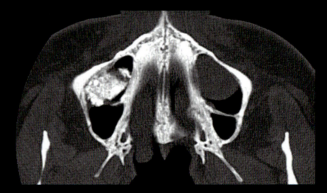

Axial section

24 Anatomical Variations
Palate: Ectopic tooth within the hard palate

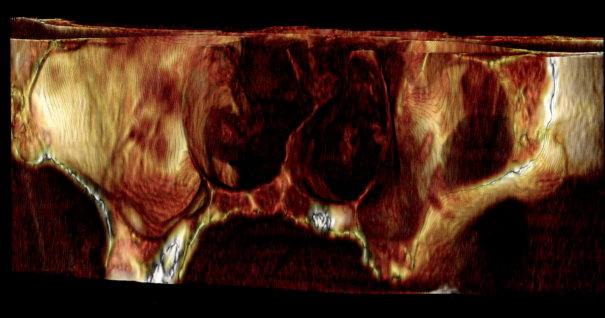

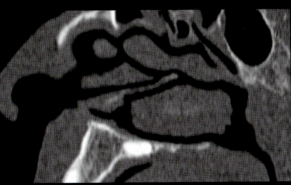

Sagittal section

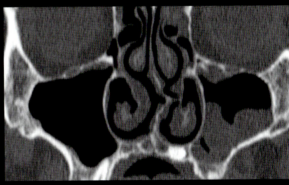

Coronal section

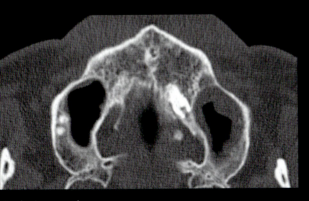

Axial section

25 Anatomical Variations
Nasal cavity

Deflection of the septum towards the left with maxillary sinus septa with an effect on the middle meatum, determining a turbinate-septum contact and air-volume reduction of the ipsilateral nasal cavity. Moreover, there is a partial bilateral opacity of the maxillary and anterior ethmoid sinuses.

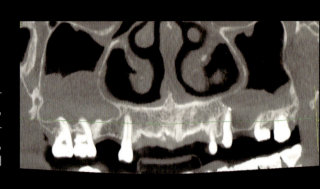

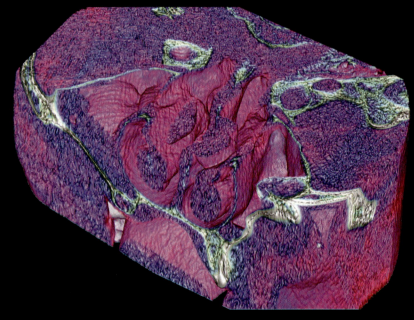

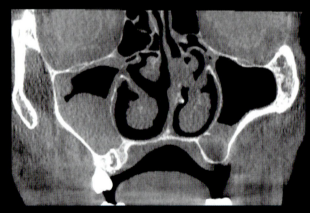

Coronal section

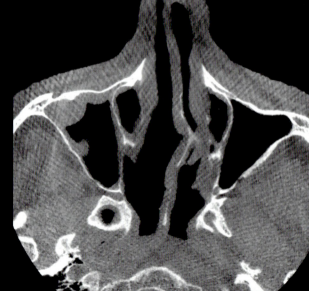

Axial section

26 Anatomical Variations
Nasal cavity

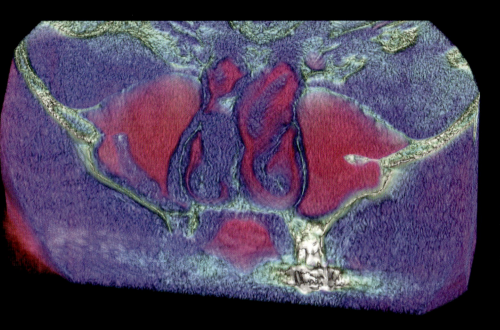

Deflection of the septum towards the right with ipsilateral middle-meatal crests and septum–middle turbinate contact.

Coronal section

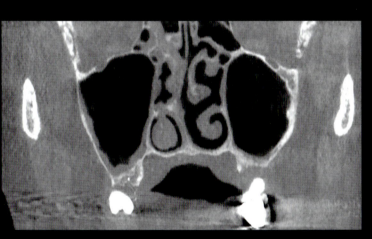

Axial section

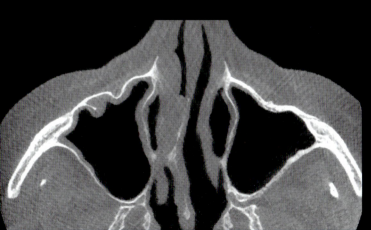

27 Anatomical Variations
Mandibular symphysis

Radiologic evidence of the course of the anastomotic branch between the sublingual artery and the incisive branches coming from the mandibular canal. These foramina have a variable position both vertically and horizontally. They can be found along the median line or symmetrically to it. In this case, two median foramina are visible, one of them in correspondence to the mandibular edge and the other one in a more cranial position.

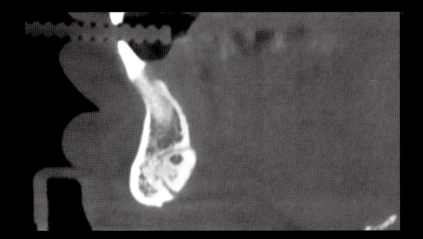

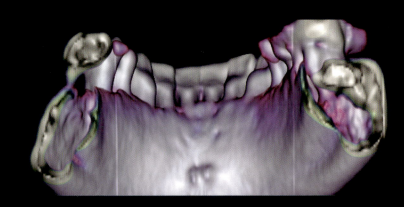

28 Anatomical Variations

Third molars: Contiguity of the maxillary third molar with the maxillary sinus

The radiologic examination shows the relationship between third molar, second molar, and maxillary sinus. Periodontal probing distal to the second molar leads the clinician to the third molar extraction.

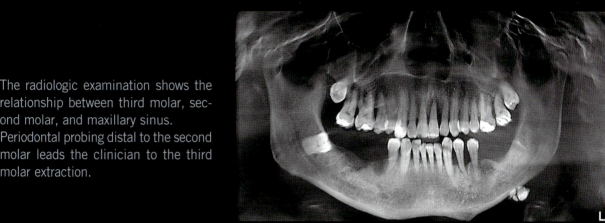

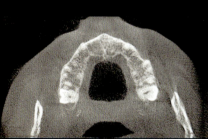

Axial section

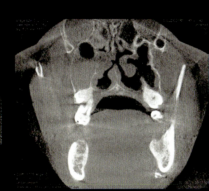

Coronal section

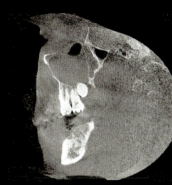

Sagittal section

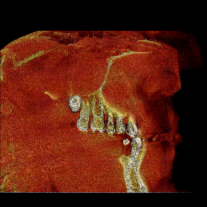

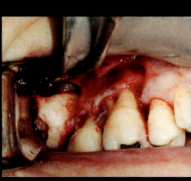

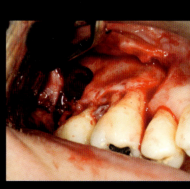

Once the tooth is extracted, the maxillary sinus membrane becomes visible.

29 Anatomical Variations

Third molars: Proximity of the third molar roots to the inferior alveolar canal

The axial and coronal reconstructions show the direct relationship between the anatomical structures.
The radiographic and clinical images show, after the extraction, the neurovascular bundle in correspondence to the root apex.

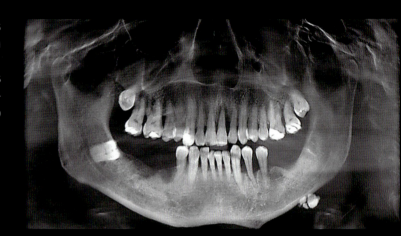

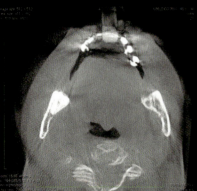
Axial section

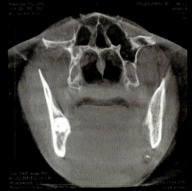
Coronal section

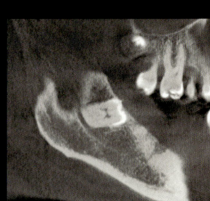
Sagittal section

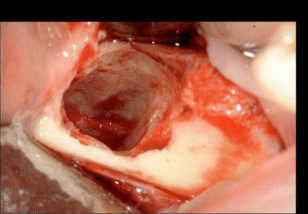

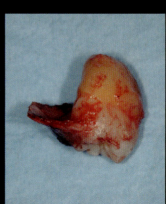

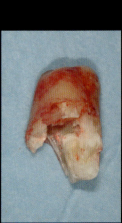

30 Pathologic or Iatrogenic Anatomical Variations
Crestal dehiscence and bone dehiscence of the crestal area of the alveolar process

These fenestrations of the maxillary sinus may be the consequence of inflammatory processes or traumatic tooth extraction.
In treatment planning a surgical intervention in this area, their positions must be carefully evaluated.
A crestal incision may allow the penetration of the scalpel through the fenestration, causing a laceration of the sinus membrane. In these patients, a partial-thickness flap must be used.

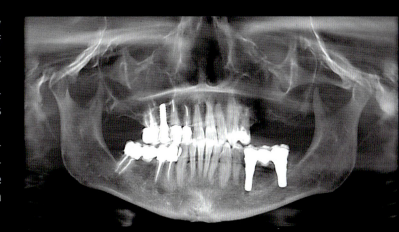

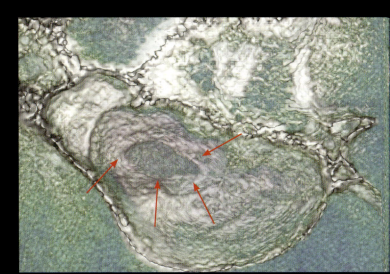

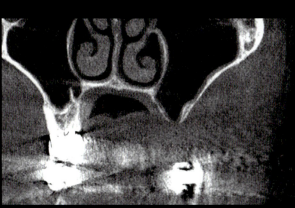

Coronal section

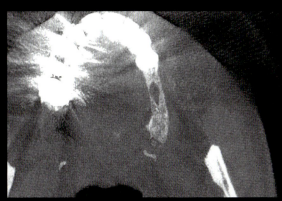

Axial section

31 Pathologic or Iatrogenic Anatomical Variations

Nasal cavity: Absence of the lateral wall of the nose

The CT sections highlight an alteration in correspondence to the left maxillary sinus. The lateral wall of the nose/medial wall of the maxillary sinus is absent, with a direct communication between maxillary sinus and nasal cavity.
The maxillary sinus mucosa appears thickened.

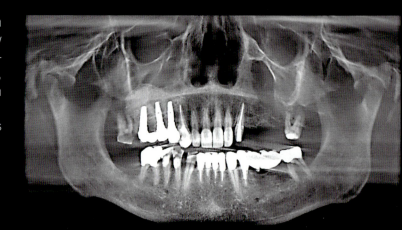

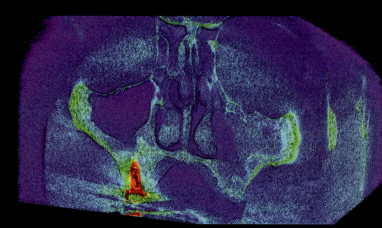

Sagittal section

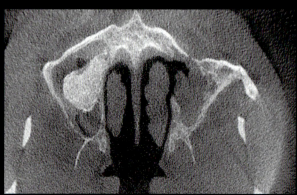

Coronal section

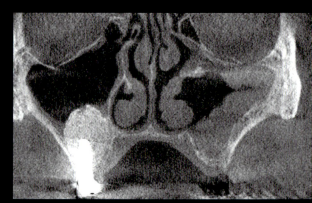

Axial section

32 Pathologic or Iatrogenic Anatomical Variations

Crestal dehiscence: Dehiscence of the palatal wall of the alveolar crest

This interruption is the result of a traumatic tooth extraction.
In such patients, a maxillary sinus elevation must be performed with great care because the adherence between the palatal mucosa and the sinus membrane during the elevation may cause a laceration, increasing the difficulty of the procedure.

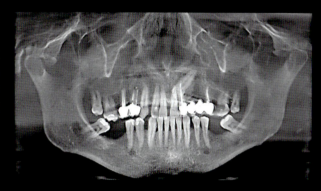

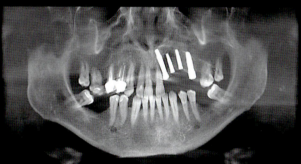

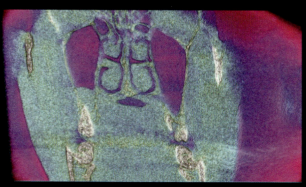

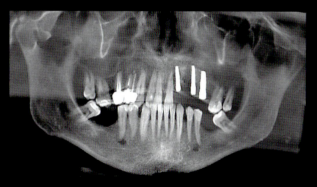

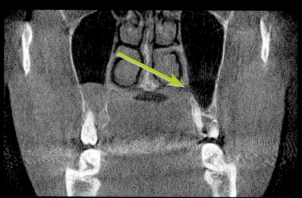

Coronal section

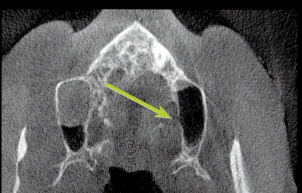

Axial section

33 Pathologic or Iatrogenic Anatomical Variations
Crestal dehiscence

Interruption of the maxillary sinus floor. There is evidence of a wide collapsing area between the sinus mucosa and the oral mucosa. The execution of a partial thickness flap is the only solution that will avoid laceration of the sinus membrane. If not managed in the proper way, these dehiscences can result in oroantral fistulas.

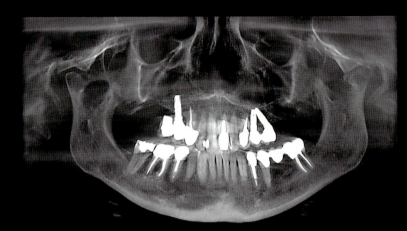

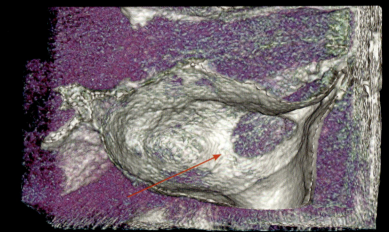

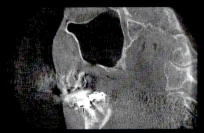
Sagittal section

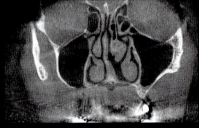
Coronal section

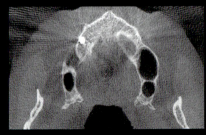
Axial section

34 Pathologic or Iatrogenic Anatomical Variations
Maxillary sinus: Maxillary sinus radiopacity

The radiologic appearance corresponds to the root of a premolar that was accidentally dislodged into the maxillary sinus during a traumatic extraction.

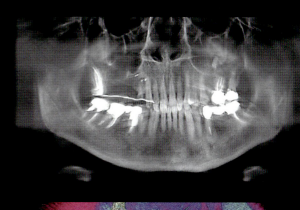

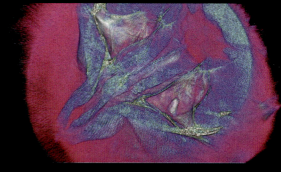

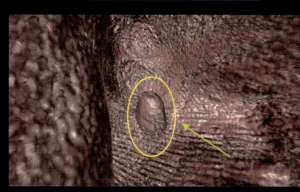

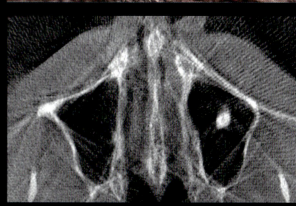

Coronal section   Axial section

35 Pathologic or Iatrogenic Anatomical Variations

Maxillary sinus: Radiologic evidence of aspergillosis of the maxillary sinus

The diagnosis of mycotic infection has been confirmed by the radiologic examination. The maxillary sinus appears completely obliterated by the hypertrophy of the membrane.

A crestal dehiscence is also present, placing the oral cavity mucosa in contact with the sinus mucosa. After treatment by an ENT, the sinus appears ventilated.

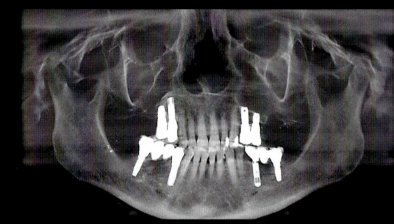

	Sagittal section	Coronal section	Axial section
Preoperative	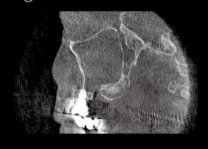	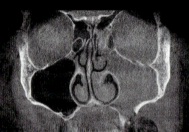	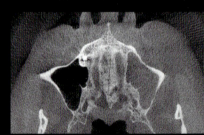
Postoperative	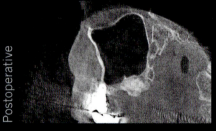	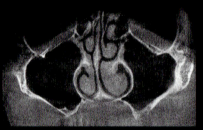	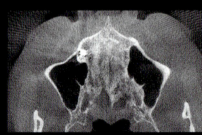

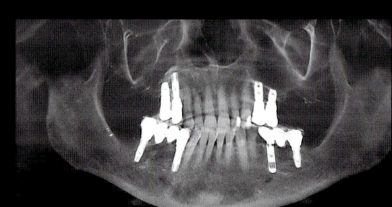

36 Pathologic or Iatrogenic Anatomical Variations

Maxillary sinus: Radiopacities in the maxillary sinus related to multiple mucosal cysts

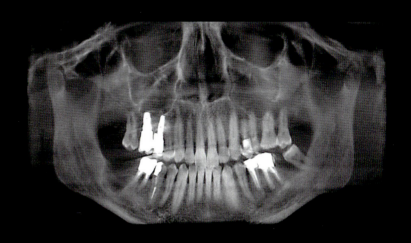

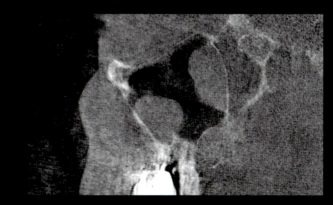

Sagittal section

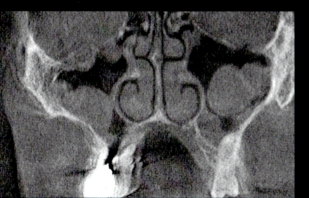

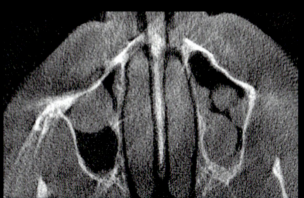

37 Pathologic or Iatrogenic Anatomical Variations

Maxillary sinus: Maxillary sinusitis with bilateral obliteration of maxillary sinuses

The inflammatory process involved the contiguous paranasal sinuses also. It is present as an ethmoiditis with further opacification of the sphenoid sinus.
After treatment by an ENT, the complete rehabilitation of the ventilation of the paranasal sinuses is evident.

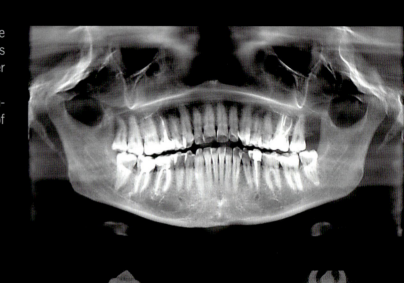

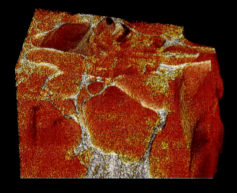

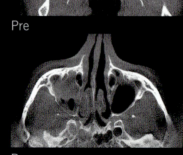
Pre

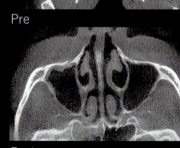
Pre

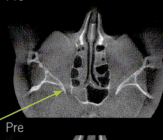
Pre

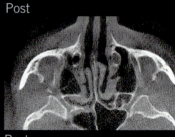
Post

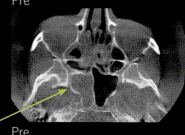
Pre

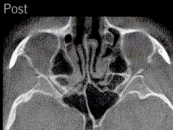
Post

38 Pathologic or Iatrogenic Anatomical Variations

Maxillary sinus: Sinusitis caused by the crestal elevation of the maxillary sinus

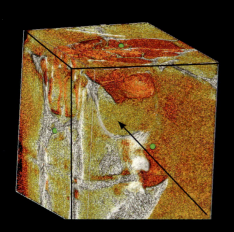
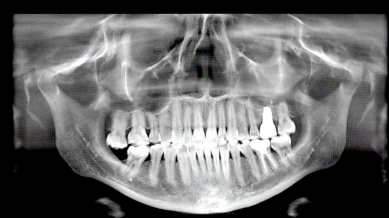

The case shows a complication of the crestal elevation of the sinus. The sinus mucosa appears thickened with partial obliteration of the maxillary sinus.

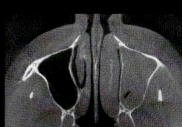

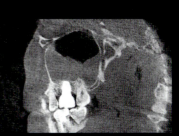

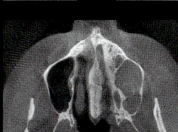

Sagittal section

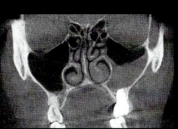

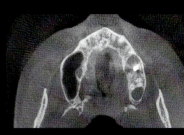

Axial section

Coronal section

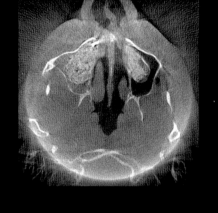
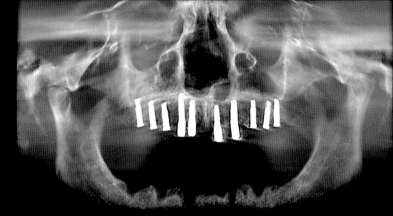

Coronal section

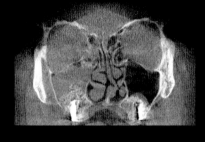
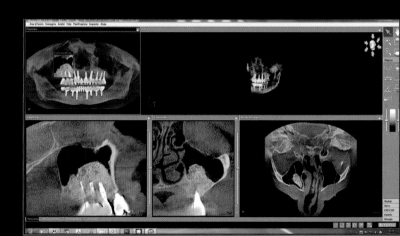

40 Pathologic or Iatrogenic Anatomical Variations
Maxillary sinus: Result of treatment by an ENT

The case shows a complication of the sinus elevation procedure.
The mucosa appears thickened with partial obliteration of the sinus. After treatment, the restoration of the normal sinus air volume is evident.

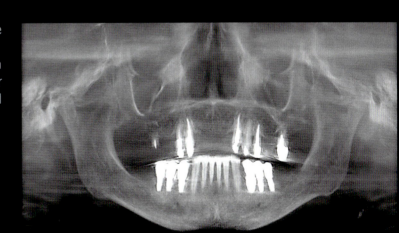

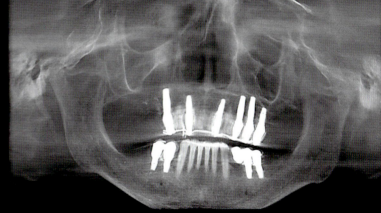

Axial section

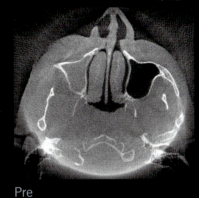 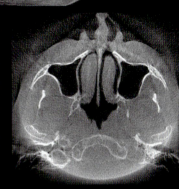

Pre Post

Coronal section

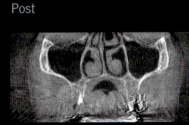

Pre Post

41 Pathologic or Iatrogenic Anatomical Variations

Maxillary sinus: Failure of treatment by an ENT

The patient underwent treatment for maxillary sinusitis. The expected results were confirmed by CT preceding the maxillary sinus elevation, confirming the resolution of the sinusitis. However, after the maxillary sinus elevation procedure, the sinus once again developed a sinusitis, as evidenced by the following examination performed after 6 months.

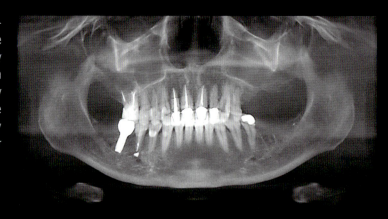

Preoperative

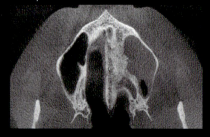 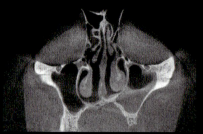 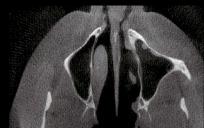

Postoperative

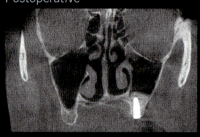 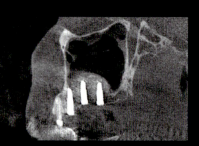

6-month follow-up

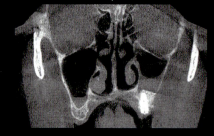 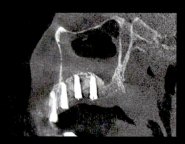 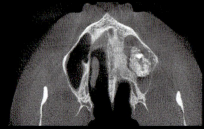

Coronal section   Sagittal section   Axial section

42 Pathologic or Iatrogenic Anatomical Variations

Maxillary sinus: Implant-prosthetic rehabilitation of the posterior maxilla

Note that two different surgical approaches were used, maxillary sinus elevation (maxillary left) vs short implants (maxillary right). On the right, a generalized thickening of the maxillary sinus membrane is visible, with a complete obliteration of the air space. A consultation with an ENT contraindicated the maxillary sinus elevation. Consequently, the left side was treated with short implants.

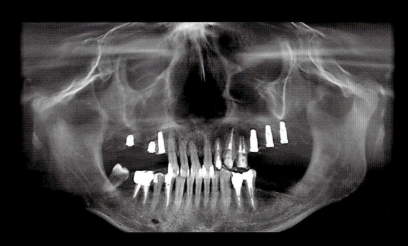

Sagittal sections

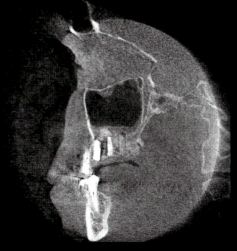 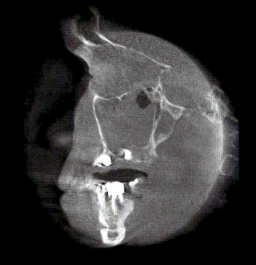

Coronal section

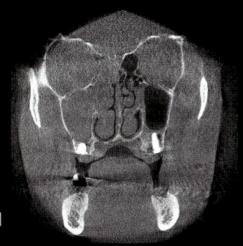 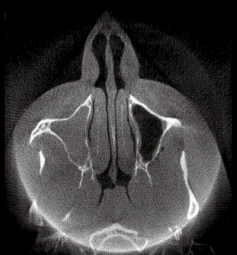

Axial section

43 Pathologic or Iatrogenic Anatomical Variations
Maxillary sinus

Results of previous apicoectomy. The material for the retrograde filling appears to be in correspondence with the maxillary sinus floor and enveloped in the antral mucosa, which presents a secondary slightly diffuse thickening of the maxillary sinus walls.

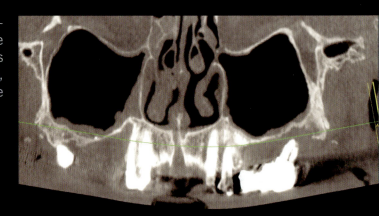

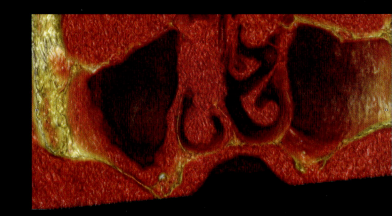

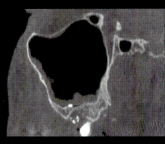

Sagittal section

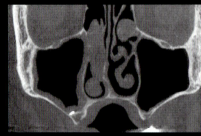

Coronal section

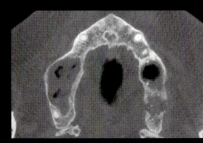

Axial section

44 Pathologic or Iatrogenic Anatomical Variations
Paranasal sinuses

Reconstruction of the airways in patients affected by pathologic processes of the maxillary sinus.
It is possible to note the much larger volume of the open sinus cavity compared to the contralateral sinus.

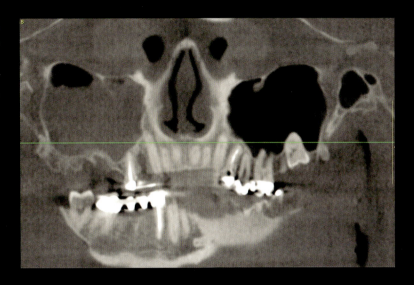

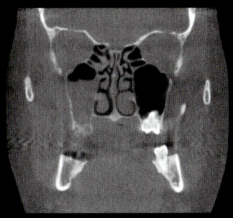

Coronal section

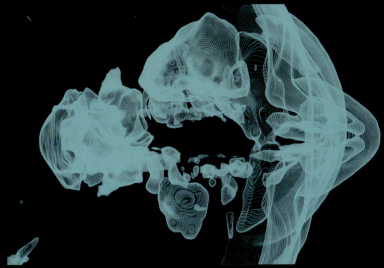

45 Pathologic or Iatrogenic Anatomical Variations
Maxillary sinus

Subtotal opacification of the left maxillary sinus in spite of the patency of the osteomeatal complexes, as evident in the 3D reconstructions. It is possible to observe the calcified area peripheral to the formation.

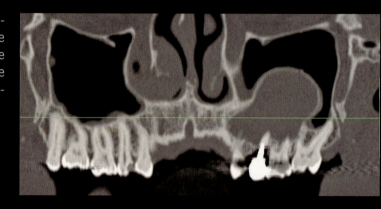

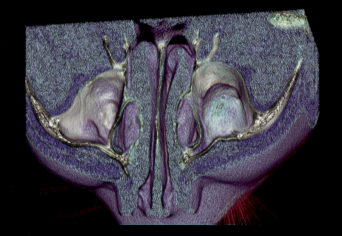

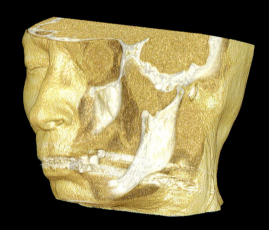

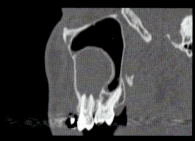

Sagittal section

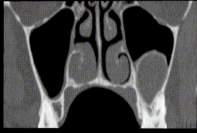

Coronal section

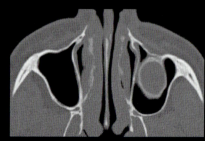

Axial section

46 Pathologic or Iatrogenic Anatomical Variations
Maxillary sinus

Thickening of the mucosa of the floor, with ossified outline, corresponding to the maxillary right premolar roots. There is also a formation similar to a mucosal cyst at the root of the maxillary right first molar. The tooth is carious and does not react to the vitality test. Such findings suggest an odontogenic etiology in the maxillary sinus.

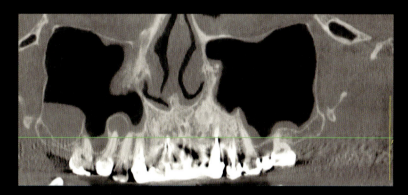

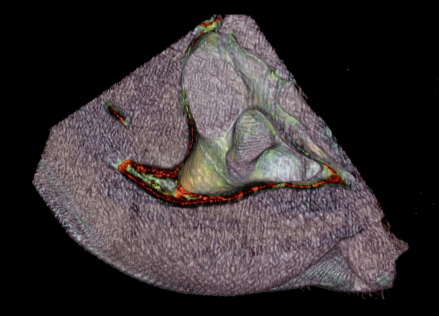

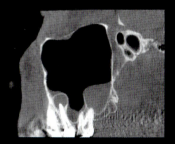
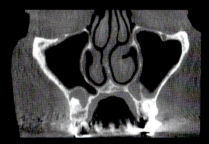
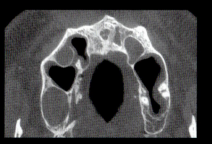

47 Pathologic or Iatrogenic Anatomical Variations
Maxillary sinus

Pinnacle formation in the left maxillary sinus corresponding to a previously endodontically treated tooth.
The radiologic finding presents a marked bone formation along the edge with nonossified content.
Further evaluation by an ENT will be necessary. In the 3D reconstruction it is possible to evaluate the extension of bone formation within the maxillary sinus.
In this patient, the importance of 3D examinations for the diagnosis of maxillary sinus pathology is placed in evidence.

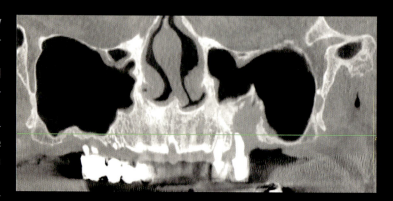

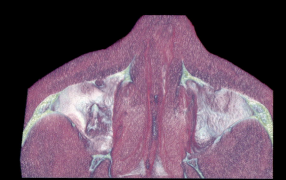
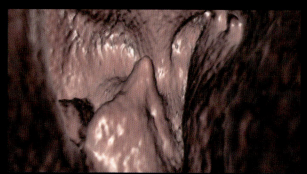

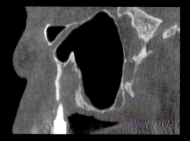
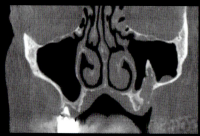
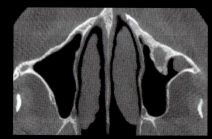

Sagittal section   Coronal section   Axial section

48 Pathologic or Iatrogenic Anatomical Variations
Maxillary sinus: Implant located in the maxillary sinus

The loss of primary stability caused the dislodgment of the implant into the sinus. The 3D reconstructions highlight its sloping position within the maxillary sinus and the reactive thickening of the sinus mucosa.

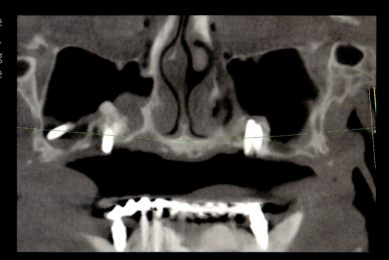

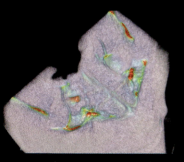
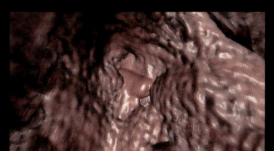
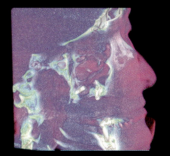

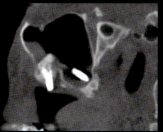
Sagittal section

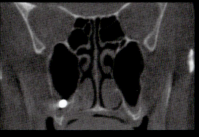
Coronal section

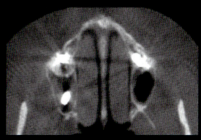
Axial section

49 Pathologic or Iatrogenic Anatomical Variations
Maxillary sinus: Total bilateral opacification

Extended bilateral radiopacity of the maxillary sinus. The inflammatory process is affecting, to the extent that it is possible to evaluate, both sinuses almost completely; moreover, a suspected area of periapical pathology in continuity with the antral floor is visible. However, the sections shown here do not allow evaluation of the osteomeatal complex area.
Therefore, it is advisable to always specify extension of the acquisition plane in order to include the middle-meatal region and the osteomeatal complex.

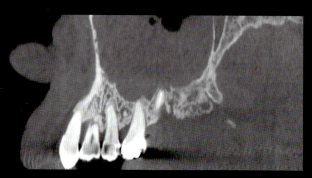
Sagittal section

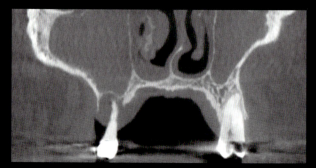
Coronal section

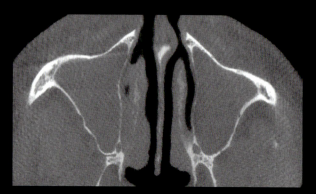
Axial section

50 Maxillary sinus

Pathologic or Iatrogenic Anatomical Variations

Left maxillary sinus opacification with presence of a tooth.
Loss of the delimiting bone wall of the maxillary sinus and invasion of the nasal space. (Courtesy of Dr Francesco Grecchi, Maxillofacial Surgery Department, Galeazzi Hospital, Milan, Italy.)

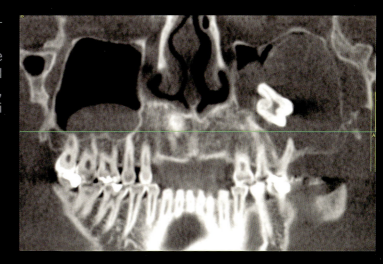

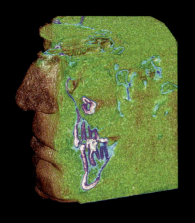 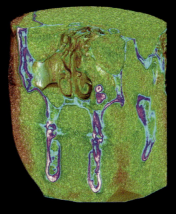 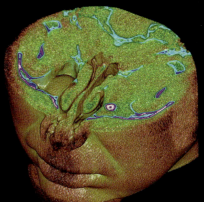

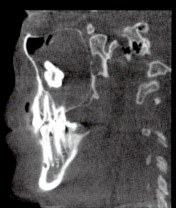 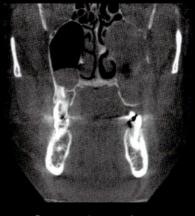 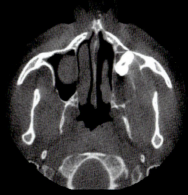

Sagittal section · Coronal section · Axial section

51 Pathologic or Iatrogenic Anatomical Variations
Maxillary sinus: Sinus elevation complication

The patient underwent left maxillary sinus elevation. The sinus appeared to be well ventilated, with a patent osteomeatal complex and absence of sinus mucosa thickening. After 7 days, the patient still had evidence of swelling in the operative area. Consequently, another CT examination was prescribed, showing a diffuse sinus opacification. The graft appears to be dispersed into the maxillary sinus, with complete obliteration of the sinus space.

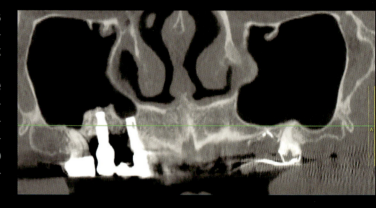

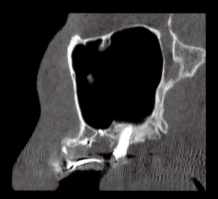
Sagittal section

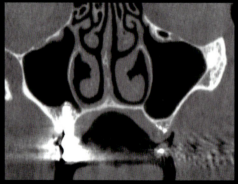
Coronal section

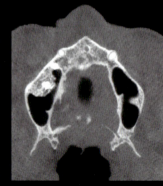
Axial section

The patient underwent a surgical intervention to reevaluate the maxillary sinus and to remove the graft.

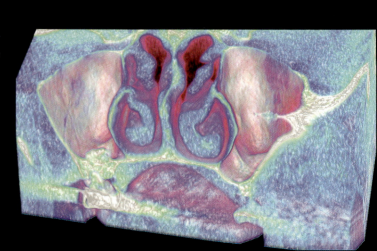

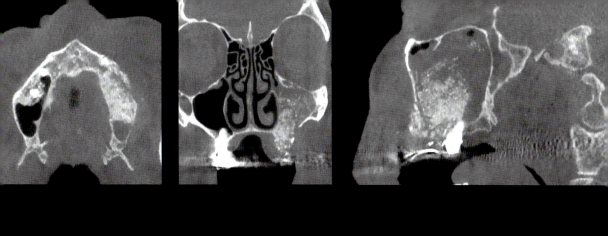
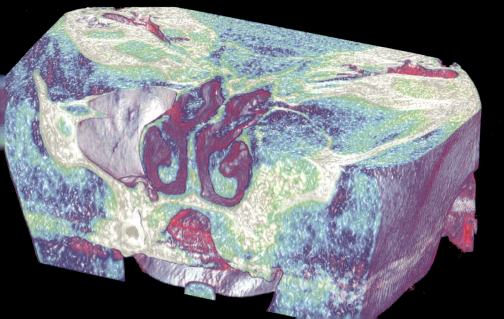

52 Pathologic or Iatrogenic Anatomical Variations
Maxillary sinus: Radiologic finding of turbinectomy

The increased space in the inferior meatus is evident.
The ventilation of the sinus appears to be optimal.

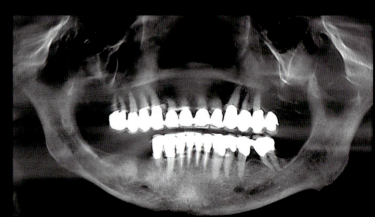

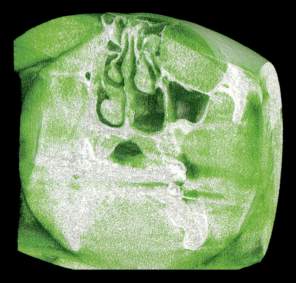

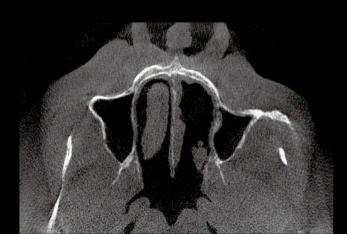

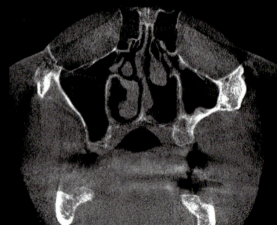

53 Pathologic or Iatrogenic Anatomical Variations
Maxillary sinus: Diffuse opacification of right maxilla

It is possible to evaluate the total obliteration of the sinus cavity and the disappearance of the bone delimiting the nasal cavity in the posterior superior area.

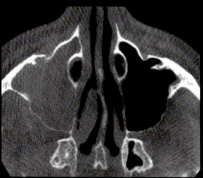
Axial section

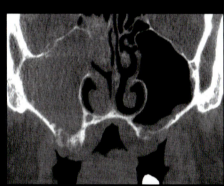
Coronal section

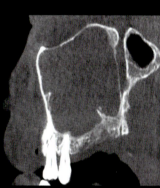
Sagittal section

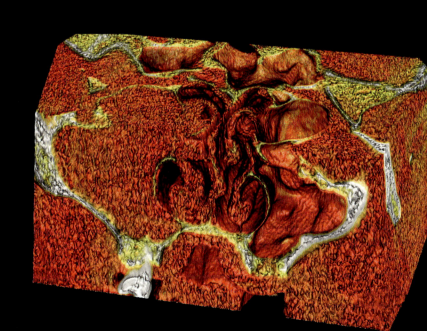

54. Maxillary sinus: Rhinolith of the nasal cavity

In the panoramic image of the patient, a radiopacity in the right nasal region is evident. A more accurate medical examination revealed altered respiration in the ipsilateral nostril.

The clinical examination highlighted the presence of an exophytic formation.

The CBCT examination revealed a rhinolithic formation located inferior to the inferior turbinate, with an almost total obliteration of the inferior meatus. Moreover, there was a thickening of the nasal mucosa.

In the surgical phase, the rhinolithic formation was eliminated, and an inferior turbinectomy was performed. The CBCT scan taken 1 year after treatment shows optimal ventilation of the nasal cavity with a normal thickness of the mucosa.

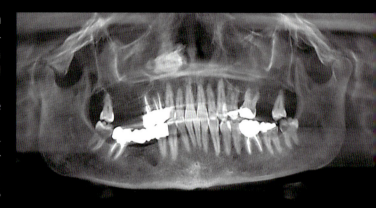

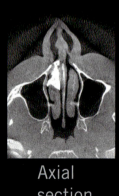

Axial section

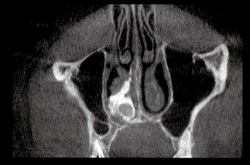

Coronal section

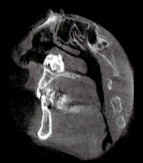

Sagittal section

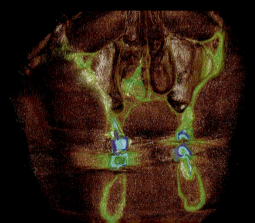

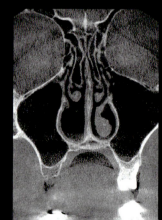

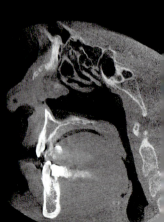

55 Pathologic or Iatrogenic Anatomical Variations
Nasal cavity

Evident hypertrophy of the right nasal mucosa, with reduction of air patency compared to the contralateral nasal cavity, as shown in the 3D reconstructions; moreover, there is evidence of a pneumatization (concha bullosa) of the left middle turbinate, which did not determine the dysventilation of the infundibular region.

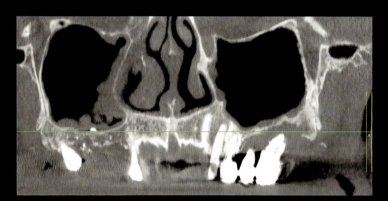

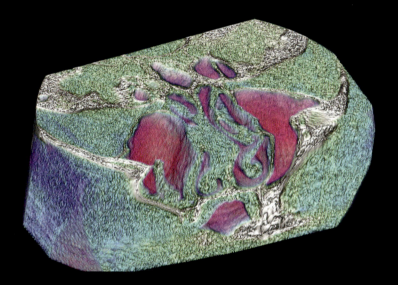

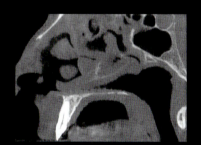
Sagittal section

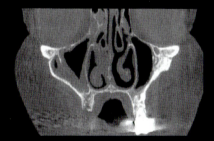
Coronal section

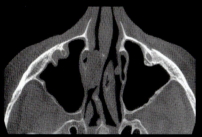
Axial section

56 Pathologic or Iatrogenic Anatomical Variations

Mandibular symphysis: Osteonecrosis of mandibular symphysis with pathologic fracture and osteomyelitis of the inferior mandibular edge from canine to canine, caused by an untreated peri-implantitis

Discontinuity of the mandibular edge, with diffuse radiolucency in the symphysis area extending posteriorly along the apical area of the premolars.
The treatment included the surgical treatment of the inflammatory process with concomitant removal of bony sequestra and subsequent hyperbaric oxygenation.[23] (Courtesy of Dr Francesco Grecchi, Maxillofacial Surgery Department, Galeazzi Hospital, Milan, Italy.)

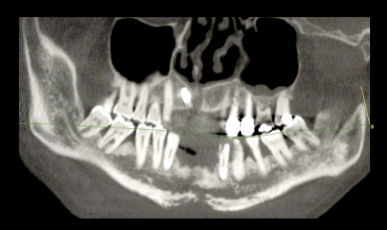

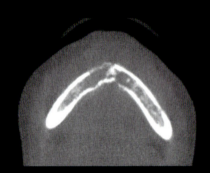

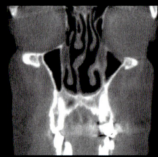

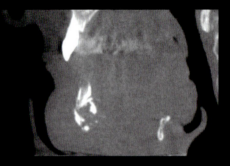

Axial section   Coronal section   Sagittal section

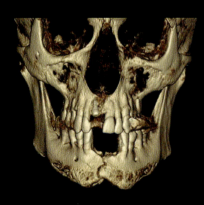

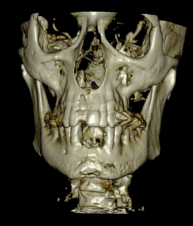

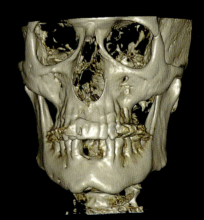

57 Pathologic or Iatrogenic Anatomical Variations

Mandible

Radiologic findings of multiple cystic formations corresponding to teeth, with presence of intracerebral calcifications referring to Gorlin-Goltz syndrome. (Courtesy of Dr Francesco Grecchi, Maxillofacial Surgery Department, Galeazzi Hospital, Milan, Italy.)

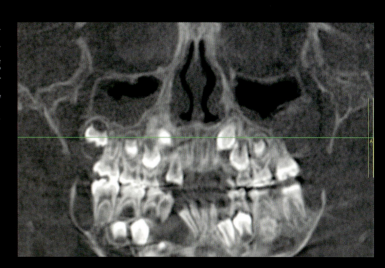

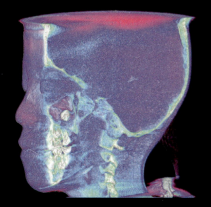
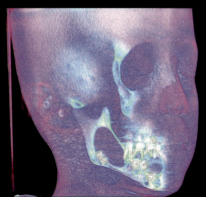
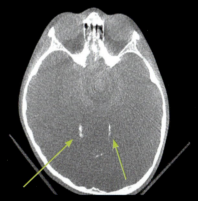

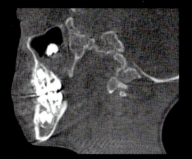
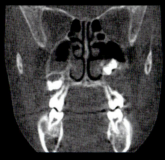
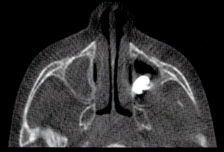

Sagittal section   Coronal section   Axial section

58 Pathologic or Iatrogenic Anatomical Variations
Mandible: Mandibular osteolytic neoformation

Radiolucent lesion of likely cystic type, which developed following apical periodontitis of the mandibular left first molar.
The radiolucency has completely filled the mandibular medullary space and modified the mandibular canal pathway.
In the 3D reconstruction it is possible to visualize the mesial root of the tooth within the radiolucent area.

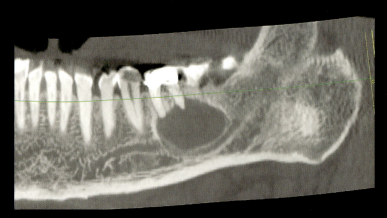

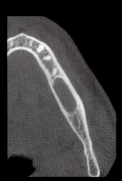

Axial section

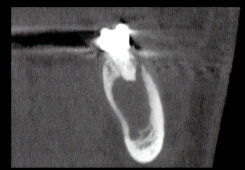

Paraxial section

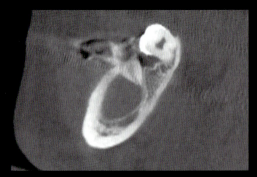

Sagittal section

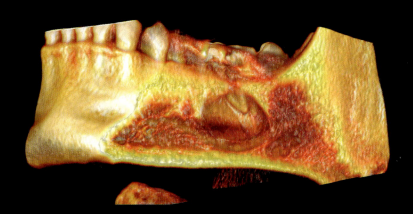

59 Pathologic or Iatrogenic Anatomical Variations

Third molars: Pathology of third molars with pericoronal radiolucency

The root of the mandibular left third molar emerges from the lingual cortex and, more cranially, the lingual cortex seems to be resorbed.
In the other CBCT sections it is evident that the root of the tooth is in direct contact with the mandibular canal.

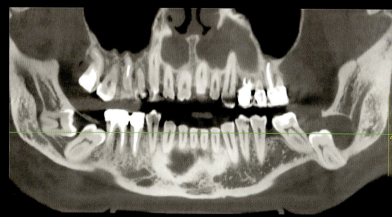

Axial section

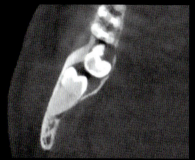 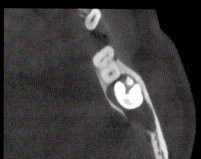

Paraxial section

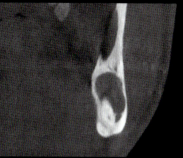

Sagittal section

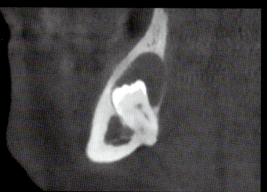 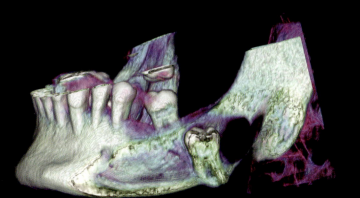

60 Pathologic or Iatrogenic Anatomical Variations

Mandible: Odontogenic cyst associated with mandibular right canine impaction

CBCT sections highlight the invasion of medullary spaces by the cyst, with buccal expansion of the cortical bone.

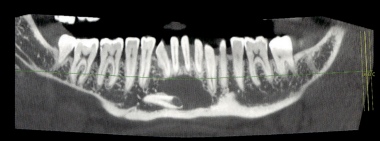

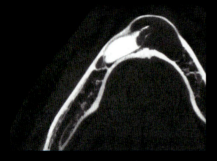
Axial section

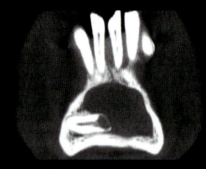
Coronal section

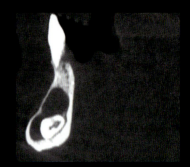
Sagittal section

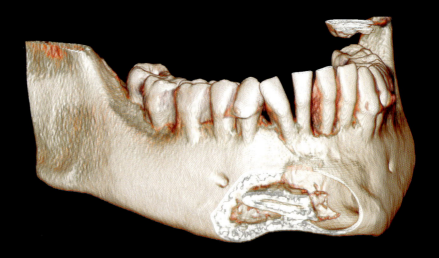

61 Pathologic or Iatrogenic Anatomical Variations

Maxillary sinus: Radiopacity of the left maxillary sinus with inclusion of a tooth

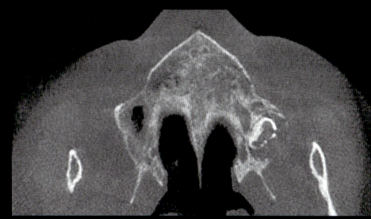

Axial section

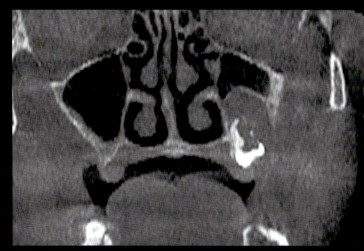

Coronal section

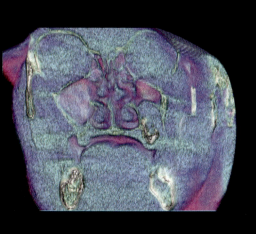

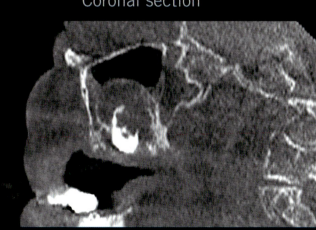

Sagittal section

62 Pathologic or Iatrogenic Anatomical Variations

Maxillary sinus: Dental implant dislodgment in the maxillary sinus

The patient reported a previous crestal maxillary sinus elevation.
The CBCT evaluation highlights the presence of a foreign body with reactive thickening of the sinus membrane.
The implant appears to still be located along the axis of the osteotomy, with the healing abutment attached.
A probable explanation is that the loss of primary stability is a consequence of crestal bone remodeling, a phenomena occurring

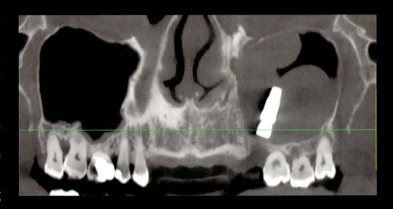

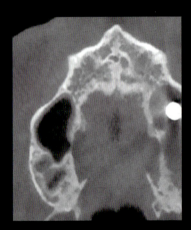
Axial section

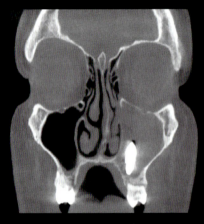
Coronal section

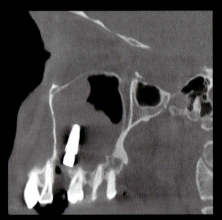
Sagittal section

when the implant is exposed to the oral environment.
The creation of biologic width led to crestal bone remodeling.

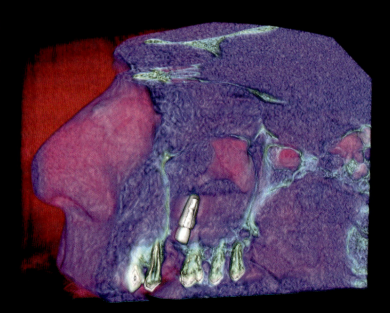

63 Pathologic or Iatrogenic Anatomical Variations
Nasopalatal region: Radiolucent formation

The lesion, probably a cyst, invaded the nasal cavities, with bone resorption of the hard palate and the buccal cortex.

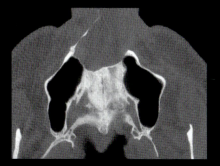
Axial section

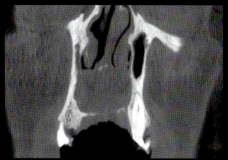
Paraxial section

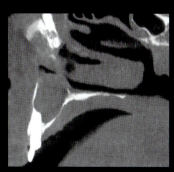
Sagittal section

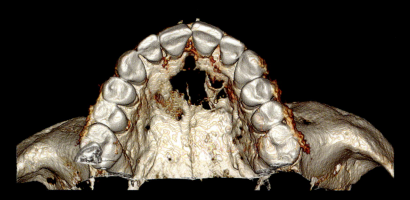

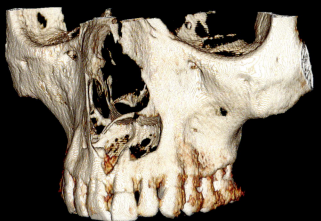

64 Pathologic or Iatrogenic Anatomical Variations

Maxillary sinus: Radiolucent formation medial to the grafting material after sinus elevation

During its development, the lesion involved the palatal cortical bone, creating a convexity along the palatal vault.

The reduced osseointegration of the implants in contact with the lesion is clearly evident.

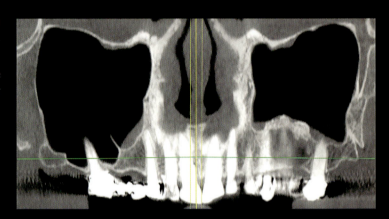

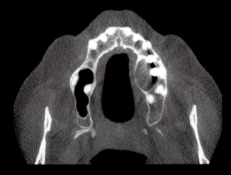

Axial section

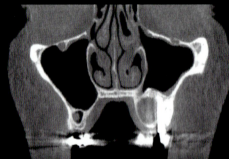

Coronal section

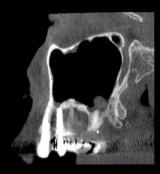

Sagittal section

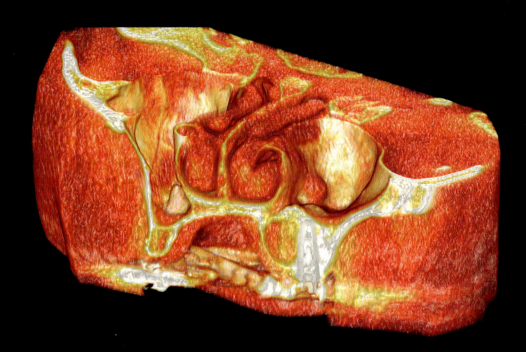

65 Pathologic or Iatrogenic Anatomical Variations

Maxillary sinus: Complication following a traumatic extraction

Oroantral fistula, following resolution, with formation of an intralesion gaseous bulla and incomplete thin calcified shell.
The relationship between the edentulous area, the interruption along the alveolar crest, and the lesion location are visible.
A follow-up of the healing process after 3 months via CT is recommended.

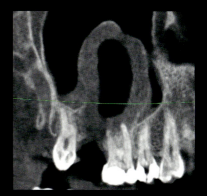

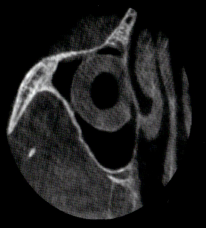

Axial section

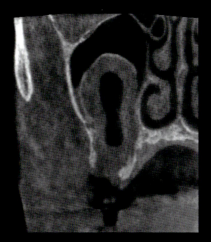

Paraxial section

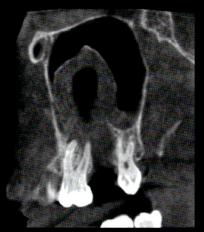

Sagittal section

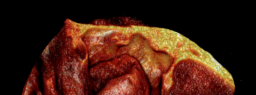

References

1. Harris D, Horner K, Gröndahl K, et al. E.A.O. guidelines for the use of diagnostic imaging in implant dentistry 2011. A consensus workshop organized by the European Association for Osseointegration at the Medical University of Warsaw. Clin Oral Implants Res 2012;23:1243–1253.
2. Ludlow JB, Ivanovic M. Comparative dosimetry of dental CBCT devices and 64-slice CT for oral and maxillofacial radiology. Oral Surg Oral Med Oral Pathol Oral Radiol Endod 2008;106:106–114.
3. Chau AC, Fung K. Comparison of radiation dose for implant imaging using conventional spiral tomography, computed tomography, and cone-beam computed tomography. Oral Surg Oral Med Oral Pathol Oral Radiol Endod 2009;107:559–565.
4. Davies J, Johnson B, Drage N. Effective doses from cone beam CT investigation of the jaws. Dentomaxillofac Radiol 2012;41:30–36.
5. Loubele M, Maes F, Jacobs R, van Steenberghe D, White SC, Suetens P. Comparative study of image quality for MSCT and CBCT scanners for dentomaxillofacial radiology applications. Radiat Prot Dosimetry 2008;129:222–226.
6. Mozzo P, Procacci C, Tacconi A, Martini PT, Andreis IA. A new volumetric CT machine for dental imaging based on the cone-beam technique: Preliminary results. Eur Radiol 1998;8:1558–1564.
7. Liang X, Jacobs R, Hassan B, et al. A comparative evaluation of Cone Beam Computed Tomography (CBCT) and Multi-Slice CT (MSCT). Part I. On subjective image quality. Eur J Radiol 2010;75:265–269.
8. Cho SC, Wallace SS, Froum SJ, Tarnow DP. Influence of anatomy on Schneiderian membrane perforations during sinus elevation surgery: Three-dimensional analysis. Pract Proced Aesthet Dent 2001;13:160–163.
9. Torretta S, Mantovani M, Testori T, Cappadona M, Pignataro L. Importance of ENT assessment in stratifying candidates for sinus floor elevation: A prospective clinical study. Clin Oral Implants Res 2011;24:57–62.
10. Pignataro L, Mantovani M, Torretta S, Felisati G, Sambataro G. ENT assessment in the integrated management of candidate for (maxillary) sinus lift. Acta Otorhinolaryngologica Ital 2008;28:110–119.
11. Prasanna LC, Mamatha H. The location of maxillary sinus ostium and its clinical application. Indian J Otolaryngol Head Neck Surg 2010;62:335–337.
12. Rosano G, Taschieri S, Gaudy JF, Weinstein T, Del Fabbro M. Maxillary sinus vascular anatomy and its relation to sinus lift surgery. Clin Oral Implants Res 2011;22:711–715.
13. Testori T, Rosano G, Taschieri S, Del Fabbro M. Ligation of an unusually large vessel during maxillary sinus floor augmentation. A case report. Eur J Oral Implantol 2010;3:255–258.
14. Parenti ADM, Fumagalli L, Capelli M, et al. Variazioni anatomiche: Anatomia normale e variabilità clinica; utili nozioni per valutare attentamente lo spessore osseo a livello mandibolare. Quinessenza Int 2010;26:39–44.
15. Rosano G, Taschieri S, Gaudy JF, Testori T, Del Fabbro M. Anatomic assessment of the anterior mandible and relative hemorrhage risk in implant dentistry: A cadaveric study. Clin Oral Implants Res 2009;20:791–795.
16. Gaudy J. Atlas d'anatomie implantaire. Issyles-Moulineaux: Elsevier Masson, 2006.
17. Weinstein T, Parenti A, Fumagalli L, et al. Il nervo alveolare inferiore, il forame mentoniero e il canale incisale: Anatomia e variabilità anatomica ed esami strumentali per evidenziare lesioni neurologiche. Quintessenza Int 2011;27:11–19.
18. Maqbool A, Sultan AA, Bottini GB, Hopper C. Pain caused by a dental implant impinging on an accessory inferior alveolar canal: A case report. Int J Prosthodont 2013;26:125–126.
19. von Arx T, Hanni A, Sendi P, Buser D, Bornstein MM. Radiographic study of the mandibular retromolar canal: An anatomic structure with clinical importance. J Endod 2011;37:1630–1635.
20. Shelley AM, Rushton VE, Horner K. Canalis sinuosus mimicking a periapical inflammatory lesion. Br Dent J 1999;186:378–379.

21. Neves FS, Crusoe-Souza M, Franco LC, Caria PH, Bonfim-Almeida P, Crusoe-Rebello I. Canalis sinuosus: A rare anatomical variation. Surg Radiol Anat 2012;34:563–566.
22. de Oliveira-Santos C, Rubira-Bullen IR, Monteiro SA, Leon JE, Jacobs R. Neurovascular anatomical variations in the anterior palate observed on CBCT images. Clin Oral Implants Res 2013;24:1044–1048.
23. Grecchi F, Zollino I, Candotto V, et al. A case of mandible osteonecrosis after a severe periimplant infection. Dent Res J (Isfahan) 2012;9:S233–S236.

G Perrotti
M Politi

4

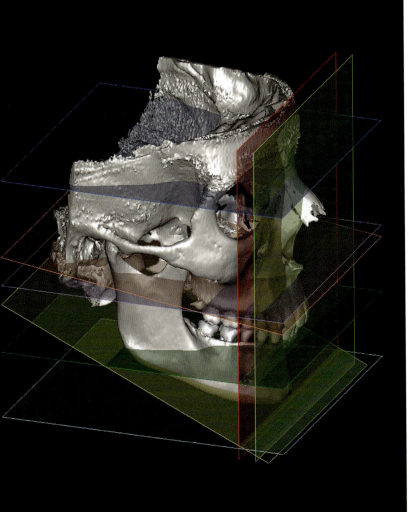

Three-dimensional radiology has provided an ideal tool to assess skull morphology anthropometrically. For over 50 years, two–dimensional (2D) cephalometry has given oral and maxillofacial surgeons and orthodontists a way to measure facial proportions and to use standard values as a reference to plan remodeling and repositioning of basal bones and teeth, and this is still the most commonly used technique in orthodontics.

Skeletal malocclusions are subdivided into Class I, II, and III, setting a clear standard that can be used and understood internationally. The advent of cone beam computed tomography (CBCT) is slowly but inexorably replacing conventional 2D radiology. Moreover, the vision of facial proportions is transforming as the technical approach—ie, the method of analysis—also evolves, changing from linear to multiplanar and leading to a different result in the analysis itself.

The classifications are being updated as three–dimensional (3D) rendering reproduces skeletal morphology in greater detail. Measurement becomes more accurate and the field of study broader.

This chapter shows the investigation approach of the authors who, through multiplanar cephalometry, have developed a system to classify malocclusions using 3D images.

Evolution of Cephalometry

Concepts of Cephalometry

The study of morphologic relationships has been evolving from early-stage craniometry, a 2D anthropometric method to measure the head and skull, to analysis of cephalometric radiographs, a 2D radiologic examination of the skull.

For orthodontists, it is necessary to know the reciprocal relationships of the most important functional units of the face (skull base, maxilla, mandible, teeth). Cephalometric analysis is used to compare patients with general averages derived from a sample population.

The aim is to compare a patient with a normal control population so as to detect any difference between the dentofacial relations in that patient and in individuals belonging to the same race or ethnic group. It can be useful to imagine that the aim of cephalometric analysis is the evaluation of horizontal and vertical relations of the five most important facial components. In regard to the kind of cephalometric analysis applied, the result of analysis can change depending on the method used to locate structures in the facial skeleton, the selection of landmarks, and the reference values used to compare measured values. The terms used for comparison or predefined data can be named in many ways—ideal, normal, mean, standard—and the choice of one term over the other does not influence the underlying concept.

Several analyses have been introduced to assess dysgnathic individuals and to understand the implications these analyses can have on planning orthodontic treatment and on its outcome.

Each method allows the clinician to understand the limitations and opportunities of planning an ideal treatment for an individual patient. The dilemma has always been to understand which analysis is the best to quantify, in objective terms, the spatial relations in the context of craniofacial and dentofacial complexes.

It is often necessary to combine analyses for the sake of completeness, as in most cases a single analysis does not include all the desired interrelations. None of the tracings currently available is exempt from criticism and limitations that may be more or less severe, even if a tracing is adequate to the needs of standard clinical practice. No single measurement is suitable for the analysis; only the sum of measurements will provide the clinician a clearer picture of the skeletal and dental problems of a patient without suggesting how to combine values from the various measurements to obtain accurate indications for diagnosis and treatment.

Only after a global assessment, including the collection of the patient's medical and stomatologic history, clinical examination, study of dental casts, intraoral and extraoral photographs, and radiographs (panoramic, lateral cepholmetric, and posteroanterior [PA]) can a final diagnosis can be made to plan the best treatment for the patient under investigation.

Therefore, it should always be considered that cephalometric analysis alone is not sufficient for a complete diagnosis of orthodontic patients; it is only one element in a complete diagnostic work-up.

Introduction to Radiology in Orthodontics

Cephalometric radiography, introduced in 1931 by Holfrath in Germany and by Broadbent in the United States, has provided a clinical investigation tool to study skeletal malocclusions and disharmonies. Cephalometry has undoubtedly been the most frequently used technique in the orthodontic research literature to compare, differentiate, and describe different samples of individuals in statistical trials.

The first goal of this method was to study the laws regulating craniofacial growth patterns under normal circumstances, but it soon became evident that radiographic images could be used to analyze dentofacial proportions and to clarify the anatomical basis for malocclusions, which are due to the interaction between the position of the maxilla and mandible and the teeth after eruption.

The reason why cephalometric tracings are used probably lies in the fact that they help operators to make a better diagnosis, leading to an accurate treatment plan and a more stable outcome.

Most of the cephalometric analyses described in the literature are quantitative. They assess the craniofacial skeleton through absolute measurement of the following:

- Volumetric comparisons
- Angles
- Width and height
- Relationships

There are fundamental characteristics that a tracing must have, according to most authors:

- Simple and essential execution with the use of clearly defined and easy-to-locate landmarks
- Reliability and clinical significance of the information obtained with skeletal and dentoalveolar evaluations on different planes (sagittal, vertical, and transversal)
- A limited number of possible measurements so as to maintain a general vision of the situation at any time
- An immediate understanding of the case due to a graphic layout promoting dialogue with colleagues from other specialties and with patients
- Methodologic reliability obtained by considering different reference bone planes, as these planes are already subject to variations[1]

To obtain a highly reproducible cephalometric analysis, it is necessary to define standards for acquiring radiographic images. To meet this need, Broadbent in 1931 introduced the cephalostat or cephalometer, which, though modified, is still based on its early principles.

After the advent of cephalometry, orthodontists have started relying on lateral cephalometric radiographs as a primary source of information on skeletal and dentoalveolar anatomy. Nevertheless, PA cephalometric radiographs and their related analyses provide a major contribution to the qualitative and quantitative assessment of the dentofa-

cial region.[1] In many cases the presence and severity of facial asymmetry can be diagnosed using PA cephalometry.[2,3]
Detection of structural problems is extremely important in planning treatment. Unfortunately, PA cephalometry does not always give accurate information, even with the aid of lateral and submentovertex projections.

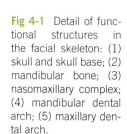

Fig 4-1 Detail of functional structures in the facial skeleton: (1) skull and skull base; (2) mandibular bone; (3) nasomaxillary complex; (4) mandibular dental arch; (5) maxillary dental arch.

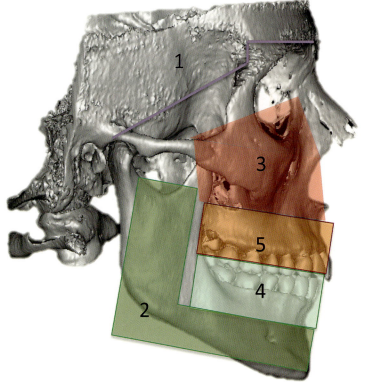

Advantages of Cephalometric Analysis

Cephalometry has been and is still, to some extent, the only method available to study spatial relationships between the skull and superficial and dental structures.[4]
Today cephalometric analysis is usually performed with the following objectives:

- Studying mechanisms of physiologic and pathologic facial growth
- Identifying the type of structural alteration and etiology in patients with craniofacial dysgnathia/dysmorphia with consequent skeletal classification of a facial model, a necessary step in orthodontic cases
- Developing a method to forecast growth in terms of quantity and direction to provide information that, combined with the treatment goals, gives a reliable forecast of the outcome at the end of treatment
- Monitoring the actual changes obtained at the skeletal and dental levels at the end of treatment by using adequate techniques to compare cephalometric tracings

It is useful to think of cephalometric analysis as the evaluation of the horizontal and vertical relationships of the six most important facial components (Fig 4-1):

- Skull and skull base
- Mandibular bone base
- Maxillary bone base
- Mandibular teeth with their alveolar processes[5]
- Maxillary teeth and their alveolar processes
- Soft tissues[6]

In this perspective, every cephalometric analysis is a procedure to provide a description of relationships among these functional units. Also the PA projection gives a second image of the skull base in two orthogonal projections. It is so-called because the beam of x-rays crosses the skull in the posteroanterior direction (Fig 4-2). This projection is used to study the following:

- Dentoalveolar and facial asymmetries
- Dental and skeletal crossbites
- Functional mandibular dislocation
- Development abnormalities
- Traumas

Diagnostic casts provide more detailed information on dental structures, and extraoral photos give more complete information on surface characteristics, but only cephalometric images deliver accurate information on spatial relationships between superficial and deep structures.

To some extent, CT, magnetic resonance imaging (MRI), and ultrasonography also depict superficial and deep structures simultaneously. Nevertheless, all of these techniques, at least today, involve a higher economic and/or physiologic price and provide information with lower spatial resolution in the projections that are of paramount interest for craniofacial biology, ie, the sagittal and frontal views.

It is therefore appropriate to state that conventional 2D radiology, compared with other methods available, is relatively noninvasive and nondestructive; it provides fairly extensive information at a relatively low physiologic price.[1]

One of the most important uses of cephalometry consists in acknowledging and assessing changes during orthodontic treatment. By superimposing a set of cephalometric images obtained before, during, and after treatment, it is possible to study retrospectively the modifications in basal bone and tooth positions (Fig 4-3).

The changes observed are the combined result of growth and treatment (except for adults).[5]

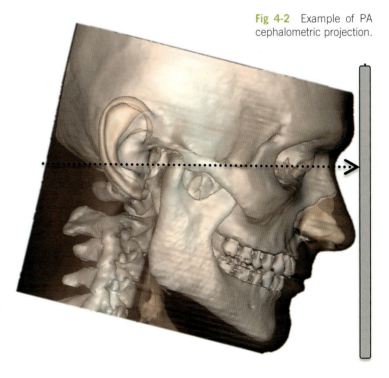

Fig 4-2 Example of PA cephalometric projection.

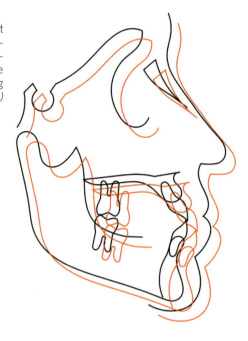

Fig 4-3 The two most important cephalometric images are superimposed to show the same patient at the beginning of treatment (black line) and later (red line).[5]

As opposed to diagnostic procedures like measurement with a caliper, palpation, auscultation, probing, and oral history collection, an additional benefit of 2D radiographic images analyzed with cephalometric systems is tangible and long-lasting documentation. Its value greatly depends on the sensitivity of the specialist in interpreting it and on the reliability of his/her judgment.[1,7]

Limitations of Cephalometric Analysis

Like other diagnostic modalities, cephalometric analysis offers both the benefits described so far as well as some limitations, which are partly interconnected. These limitations mainly derive from the fact that many of the above advantages are relative rather than absolute. Although the information obtained outweighs the physiologic costs, it is always worth assessing radiation exposure when a cephalometric radiograph is taken. Even if the quantity of radiation absorbed by a patient in a cephalometric radiograph is well below the maximum values set for the population (the average dose of rays for each of these radiographs is slightly higher than the dose for an intraoral radiograph), it is not acceptable to take cephalometric radiographs that are not useful for diagnosis or treatment purposes. On the other hand, orthodontics needs to develop a realistic vision of the cost-benefit ratio associated with cephalometry. Radiation risk is always present, though very limited.[1]

The use of angular rather than linear measurements avoids problems related to mag-

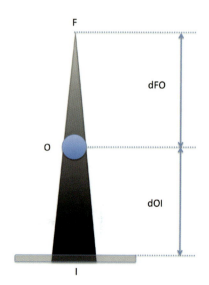

Fig 4-4 The size of the image (I), which is the projection of the object (O) onto the film, is directly proportional to the distance (dOI) between the object and the film, and it is inversely proportional to the distance (dFo) between the ray-emitting tube (F) and the object.

nification because angular measurements remain constant irrespective of the magnification factor.

In side-to-side cephalometric radiographs, paired structures are magnified differently, with the side closer to the source of rays appearing larger than the equivalent structure closer to the film. The problems with locating bilateral structures undergoing different magnification can be somewhat mitigated by recording intermediate points between these structures.

Distortion occurs because of different x-ray angles. It is well known that x-ray beams are not parallel; they are projected in a fanlike shape, inducing distortion of anatomical structures except for those that are along the central beam (Fig 4-4). Therefore, both angular and linear measures will be impaired to some extent (Fig 4-5). Poor alignment or tilting of cephalometric components such as the cephalostat or film or rotation of the patient's head on any spatial plane will introduce another factor of distortion (Fig 4-6).

Incorrect positioning of the patient in the cephalostat causes asymmetric distortion both of angular and of linear measures in lateral cephalograms.[8] In many clinical trials radiographic limitations have nevertheless turned out to be minor; hence, the errors introduced in this phase can be considered as negligible for routine purposes.[9,10]

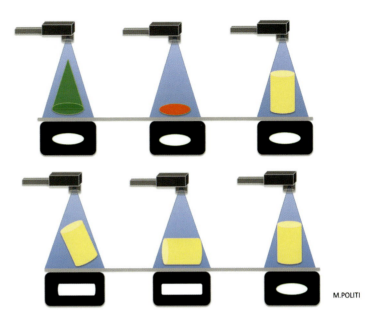

Fig 4-5 Distortion and magnification in cephalometric radiographs.

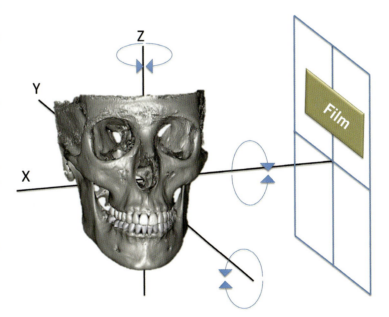

Fig 4-6 Axial directions of potential misalignments of the patient's head.

Intrinsic Errors in the Measurement System

Errors can occur in conventional cephalometry because of traditional manual tools of measurement. Many studies have shown that the alertness and experience of the operator as well as the working conditions and the instruments in use all play an important role in determining the range of error in cephalometric measurements. It is doubtless that computed cephalometric systems make data collection faster and less bothersome and also reduce errors.[9–11]

Errors in Landmark Identification

Wrong placement of landmarks is considered as the first source of errors in cephalometry.
The factors implied are listed below.

Quality of Radiographic Images

Quality of images influences the degree of accuracy in cephalometric analysis. A radiograph is considered to be acceptable from a diagnostic point of view by examining the following features:

- *Contrast:* the difference between structures having different (dark or light) shades. An increase in contrast improves the subjective perception of sharpness. Conversely, excessive contrast results in loss of details because of darkening of low-absorption areas as compared to areas of high absorption.
- *Sharpness:* perception of contour definition of a structure. It is associated with blurring (change in optical density between the contours of a structure and its surroundings).
- *Background noise:* refers to all disturbance factors present in a radiograph. It can be due to radiographic complexity of the area, ie, radiographic superimposition of anatomical structures at different levels of depth. This is known as structural noise, which may depend on intrinsic equipment features; for example, the x-ray detector (in the broadest sense, ie, film, electronic sensors, etc) can introduce a so-called quantic noise (depending on the number of radiosensitive grains in the film or on the resolution of the electronic sensor). These kinds of errors can be minimized by using high-resolution and high-quality films and sensors.

Grummons et al[12] have established that, for PA cephalometric radiographs, 2D cephalometric measurements should be used for a comparative rather than a quantitative analysis as they are subject to distortion because of the projection technique.
Nowadays the application of digital technology to conventional radiography has changed the quality of radiographic images, improving their sharpness and reducing their background noise at the same time.
It has been observed that the main benefit of digital radiography lies in a reduction of the radiation dose associated with shorter exposure times.[6]

Accuracy in Defining Landmarks and Reproducibility of Their Location

Cephalometric reliability is strongly influenced by correct definition of landmarks, which has to be clear and nonambiguous. It should also be taken into consideration that often the identical cephalometric point is identified using different abbrevations, which can cause problems, confusion, errors, and waste of time. Therefore, it would be useful to have an international standardized list of landmarks.

Definitions like "the most prominent" or "the highest" must always be accompanied by reference planes. If the conditions required for radiographic recording (eg, lips in resting position, centric occlusion, or head positioning) are not precise, errors can be introduced in measuring. According to some experts,[1] certain landmarks can be located less accurately than others.

Geometrically constructed landmarks and those identified as points of transition from convexity to concavity prove to be extremely unreliable. Moreover, the radiographic complexity of a specific area greatly influences accuracy, thus making some landmarks more difficult to identify and creating incorrect cephalometric angular and linear measurements. This is the reason why the actual value of some landmarks has been often questioned.[1]

Operator and Recording Procedure

In interpreting the radiographic images of dentofacial and cranial structures, it is necessary to know these structures very well; otherwise, radiographic interpretation, rather than being based on a cephalometric method, is left to chance. Furthermore, scientific knowledge should be integrated with good dexterity so that accurately identified structures are correctly traced. In cephalometric studies, the operator-specific level of error needs to be defined if meaningful consequences must be drawn from the data available. The operator can introduce two kinds of errors depending on the aim of the study:

- Intraoperator variability, which might imply disagreement among observers in identifying a reference point as well as an operator's intrinsic variability over time due to changes in his/her identification procedure
- Errors introduced unconsciously due to the observer's expectations when assessing the outcome of scientific investigation. To mitigate this bias, one can use randomization of the measures gathered or double-blind trials

The different values obtained among several measurements can reflect normal, casual variation, but sometimes the variation can also be due to incorrect identification of a landmark or improper recording on the part of an instrument.

In experimental studies, it is often reported that accurate (with no systemic errors) and precise (not affected by casual errors) measures are difficult to obtain.

Accuracy of a measurement procedure is the property whereby the recorded measurements coincide with the values actually measured. Accuracy is achieved by repeating the measurement of a fixed and known quantity under constant conditions. Precision of a measurement procedure is the property whereby the repeated measures obtained are very similar (or, even better, they are identical) to their mean value.

In a specific study or procedure, two kinds of errors can be identified with reference to accuracy and precision:

- *Systemic error (bias):* the degree of inaccuracy of a measurement procedure; ie, the same error is present in all measurements
- *Random error:* the degree of imprecision of a procedure; ie, accidental deviation in measuring a constant entity due to chance

Random errors can be reduced if measurements are repeated and their values are weighted around the mean. The more repeated measurements, the lower the impact of random error, even if there is a practical limit to the number of repeated measurements possible for each cephalometric radiograph, especially in clinical practice. Also, for scientific research purposes, if serial measurements of two groups have to be compared, two measurements will be sufficient. Imprecision can also be reduced by improving quality in detection procedures.[13]

3D Cephalometry

Since the development of cephalometric radiology, several analyses have been proposed that are useful in describing how much a patient differs from standard values derived from other studies. These analyses allow clinicians to speak a common clinical language. Despite the amazing nature of CBCT images, 3D cephalometric radiographs are less commonly used than 2D images. A review of literature in the last 5 years shows that 3D cephalometric investigation has aroused the interest of several orthodontic and maxillofacial surgical schools.

The first phase of study has been devoted to verifying the accuracy and repeatability[14-16] of linear and/or angular measurements obtained from axial, coronal, and sagittal images or 3D-rendered images, as compared to conventional systems and anthropometric assessments.

Swennen and Schutyser[15] published a paper in 2006 on cephalometric analysis, comparing the values obtained from images reconstructed from spiral CT and CBCT with an emphasis on benefits, potentials, and drawbacks of 3D analysis. In the same year, the authors also published *Three-Dimensional Cephalometry: A Color Atlas and Manual*,[17] proposing a 3D analysis of hard and soft tissues using linear, angular, orthogonal, and proportional measures among planes and points/planes but without providing standard values.

Jacobson[18] developed a new anthropometric analysis both for hard and soft tissues based on a multiplanar system with four primary reference planes (anterior facial plane, lower facial plane, superior facial plane, and midsagittal plane) and four additional planes. In this study the sample consisted of 40 men and 40 women, all North Americans, aged 20 to 40 years with normal occlusion as assessed by a 50-member jury (25 men and 25 women) of different races and social classes, who selected only the "most attractive" individuals.

All measures on hard tissues were adjusted to the actual physical sizes, first adapting magnification using lateral and frontal radiographs of dry skulls with metal markers and then taking measurements directly on skulls. The values obtained by the authors are anthropometric, therefore actual, as they do not include individual measurements, and they include ratios in facial proportions.

The model of analysis by Gateno et al[14] aimed at preserving the benefits of 2D cephalometry by overcoming its now evident limitations. He outlined a new cephalometric system subdivided in six modules: symmetry, transversality, verticality, pitch, anteroposteriority, and shape. The sequence in discussing the modules aims at reflecting the ideal theoretical sequence in developing a 3D plan of surgical treatment:

- *Dimension:* measured as linear distance in 3D space
- *Form:* measured by projecting landmarks onto the midsagittal plane of a local system of coordinates for each facial unit
- *Position:* measured differently according to the measurement direction
- *Transversality:* measured as linear distance between the landmarks used and

the midsagittal plane of the global system of coordinates
- *Vertical and anteroposterior position:* measured after all landmarks used have been projected onto the midsagittal plane of the global system of coordinates
- *Orientation:* calculated as pitch, roll, and yaw separately for each facial unit

In his paper, Gateno underlined the problem associated with measures taken directly in 3D and outlined strategies to resolve them; in particular, he developed two systems of coordinates, a local and a global system, to allow correct measurement values to be obtained by way of comparison.

In 2010 Wu et al[16] published a paper that introduced 3D models obtained from the orthogonal projection of lateral and PA cephalometric radiographs and compared measurements obtained with 2D analysis to those taken from a 3D model. It was difficult to recognize the same landmarks in both cephalometric radiographs, and, although the 3D linear measurements were 98.8% accurate, the 3D analysis was not as complete as the conventional 2D analysis because it could only identify 15 landmarks in both cephalometric radiographs. Many other studies have been done on the accuracy of landmark definition, which is considered to be the greatest source of error in cephalometric analysis.[19] This kind of error is influenced by many factors such as quality of the radiographic image, accuracy in defining landmarks, reproducibility in their positioning, the operator, and the recording procedures.[20,21]

Oliveira et al,[22] Kusnoto et al,[23] and Medelnik et al[24] state that reproducibility in landmark identification differs on the three spatial planes (X, Y, Z). This implies that some points are easy to identify on one or two planes but difficult to detect on the third plane.

Farronato et al[25] propose a comparison between the new 3D cephalometric analysis based on the identification of 10 points and a conventional 2D Steiner analysis. The reference planes used were built starting from sella (S), which is automatically determined by the software as the intersection between the planes. Besides a comparison between the two cephalometric systems, the authors studied the volumes and centroids of maxilla and mandible to monitor growth in the three dimensions of space.

In 2012 Farronato et al[26] published a new paper in which a pool of 65 CBCT patients of Ricketts skeletal Class I were studied with dedicated software, and a cloud of points was calculated for each landmark representing the normal range. A cephalometric analysis with 18 landmarks was used in this trial.

Construction of a 3D Cephalometric Analysis Model

Reference Systems

3D cephalometry is a more complex upgrade than the simple addition of depth as a parameter in lateral cephalometric analysis.

There are several issues associated with 3D cephalometry, and one of the most important ones is certainly the selection of reference systems from which to base linear or angular measurements. Both in 2D and in 3D, there are two types of reference systems.

Internal reference systems are defined by internal landmarks such as the Frankfurt horizontal plane (FH) or the sella-nasion line (SN).

They offer the following advantages:

- They are not influenced by the position of the head
- There are standard values
- They are more popular because they have been used for a longer time[14]

They also present drawbacks:

- They can be difficult to define
- They can be distorted by craniofacial deformities or asymmetries

External reference systems are defined by external elements such as the axial and coronal planes (passing through the external auditory canals and parallel respectively to the axial and coronal planes) and the midsagittal plane (dividing the head into two halves).

There are benefits to these systems:

- They are easy to define
- They are not influenced by craniofacial deformities

They have just one drawback:

- They are only reliable if the patient's head is in the natural head position (NHP)[14]

The internal reference systems, eg, the FH plane, may not be reliable because of potential congenital asymmetries and asymmetries associated with deficit of the middle third,[27] while in external reference systems it is necessary to start by defining the NHP, ie, orientating the head of the patient in a neutral position that is not tilted, rotated, or stretched.

Several studies have aimed at building a midsagittal plane. A study by Damstra et al[28] has proved that there are clinically relevant differences between the midsagittal plane and the symmetry plane on multislice CT and CBCT images. In this paper, it was also reported that nasion has a maximum deviation from the morphometric midsagittal plane of < 0.50 mm and can be used as a reference to build the plane. Jacobson[18] defines the midsagittal plane as a midplane dividing the head sagittally through nasion when the patient, in frontal view, is in NHP. In this case, the midsagittal plane derived from NHP is based on visual perception and does not rely on internal structures.

Studying 2D radiographs of many individuals with craniomandibular asymmetries, Trpkova et al[27] concluded that the vertical lines traced as perpendiculars through middle points between pairs of bilateral orbital landmarks are more accurate and reliable than those constructed between two median points.

A significant effect on measurements starting from the midsagittal plane has been described. It has been shown how the distance between landmarks can influence the degree of error in measurements: the closer the points, the greater the error in angular measurement.[29] The great variation of midsagittal planes in apparently symmetric groups of people can be explained by the fact that "perfectly symmetric" does not exist, and a certain degree of asymmetry is intrinsic in every individual.[30–32]

Therefore, the median landmarks used in building midsagittal planes can deviate from the true symmetry plane (ideally dividing the head in two identical halves on the sagittal plane).

Furthermore, the combined effect of two or more nonmedian points, because of minor local remodeling, could induce significant deviation from the true symmetry plane. This suggests that internal structures, even if remodeled, could be irrelevant for visible facial symmetry; hence, a midsagittal plane based on median landmarks can vary among individuals and is still debatable.[33]

3D Measurements

A cephalometric analysis consists of a series of measurements that best describe various geometric parameters of a specific facial district. Four key parameters can be measured: dimension, form, position, and orientation. Currently standard 2D cephalometric radiographs are fraught with two basic problems:

1. Many crucial parameters cannot be measured on a flat cephalometric radiograph, which is limited because there is no third dimension.
2. Most of the measurements taken on cephalometric radiographs are distorted in the presence of facial asymmetries.[34]

3D measurements can be linear, like the ones taken between two points or two lines or a line and a plane, or they can be angular, like those taken between planes or lines. In the latter case, it should always be considered that the value obtained derives from three angles (pitch, roll, and yaw) around the X-, Y-, and Z- axes (Fig 4-7).

Measurements taken in the three dimensions of space are very different from 2D measurements, and attention should be paid to reading them, especially angular measurements.

A more complete description, like the one obtained from 3D reconstructions of CT scans, requires consideration of not only translation into three spatial dimensions but also rotation around three axes (pitch, roll, and yaw).

The orientation of an object is established by how it is placed in space in relation to a reference structure, which is usually specified by a Cartesian system. It can therefore be defined as the description of the rotation of an object from its initial position to the actual one.[14]

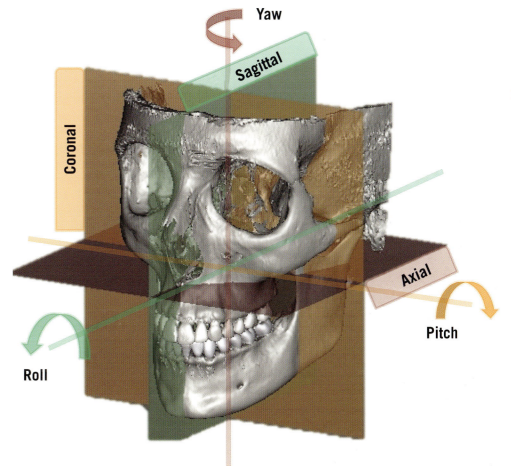

Fig 4-7 Graphic representation of pitch, roll, and yaw.

An object's orientation can be described with three angles (see Fig 4-7): the pitch, referring to rotation around the transversal axis (X); the roll, referring to rotation around the anteroposterior axis (Y); and the yaw, rotation around the vertical axis (Z).

To calculate these angles, it is necessary to separate the two reference systems that have been constructed for this purpose:

- The global reference system is used for the entire volume acquired.
- The local reference system is used for the individual structure to be analyzed.

After obtaining the same measurements in both systems, one can assess how much the structure has rotated around its axes. Based on these principles, the angular values obtained are actually values composed by pitch, roll, and yaw, as opposed to 2D radiographs, in which only pitch is measured. In Fig 4-8a the mandible presents a roll and yaw component of 0 degrees; therefore, the midsagittal plane (shown in red) is parallel to the global system, so that in both systems the value of the gonial angle will be the same. In Fig 4-8b there is a 20-degree yaw and a 0-degree roll. In this case, the local midsagittal plane is rotated

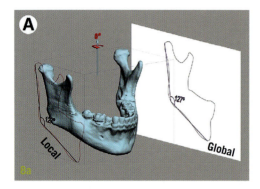

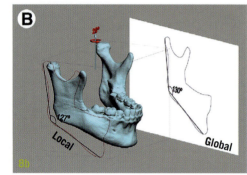

Figs 4-8a and 4-8b The local system of coordinates is represented by the cube containing the mandible, while the global system is represented by the projection on the left of the mandible.[13]

with reference to the global system but the value does not change because the mandible has rotated together with the plane in the local system. This is not the case with the global system, where the value is distorted because of the yaw component.

The local system of coordinates is represented by the cube containing the mandible, while the global system is represented by the projection on the left of the mandible.[14]

Accuracy and Repeatability of Measurements

Several studies have been done to assess the reliability of measurements taken directly in 3D. For instance, Lascala et al[35] in 2004 have recorded statistically smaller measures in 3D. Hilgers et al[36] in 2005 stated that direct measures on CBCT are accurate and reproducible. Another study has been published by Periago et al[37] in 2008 reporting differences between measures taken directly in 3D and on a dry skull (1 mm in 60% of the cases and 2 mm in 10% of the cases). The author stated that they were nevertheless accurate enough to study craniofacial structures.

More recently, Baumgaertel et al[38] reported that, even if direct CBCT measures are underestimated, they become statistically significant only if composite measures are used, ie, when the same point is positioned several times, thus adding a source of error. It should be kept in mind that the studies performed by these authors have used direct measurements on 3D renderings, which add sources of error due to the inaccuracy of the gray scale selected for the segmentation process. However, to get an accurate assessment, landmarks should be located on multiplanar reconstructions obtained with dedicated software programs.[39]

Tomographic scans (CBCT and CT) allow the clinician to obtain accurate and repeatable 3D linear measures of the craniofacial complex. Small motions in the head position away from the ideal position do not influence the accuracy of values based on 3D reconstructions.[40]

If the head is scanned in the ideal and rotated position, the difference between 3D measurements and the gold standard (corresponding to measurements on a dry skull) is relatively small (about 0.5 mm). This could be due to the rigid nature of transpositions of bony tissues caused by movement; ie, the position of image acquisition does not influence the reciprocal location of anatomical landmarks differently from what could happen with soft tissues.[41]

Accuracy of measurements in 3D images will also depend on the size of voxels. Damstra et al[42] in 2010 performed a study to test the accuracy of measurements by comparing images with 0.25- to 0.40-mm voxels and in real size (using Simplant Ortho software [Materialise]). Their result confirmed a previous study by Ballrick et al[43] that showed that there is no difference in the accuracy of measurements, especially if these refer to craniofacial structures. One can therefore say that the size of voxels necessarily depends on the kind of problem the patient has and on the treatment envisaged in that specific case. Liedke et al[44] has analyzed external root resorption through CBCT images with voxels of different sizes (0.4 mm, 0.3 mm, and 0.2 mm); although the results were practically identical, it was easier to make a diagnosis with smaller voxels.

Effects of Facial Asymmetry

There can be problems in the context of 3D measurements when examining the x-rays of patients with facial asymmetries. An abnormal pitch or roll or transversal position of a single facial unit can be deduced in patients with facial asymmetry, and measures taken directly in 3D are not realistic, most of all in assessing orientation and position.

In evaluating facial asymmetry, in particular in calculating the size of structures in the maxillofacial complex, a paper by Gateno and Teichgraeber[14] in 2011 has shown differences between 2D and 3D. The projection of a 2D image does not necessarily correspond to the object, which could be parallel to the film during scanning; if this is the case, changes in yaw would cause a distortion of the 2D value in anteroposterior measures. For instance in the Gribel et al[45] study it has been reported that the measure taken between the condylion and point A was smaller in the side-to-side teleradiography than with measures taken directly on a dry skull. Modifying the roll, the result tends to change for vertical measures. In this case, as there is no such distortion in 3D, direct measures in 3D turn out to be superior to those obtained in 2D.

CONCEPT OF NORMALITY

One of the most critical points of cephalometric analysis is the difficulty in setting the boundaries between the norm and deviation from it. Almost all methods of analysis refer to an ideal model of the facial skeleton, even though variability of the skull structure is extreme, and its architectural equilibrium can be obtained through numerous or even endless possible adaptations or variations of its components.[20]

The term normality is ambiguous because it implies a concept of an "ideal," which changes according to the evolution of knowledge, esthetic standards, treatment modalities, the concept of good health, plus a certain margin of variation within statistics. It is used with all these meanings, and it is universally acceptable.[4]

However, the concept of an ideal should not be confused with something to be idolized, as is often the case[46]; dictionaries associate "ideal" and "imaginary" and distinguish them from the word "realistic."

Orthodontists must therefore know the requirements for good occlusal function and a pleasant look in most individuals, but they should not forget that their patients are unique, sometimes very peculiar individuals, who should be treated as such. The set of conditions that apply to most of the population can be called normality. Normality is nevertheless not imposed on everyone, and it is not always necessary for good health and a pleasant look.[47]

Downs[48] says: "We can have a value for a given relation and a value for a different relation, which, considered separately, can be acceptable and combine so that one offsets the unbalance in the other and a normal face type results. But it can also happen that two values for the same relations can be acceptable if taken alone but when combined, they give origin to disharmony, ie, an abnormality." This concept has been followed by the authors in developing both analyses, which has allowed the concept of normality to be replaced with that of compensation.

Model of 3D Cephalometric Analysis

The 3D cephalometric system uses a series of landmarks, reference planes, and construction points and is therefore considered to be multiplanar. The landmarks used in the 3D analysis are identified using a multiplanar reconstruction system. The landmarks in the 3D cephalometric system are as follows:

- Nasion (N)
- Subspinale (A)
- Jugale right (JR)
- Jugale left (JL)
- Jugale median (JM)
- Anterior nasal spine (ANS)
- Condylion right (CoR)
- Condylion left (CoL)
- Gonion right (GoR)
- Gonion left (GoL)
- Gnathion (Gn)
- Menton (Me)
- Pogonion (Pog)
- Crestal point between molars right (PcmR)
- Crestal point between molars left (PcmL)

There are three reference planes:

- Coronal plane
- Sagittal plane
- Axial plane

These planes do not depend on the head posture during CT acquisition. Each point of these planes is identified on the 0.00 slice of the corresponding coronal, sagittal, and axial planes so that it is outside the skull structure, thus avoiding problems associated with, for instance, local bone remodeling.[33]

The construction planes used are:

- Anterior facial plane (AFP): plane passing through ANS parallel to the coronal plane
- Superior facial plane (SFP): plane passing through N and parallel to the axial plane
- Spinal plane (ANSPl): plane passing through ANS and parallel to the axial plane
- Mental plane (MePl): plane passing through Me parallel to the axial plane
- Maxillary plane (MxPl): plane passing through the JM point (median point between JR and JL), which is orthogonal to the coronal plane
- Pogonion plane (PogPl): plane passing by Pog parallel to the coronal plane

The analysis uses a set of linear and angular measurements obtained by calculating the distance between landmarks and between landmarks and planes built coplanarly to the three reference planes (axial, coronal, and sagittal) of the 3D system (Figs 4-9 and 4-10).

The 3D cephalometric method is subdivided into modules that are oriented to the cephalometric study of the maxillofacial structure. Four modules have been identified for the multiplanar analysis.

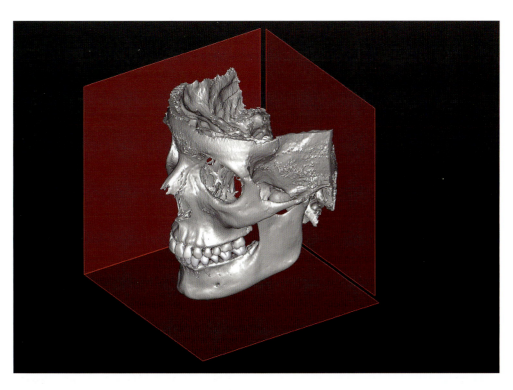

Fig 4-9 Representation of the three reference planes forming the extracranial reference system.

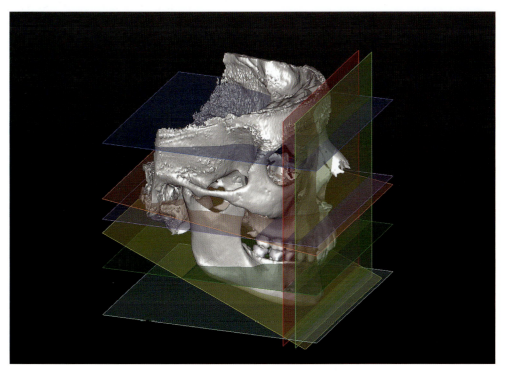

Fig 4-10 Representation of the construction planes forming the intracranial reference plane.

1. Module A: vertical dimensions
2. Module B: sagittal dimensions
3. Module C: assessment of skeletal symmetry
4. Module D: assessment of craniofacial growth expectancy

Module A: Vertical Dimensions

The study of anterior vertical dimensions as facial proportions is very important to assess proper harmony in vertical growth between the bone bases and allows the patient to be classified as a mesocephalic, brachycephalic, or dolichocephalic individual. The distance is calculated among the three construction planes, passing through one cephalometric point and parallel to the axial plane (Figs 4-11 to 4-13). There are three calculated distances

- Superior vertical dimension (S): the distance between SFP and ANS
- Inferior vertical dimension (I): the distance between ANSPl and Me
- Total vertical dimension (T): the distance between MePl and N

Module B: Sagittal Dimensions

The study of sagittal dimensions allows identification of the reciprocal relationship between the two maxillary bones, which is an extremely important piece of information in many branches of dentistry (prosthetics, orthodontics, and surgery). There are three measurements taken:

- Maxillary position (MX): the distance between A and AFP
- Mandibular position (MB): the distance between Pog and AFP
- Intermaxillary ratio (IR): the difference between MX and MB

Module C: Craniofacial Symmetry

Symmetroscopy allows detection of the presence or absence of asymmetric skeletal structures, which is extremely important in individuals undergoing orthognathic surgery. The measurements taken entail the study of several aspects (Figs 4-14 and 4-15):

- Verticality: right and left posterior facial height; the distance between the Go and SFP
- Mandible: right and left mandibular rami: the distance between Co and Go; right and left hemimandibles: the distance between Go and Gn.
- Maxilla: maxillary height (MxH); the distance between the crestal point between the molars (Pcm) point and MxPl

Each measurement must be taken on both sides so as to compare them and assess their difference:

- When the difference is 0 to 3 mm, asymmetry is slight and is often clinically invisible, as soft tissues may conceal it.
- When the difference between the two sides is > 3 mm, asymmetry becomes relevant.

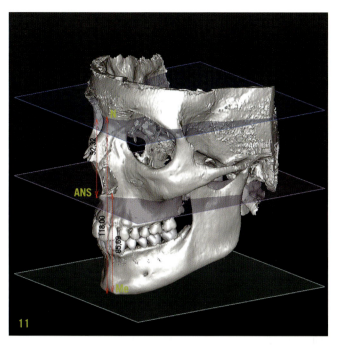
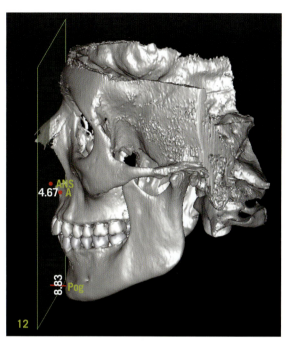

Fig 4-11 Measurements obtained as point-to-plane distances are shown.
Fig 4-12 The assessment of the sagittal dimensions are shown in terms of point-to-plane distances.

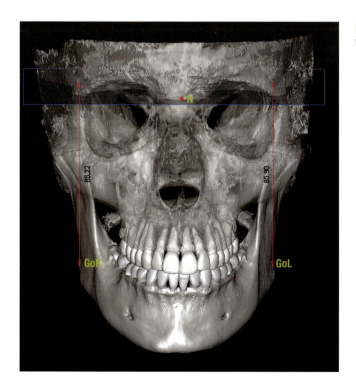

Fig 4-13 The assessment of the posterior facial height is shown as a point-to-plane distance.

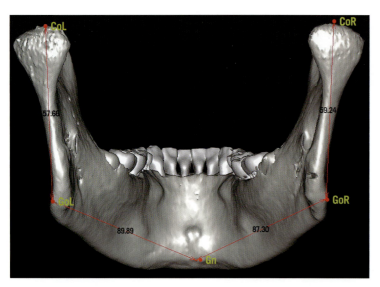

Fig 4-14 The analysis of mandibular symmetry involves the assessment of the two structural components measured as point-to-point distances.

Module D: Craniofacial Growth Expectancy

In growing individuals it is important to assess the manner in which growth is taking place and whether there is a deviation from the standard growth curve (Fig 4-16). The following measurements are taken in boys < 18 years and girls < 12 years:

- Posterior height (PH): the distance between S and (GoMPl)
- Skeletal growth pattern (SKP): % ratio between PH and T (total anterior vertical dimension)
- Mandibular tilt (MT): angle between (MbPl) and PogPl

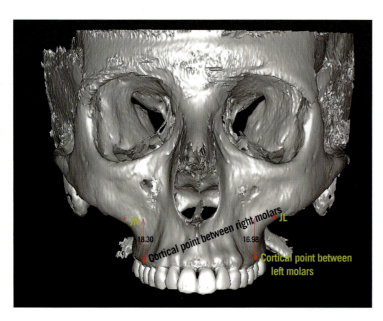

Fig 4-15 It is possible to detect alterations in the maxillary skeleton through this analysis.

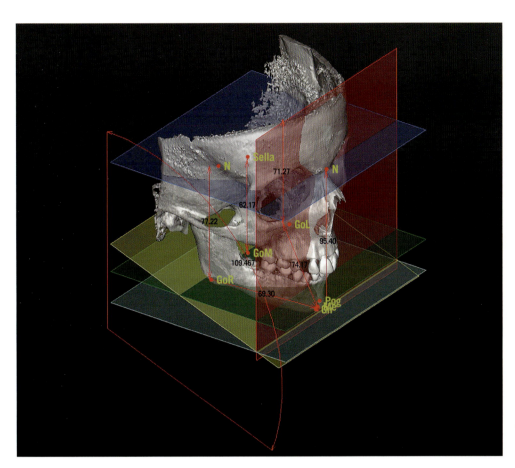

Fig 4-16 The measurements taken to gather information on growth expectancy are shown. It includes both the relationship between vertical measurements and the calculation of the angle between the two planes, focusing on the mandible.

Dysgnathic Presentations in 3D

3D Skeletal Classifications

Vertical Dimension

For each of the three measurements defined below, a specific scale of values has been developed that allows individuals to be assigned to a specific range for that specific measure in the vertical dimension. The ranges are described in Fig 4-17 and are subdivided as follows:

- Medium: ± x - σ/2 < x < x + σ/2 (including 38.2% of the population)
- Borderline: x - σ < x < x + σ (including 68.2% of the population)
- Short + or long +: x - 2σ < x < x + 2σ (including 95.4% of the population)
- Short ++ or long ++: x > ± 2σ (including the remaining 4.6% of the population).

Starting from three measurements, a diagnostic algorithm has been developed. It is based on the sum of three values: the superior vertical dimension (S), the inferior vertical dimension (I), and the total vertical dimension (T), which together form the acronym SIT.
The result of this calculation will indicate the skeletal class of the individual analyzed in terms of vertical dimension, with special attention to the total vertical dimension (T).
Seven types have been identified (Fig 4-18). Each range of values corresponds to a specific skeletal type. To assign an individual to a specific skeletal class, two of three values must fall into that category, although there are some exceptions.

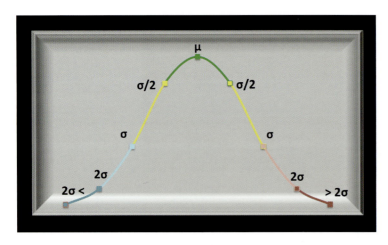

Fig 4-17 Classification of population sample based on predefined ranges.

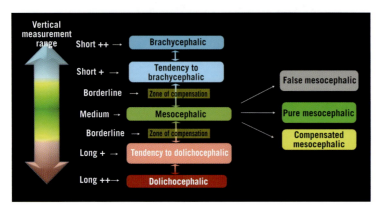

Fig 4-18 Diagnostic algorithm using the SIT values.

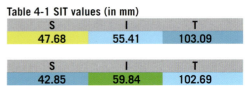

Table 4-1 SIT values (in mm)

S	I	T
47.68	55.41	103.09

S	I	T
42.85	59.84	102.69

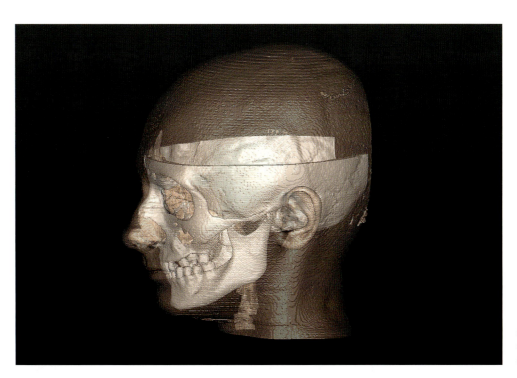

Fig 4-19a Brachycephalic individual shown in 3D reconstruction by segmentation of soft tissues (in transparence) and hard tissues.

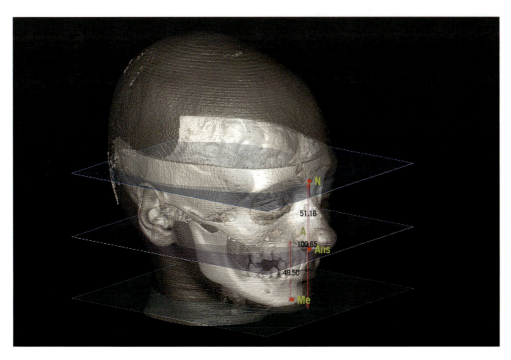

Fig 4-19b There is a significant reduction in the inferior vertical dimension.

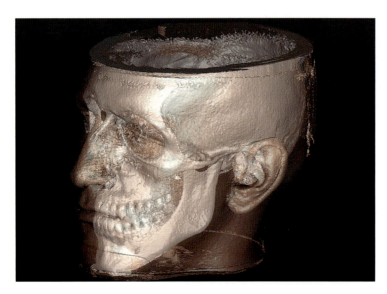

Fig 4-20a Individual tending to dolichocephaly, shown in a 3D rendering by segmentation of soft tissues (in transparence) and hard tissues.

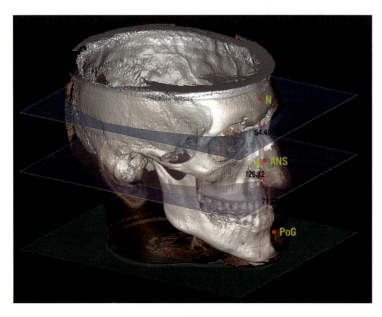

Fig 4-20b Two borderline values have lead to classification of this patient as having a tendency towards dolichocephaly in the global assessment.

Table 4-1 shows the SIT measurements of two borderline patients who are very similar yet differ in terms of the final diagnosis. In both patients, the values are in the short + and short ++ range, the discriminating factor being the dimension measured: in the first patient, the short ++ value relates to T and short + relates to I, whereas in the second patient, short ++ relates to S, and short ++ relates to T. The diagnosis of the first patient is brachycephalic (Fig 4-19) because, in the total vertical dimension, there is a further reduction in height with reference to the inferior vertical dimension (because of the borderline superior vertical dimension). In the second patient, the diagnosis is a tendency to brachycephaly, as here the total vertical dimension shows only a slight reduction in height because of a medium superior vertical dimension.

Table 4-2 SIT values (in mm)

S	I	T
46.75	56.24	102.98

S	I	T
51.48	66.13	117.61

In the patients whose values are shown in Table 4-2, the anterosuperior and anteroinferior vertical dimensions fall within the borderline category, so the skeletal type is given by the total dimension; hence, there is tendency to brachycephaly in one patient and a tendency towards dolichocephaly in the other patient (Fig 4-20) (this is caused by the partial vertical values, which are borderline; their sum has indicated a specific skeletal type).

Three subclasses have been identified for mesocephalic individuals: pure, false, and compensated.

The subdivision of mesocephalic individuals (Fig 4-21) into subclasses is based on the discrepancy in the relationship of the three values.

PURE MESOCEPHALIC: At least two of three values fall into the medium range, and one of these values must be the total vertical dimension (Table 4-3).

Table 4-3 SIT values (in mm)

S	I	T
49.71	68.46	118.17

S	I	T
48.85	71.43	120.28

COMPENSATED MESOCEPHALIC: Two of three values are in the borderline range. There are some exceptions, which are special cases of compensated mesocephalic individuals.

Table 4-4 SIT values (in mm)

S	I	T
44.89	71.79	116.68

S	I	T
57.89	64.23	122.12

The patient measurements shown in Table 4-4 are an exception to the rule of referring to total dimension when the first two values (superior and inferior) are different. The individual cannot be defined as pure mesocephalic, because that classification requires that two values must be medium (one of them being the total vertical dimension). Nevertheless, considering this is a medium total dimension and that there is a borderline value, the individual is considered to be compensated mesocephalic.

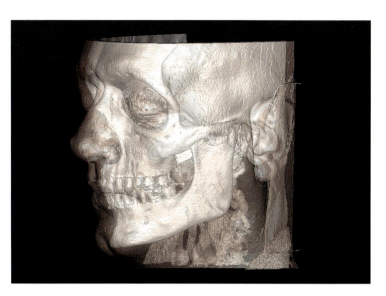

Fig 4-21a Mesocepalic compensated individual: 3D reconstruction by segmentation of soft tissues (in transparence) and hard tissues.

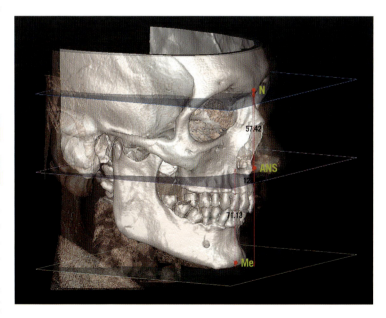

Fig 4-21b Three values are shown: superior and inferior vertical dimensions are borderline values while the total vertical dimension is a medium value.

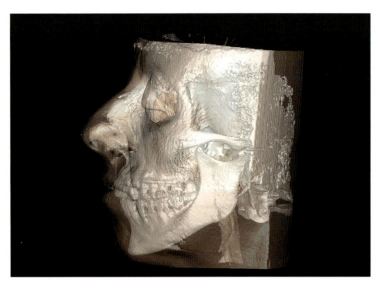

Fig 4-22a False mesocephalic individual: 3D rendering by segmentation of soft tissues (in transparence) and hard tissues.

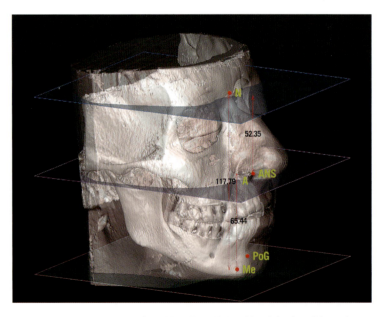

Fig 4-22b The relationship of the basal bone bases is correct, even if the maxilla and mandible, taken individually, are not in the ideal position.

Table 4-5 SIT values (in mm)

S	I	T
55.79	67.89	123.85

S	I	T
52.18	61.47	113.65

When, as shown in Table 4-5, there are three different values, with either the superior or inferior vertical dimension being medium and the total vertical dimension being borderline, the individual is classified as compensated mesocephalic.

FALSE MESOCEPHALIC: The value of the total vertical dimension falls into the medium or borderline range while the values of superior and inferior vertical dimension fall into completely opposite ranges (Fig 4-22).

Table 4-6 SIT values (in mm)

S	I	T
53.24	60.35	113.59

S	I	T
53.01	54.7	107.71

The two sets of patient measurements shown in Table 4-6 are emblematic of this skeletal type: the total dimension is medium/borderline and the other two measurements fall into opposite categories.

Sagittal Dimension

The choice of Pog rather than point B to represent the mandible in the sagittal assessment is driven by a very good reason: anthropology has shown us that human evolution and civilization have lead to a reduction in the size of the chewing apparatus.

This can be easily seen in the morphologic changes of the mandible in relation to progressive chin development as the teeth became smaller and the arches shorter, because the shortening of the mandible is limited; otherwise, the lever arm for the masticatory muscles eventually would not be sufficient. If the genial tubercles are considered as a constant, it is easy to confirm that it is actually the dental arch that moves posteriorly and not the round anterior edge of the mandible that moves anteriorly.[49]

Therefore, in line with anthropologic studies, Pog has been taken as a landmark, as it will remain constant, rather than point B, which is susceptible to posterior movement. Referring to the basic concepts in the earlier section Concept of Normality, a new skeletal class of reference can be introduced, called balanced rather than Class I; skeletal Classes II and III remain.

The choice of the term *balanced* is driven by the ideas inspiring this analysis, which attempt to overcome the main problem associated with many cephalometric systems, ie, basing classifications on individual measurements, while in fact, any measurement is influenced by other values in the same craniofacial structure. It is evident that not only do measurements depend on one another, but that an altered measure may be partially or completely compensated by others. This happens both in skeletal and in dental relationships and can often lead to an incorrect assessment if this compensation is not recognized.[50]

Another new class proposed is top balanced, which includes individuals who have reached an ideal degree of balancing.

Diagnostic Algorithm: Two of Three Values

The ranges obtained for skeletal Classes II and III have been taken into account and integrated with the ranges for balanced class. *Intermaxillary ratio* (IR) identifies the reciprocal position of the maxilla and mandible on the sagittal plane (Fig 4-23):

- < –1.5 mm indicates a Class II value
- > 2.6 mm indicates a Class III value
- A value between –1.5 and 2.6 mm indicates a balanced value

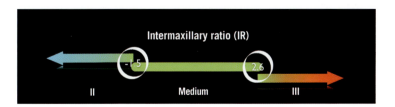

Fig 4-23 Ranges for the intermaxillary ratio.

MAXILLARY POSITION (MX) identifies the position of the maxilla on the sagittal plane:

- < 3.2 mm indicates a Class II value;
- 3.2 to 4 mm indicates an intermediate MX value between Class I and II
- 4 to 6 mm is defined as mixed value, where all three classes "coexist"
- > 6 mm indicates a Class III value

Fig 4-24 Ranges for the MX value. See also Table 4-7.

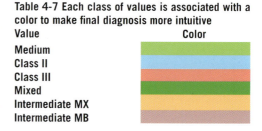

Table 4-7 Each class of values is associated with a color to make final diagnosis more intuitive

Value	Color
Medium	
Class II	
Class III	
Mixed	
Intermediate MX	
Intermediate MB	

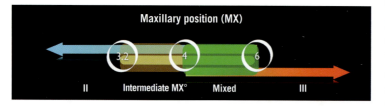

MANDIBULAR POSITION (MB) indicates the position of the mandible in the sagittal plane:

- < 0.6 mm indicates a Class III value
- 0.6 to 3.2 mm indicates an intermediate MB value between Class I and III
- 3.2 to 5.0 mm indicates a medium value
- > 5 mm indicates a Class II value

Fig 4-25 Ranges for the MB value. See also Table 4-7.

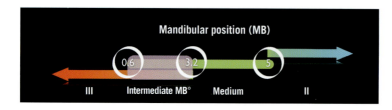

The analysis develops from concepts that had been expressed earlier by Wylie[51] in a similar form. In his cephalometry, he used five linear distances for sagittal skeletal diagnosis, stating that the coexistence of standard values for the five measurements will result in a facial skeleton that is well balanced and ideally proportioned.

Nevertheless, when the measurements of the five distances do not correspond to these values, it is not said that there is an abnormality present, as all dimensions may be greater or smaller. If variance in dimensions occurs proportionally, it is obvious that the overall balance of components is not impaired. Moreover, it is also possible that the values of the various distances are in different reciprocal relationships from those existing between standard values without resulting in an abnormality, as compensations can occur between changes in dimensions.[20]

Treasured concepts expressed by Wylie,[51] Downs,[48] and Enlow[52] in the sagittal cephalometry method state that diagnosis can be derived from the sum of three measurements; the general rule is that two values out of three identify the skeletal class, hence the term two of three.

As in vertical cephalometry, in the sagittal dimension some exceptions have been identified.

The top balanced class (Table 4-8) is identified by medium IR and MB (Pog-AFP distance) values, while the MX value (A-AFP distance) is mixed.

Table 4-8 Sagittal dimensions for a top balanced patient (in mm)

IR	MX	MB
0.91	4.19	3.28

If MX and MB are different, the IR value will determine the skeletal class.

Table 4-9 Sagittal dimensions for a balanced patient (in mm)

IR	MX	MB
0.13	6.7	6.57

Table 4-9 shows an example of a former skeletal Class I individual, who now is classified as skeletally balanced: MX and MB diverge and belong to two different and opposite classes when taken individually. However, when combined, they define an individual with an acceptable, standard relationship between the maxilla and mandible (Fig 4-26).

Table 4-10 Sagittal dimensions for balanced patients (in mm)

IR	MX	MB
0.89	13.5	2.61

IR	MX	MB
1.8	4.41	2.61

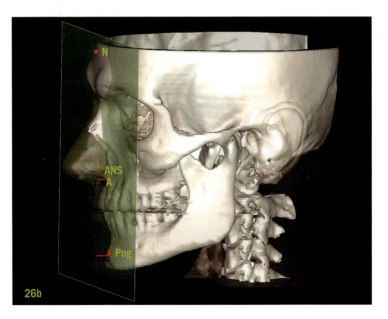

Figs 4-26a and 4-26b Balanced individual. The relationship between the maxillary and mandibular basal bone is appropriate, or within the standard, although the maxilla and mandible taken individually present opposite values.

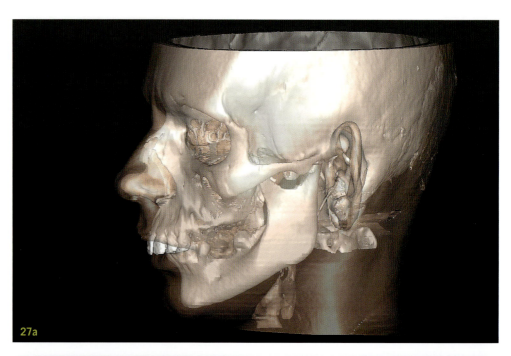

Figs 4-27a and 4-27b Skeletal Class II patient.

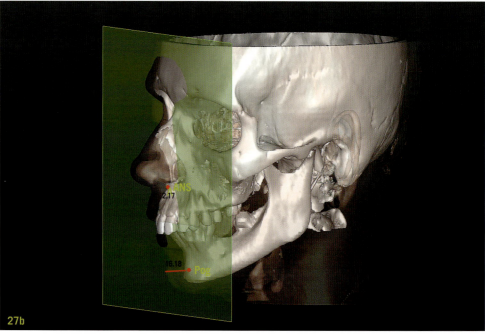

Table 4-10 shows sagittal dimensions of two skeletally balanced individuals. In the first example there are intermediate MX and MB values, while in the second patient there is a mixed MX value and an intermediate MB value; however, in both patients the resulting IR is medium.

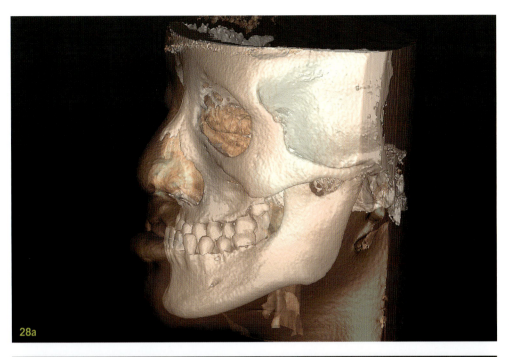

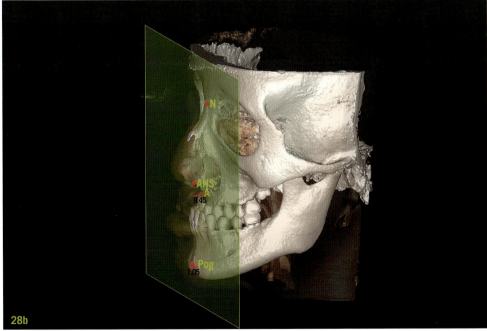

Figs 4-28a and 4-28b
Skeletal Class III patient.

The patients shown in Figs 4-27 and 4-28 are typical skeletal Class II and III individuals in whom two of three values fall into the diagnosed class (based on the IR).

Consideration should be made on values as taken individually, especially a mixed value, deriving from the fact that all three classes converge into the MX measurement. This can be explained as follows:

- The maxilla is a bone connected by sutures to the rest of the skull. Its position does not change markedly (this would explain the range of values belonging to all classes).
- On the contrary, the mandible articulates with the skull through its condylar process; therefore, it does not have many structural constraints, and this is the reason why it can change its development pattern during growth. This allows one to understand why the same rule does not apply to the maxilla.

The sagittal and vertical cephalometric analyses presented in this book represent a completely different approach to the diagnostic problem compared to standard cephalometric methods. It is based on a new way of conceiving skeletal structures in their mutual relationships. This makes it very flexible, dynamic, and capable of assessing the various bony structures, not only individually but also in relation to others.

Assessment of Asymmetry

Assessment of asymmetry with 3D multiplanar cephalometry entails taking several measurements:

- Mandibular ramus
- Mandibular body
- Posterior facial height
- Maxillary height

The difference, quantitatively and qualitatively, between 2D and 3D in detecting the presence or absence of asymmetric structures is very important. Symmetroscopy using the new 3D method becomes a valuable tool for the clinician in planning an ideal treatment plan both in orthodontics and in maxillofacial surgery.

The introduction of 3D imaging has posed a new challenge in developing practical solutions applicable in day-to-day clinical practice (Fig 4-29). Because of more accurate identification of landmarks and more accurate measurements, cephalometry can be reviewed in light of the underlying concept of normality.

In the past, researchers such as Downs, Wylie, and Enlow introduced the concept

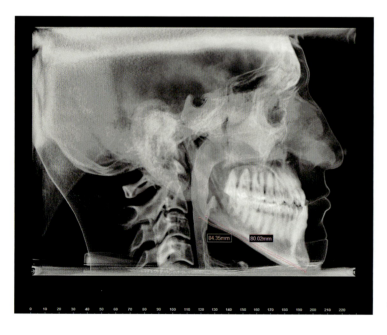

Fig 4-29a Lateral cephalometric radiograph aligned along the linear measurements of the two mandibular hemiarches.

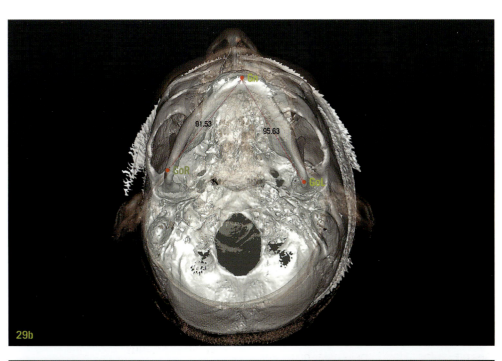

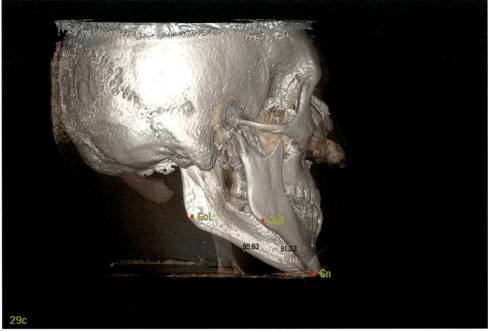

Figs 29b and 29c 3D measurements of the mandible in *(b)* axial and *(c)* ¾ lateral view.

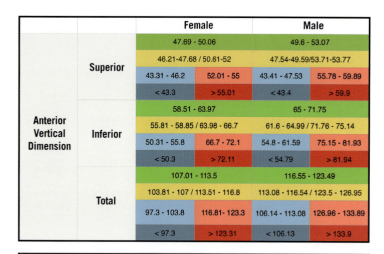

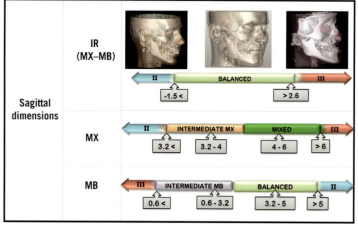

Fig 4-30 Diagnostic record.

of compensation, ie, considering measurements as a whole and relating them one to the other rather than considering them as absolute values or separate entities.

The present analysis is based on the concept of balance among the various structures, without setting rigid boundaries between normality and abnormality in the values measured for each individual patient.

The "ideal" model of reference used in most cephalometric analyses is very abstract, as the most significant feature of human beings is their uniqueness.

There is extreme variability in the structure of the head, and its architectural balance can be obtained through many, if not endless, possibilities of adaptation among the variations in its components.

Each individual must be analyzed in a different way; the goal is a case-specific evaluation interpreting craniofacial structure in all its components, not taken individually but in their mutual relationships.

The use of this new method has led to the development of diagnostic records (Figs 4-30 and 4-31) to register the values obtained with multiplanar cephalometry and a key to symbols allowing the clinician to associate a measurement with a specific diagnostic value.

TREATING PHYSICIAN: ....

Patient: ....

Age: ..../........./.......... Gender: ☐ M ☐ F

DATE: ..../........./........

			Value	Diagnosis
Anterior Vertical Dimension		S		
		I		
		T		

			Value	Diagnosis
Sagittal Dimension		DR		
		MX		
		MB		

			Value	Diagnosis
Asymmetry	Mandibular ramus	R		☐ Ramus
		L		
	Mandibular body	R		☐ Hemimandible
		L		
	Maxillary height	R		
		L		
	Posterior height	R		☐ Reduced
		L		☐ Increased

Fig 4-31 Diagnostic record.

3D IMAGING AND DENTISTRY

References

1. Athanasiou AE. Cefalometria Ortodontica. Bologna: Martina, 2000.
2. Hwang HS, Lee KH, Park JY, Kang BC, Park JW, Lee JS. Development of posterior anterior cephalometric analysis for the diagnosis of facial asymmetry. J Korean Dent Assoc 2004;42:219–231.
3. Letzer GM, Kronman JH. A posterioranterior cephalometric evaluation of craniofacial asymmetry. Angle Orthod 1967;37:205–211.
4. Graber TM. Orthodontics: Principles and Practice. Philadelphia: Saunders, 1969.
5. Fields HW Jr, Proffit WR, Sarver DM. Ortodonzia Moderna. Milan: Elsevier Masson, 2008.
6. Giannì E. La Nuova Ortognatodonzia. Milan: Piccin, 1986.
7. Arnett GW, Bergam RT. Facial keys to orthodontic diagnosis and treatment planning. Part I. Am J Orthod Dentofacial Orthop 1993;103:299–312.
8. Baumrind S, Frantz RC. The reliability of head film measurements. 1. Landmark identification. Am J Orthod 1971;60:111–127.
9. Johnson EL. The Frankfort-mandibular plane angle and the facial pattern. Am J Orthod 1950;36:516–533.
10. Nolte K, Muller B, Dibbet J. Comparison of linear measurements in cephalometric studies. J Orofac Orthop 2003;64:265–274.
11. McIntyre GT, Mossey PA. Size and shape measurement in contemporary cephalometrics. Eur J Orthod 2003;25:231–242.
12. Grummons DC, Kappeyne va de Coppello MA. A frontal asymmetry analysis. J Clinic Orthod 1987;21:448–465.
13. Bossi A, Cortinovis I, Marubini E. Introduzione alla Statistica Medica. Rome: NIS, 1991.
14. Gateno J, Xia J, Teichgraeber JF. Effect of facial asymmetry on 2-dimensional and 3-dimensional cephalometric measurements. J Oral Maxillofac Surg 2011;69:655–662.
15. Swennen GRJ, Schutyser F. Three-dimensional cephalometry: Spiral multi-slice vs cone-beam computed tomography. Am J Orthod Dentofacial Orthop 2006;130:410–416.
16. Wu MC, Cheng KS, Chen YT, Liu JK, Ting WH. Three-dimensional analysis of biplanar cephalograms. Euro J Orthod 2010;32:627–632.
17. Swennen GRJ, Schutyser FAC, Jausamen JE (eds). Three-Dimensional Cephalometry: A Color Atlas and Manual. New York: Springer, 2006.
18. Jacobson RL. Three-dimensional cephalometry. In: Jacobson A, Jacobson RL (eds). Radiographic Cephalometry: From Basics to 3-D Imaging, ed 2. Chicago: Quintessence, 2006:233–247.
19. Kumar V, Ludlow J, Mol A, Cevidanes L. Comparison of conventional and cone beam CT synthesized cephalograms. Dentomaillofac Radiol 2007;36:263–269.
20. Maj G. Manuale di Ortodonzia. Bologna: Pàtron, 1973.
21. Athanasiou AE. Orthodontic Cephalometry. London: Mosby-Wolfe, 1995.
22. de Oliveira AE, Cevidanes LH, Phillips C, Motta A, Burke B, Tyndall D. Observer reliability of three-dimensional cephalometric landmark identification on cone-beam computerized tomography. Oral Surg Oral Med Oral Pathol Oral Radiol Endod 2009;107:256–265.
23. Kusnoto B, Evans CA, BeGole EA, de Rijk W. Assessment of 3-dimensional computer-generated cephalometric measurements. Am J Orthod Dentofacial Orthop 1999;116:390–399.
24. Medelnik J, Hertrich K, Steinhäuser-Andresen S, Hirschfelder U, Hofmann E. Accuracy of anatomical landmark identification using different CBCT- and MSCT-based 3D images: An in vitro study. J Orofac Orthop 2011;72:261–278.
25. Farronato G, Garagiola U, Dominici A, et al. "Ten-point" 3D cephalometric analysis using low-dosage cone beam computed tomography. Prog Orthod 2010;11:2–12.
26. Farronato G, Perillo L, Bellincioni F, Briguglio F, Farronato D, Dominici AD. Direct 3D cephalometric analysis performed on CBCT. J Inform Tech Softw Eng 2012;2:107.
27. Trpkova B, Prasad NG, Lam EWN, Raboud D, Glover KE, Mjor PW. Assessment of facial asymmetries from posteroanterior cephalograms: Validity of reference lines. Am J Orthod Dentofacial Orthop 2003;123:512–520.

28. Damstra J, Oosterkamp BCM, Jansma J, Ren Y. Combined 3-dimensional and mirror-image analysis for the diagnosis of asymmetry. Am J Orthod Dentofacial Orthop 2010;140:886–894.
29. Nagasaka S, Fujimora T, Mitami T, Segoshi K. Development of a non-radiographic cephalometric system. Eur J Orthod 2003;25:77–85.
30. Gawilkowska A, Szczurwski J, Czerwinski F, Miklaszwenska D, Adamiec A, Dzieciolowska E. The fluctuating asymmetry of medieval and modern human skulls. Homo 2007;58:159–172.
31. Haraguchi S, Iguchi Y, Takada K. Asymmetry of the face in orthodontic patients. Angle Orthod 2008;78:421–426.
32. Klingenberg CP, Barluenga M, Meyer A. Shape analysis of symmetric structures: Quantifying variation among individuals and asymmetry. Evolution 2002;56:1909–1920.
33. Damstra J, Fourie Z, De Wit M, Ren J. A three-dimensional comparison of a morphometric and conventional cephalomeric midsagittal planes for craniofacial asymmetry. Clin Oral Investig 2012;16:285–294.
34. Xia J, Gateno J, Teichgraeber JF. New clinical protocol to evaluate craniomaxillofacial deformity and plan surgical correction. J Oral Maxillofac Surg 2009;67:2093–2106.
35. Lascala CA, Panella J, Marques MM. Analysis of the acuracy of linear measurements obtained by cone beam computed tomography (CBCT-NewTom). Dentomaxillofac Radiol 2004;33:291–294.
36. Hilgers ML, Scarfe WC, Scheetz JP, Farman AG. Accuracy of linear temporomandibular joint measurements with cone-beam computed tomography and digital cephalometric radiography. Am J Ortho Dentofacial Orthop 2005;128:803–811.
37. Periago DR, Scarge WC, Moshiri M, Scheetz JP, Silveira AM, Farman AG. Linear accuracy and reliability of cone beam CT derived 3-dimensional images constructed using an orthodontic volumetric rendering program. Angle Orthod 2008;78:387–395.
38. Baumgaertel S, Palomo JM, Palomo L, Hans MG. Reliability and accuracy of cone-beam computed tomography dental measurements. Am J Orthod Dentofacial Orthop 2009;136:19–25.
39. Grauer D, Cevidanes LSH, Proffit WR. Working with DICOM craniofacial images. Am J Orthod Dentofacial Orthop 2009;136:460–470.
40. Berco M, Rigali PH, Miner R Jr, DeLuca S, Anderson N, Will LA. Accuracy and reliability of linear cephalometric measurements from cone-beam computed tomography scans of a dry human skull. Am J Orthod Dentofacial Othop 2009;136:17–18.
41. Hassan B, Van der Stelt P, Sanderink G. Accuracy of three-dimensional measurements obtained from cone beam computed tomography surface-rendered images for cephalometric analysis: Influence of patient scanning position. Eur J Orthod 2009;31:129–134.
42. Damstra J, Fourie Z, Huddleston Slater JJ, Ren Y. Accuracy of linear measurements from cone-beam computed tomography-derived surface models of different voxel sizes. Am J Orthod Dentofacial Orthop 2010;137:16.e1–16.e6.
43. Ballrick JW, Paomo JM, Ruch E, Amberman BD, Hans MG. Image distortion and spatial resolution of a commercially available conebeam computed tomography machine. Am J Orthod Dentofacial Orthop 2008;134:573-82.
44. Liedke GS, da Silveira HE, da Silveira HL, Dutra V, de Figueiredo JA. Influence of voxel size in the diagnostic ability of cone beam tomography to evaluate simulated external root resorption. J Endod 2009;35:233–235.
45. Gribel BF, Gribel MN, Frazäo DC, McNamara JA Jr, Manzi FR. Accuracy and reliability of craniometric measurements on lateral cephalometry and 3D measurements on CBCT scans. Angle Orthod 2011;81:26–35.
46. Philippe J. Plans de tratement en ortho pédie dento-faciale. Paris: Prélat, 1979.
47. Benauwt A, Klingler E. Ortopedia Dento-Facciale. Milan: Masson, 1978.

48. Downs WB. Variations in facial relationships; their significance in treatment and prognosis. Am J Orthod 1948;34;812–840.
49. Capecchi V, Messeri P. Antropologia. Rome: Società Editrice Universo, 1979.
50. Nolte K, Muller B, Dibbet J. Comparison of linear measurements in cephalometric studies. J Orofac Orthop 2003;64:265–274.
51. Wylie WL. Cephalometric roentgenography and the dentist. Am J Orthod Oral Surg 1945;31:341–360.
52. Enlow DH, Moyers RE, Hunter WS, McNamara JA. A procedure for the analysis of intrinsic facial form and growth. Am J Orthod 1969;56:6–14.

G Perrotti
J Nowakowska

5

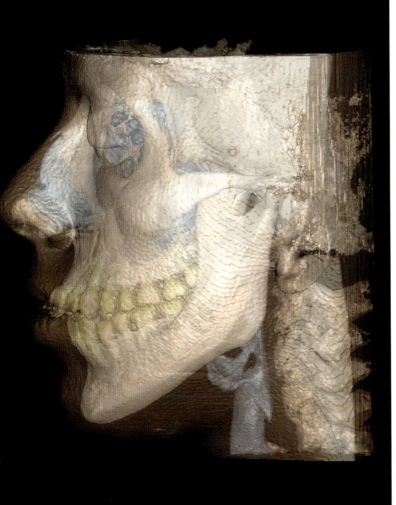

Cephalometry is the sextant of dentists, a tool to measure, classify, diagnose, plan, and, especially, to learn about and detect the details of craniofacial structures.
Orthodontists recognize the anatomy of the maxilla and the mandible through landmarks, as if they were light signals along a pathway defining how an individual is structured and will evolve during growth.
The shift from two-dimensional (2D) to three-dimensional (3D) cephalometry has made these landmarks even more accurate and detailed for the clinician. 3D techniques go deep into structures and combine images to create new forms of analysis like a grid in the third dimension.
This atlas shows the details of landmarks in the three planes of space, outlining their location in terms of both skeletal components and soft tissues.

Atlas of Cephalometric Landmarks

Introduction to Cephalometry

Cephalometry (from Greek; literally, "measure of the head") is the study of the various forms of facial profiles and bone structures making up the skull. It is performed through a radiographic examination based on the location of specific anatomical landmarks relative to structures that are considered to be fundamental.

In the past, skull radiographs in different views (lateral, frontal, and axial) were commonly used to assess the skull (or any three-dimensional body) through 2D radiographic pictures. Linear and angular measures were then compared with reference values from different schools of thought (eg, Seiner, Jarabak, Sassouni, or Ganni analysis). Unfortunately, the interpretation of some radiographic records was in doubt because of technical errors or unique anatomical configurations of patients. Needless to say, it is absolutely necessary to define anatomical structures with the greatest care so as to be able to use the analysis as a diagnostic tool. Errors in positioning the landmarks in 2D radiographs can cause significant mistakes in interpretation and clinical diagnosis. In the orthodontic literature, the most frequent cause of failure in cephalometric assessment is an error in identifying the landmarks.[1]

Recently, with the development of cone beam computed tomography (CBCT), it has become possible to obtain sagittal, axial, and coronal images passing through the landmarks both in hard skeletal tissues and in soft tissues and to identify these landmarks very accurately. Richtsmeier et al[2] have reported that the mean error in placing landmarks in 3D on CT images is always less than 0.5 mm. Nevertheless, some reference points are more difficult to reproduce than others. Olszewski et al[3] have classified reference points into four groups, from Group 1 (very high reproducibility) to Group 4 (low reproducibility). With reference to their conclusions, the critical points in soft tissues would be the soft tissue gonion (classified as Group 3) and the soft tissue zygion and pogonion (Group 4). Similarly, Williams and Richtsmeier,[4] after examining the mandible, confirmed the lower reliability of nonbiologic reference points. According to these authors, "biologic" reference points that are located on the basis of anatomy are more reliable. Conversely, reference points that are constructed or vague—ie, where the definition of the reference point includes more than a single point—are less reproducible.

Definition of Landmarks in Hard and Soft Tissues

As outlined above, an accurate definition of landmarks is crucial for correct detection. In orthodontics, after its introduction in the 1930s by Broadbent, 2D cephalometry has played a fundamental role in accurate investigation and standardization of malocclusions and skeletal dysgnathia.

Table 5-1 Landmarks: Hard tissues[5]

Figure	Abbreviation	Landmark	Definition
5-3	N	Nasion	Midpoint of the frontonasal suture
5-4	Zy	Zygion	Point of transition of the zygomaticotemporal suture
5-5	Po	Porion	Highest point on the superior edge of the bony external auditory canal
5-6	Gn	Gnathion	Obtained by construction: most posterior inferior point on angle of mandible; located at the bisector of the angle formed by two straight lines, one along the posterior of the ramus and one along the inferior edge of the mandibular body
5-7	Or	Orbitale	The lowest point in the infraorbital profile
5-8	ANS	Anterior nasal spine	The most anterior point of the maxillary profile at the level of the median palatal suture, frontal view; verify the midposition
5-9	S	Sella	Arithmetically central point of the sella turcica
5-10	Go	Gonion	Obtained by construction: the meeting point of the posteroinferior edge of the mandibular angle with the bisector of the angle formed by two straight lines, one tangent to the posterior edge of the ascending mandibular ramus, and the other tangent to the inferior edge of the mandibular body
5-11	Me	Menton	The most inferior point of the mandibular symphysis
5-12	A	Point A (subspinale)	The most posterior midpoint in the concavity of the maxilla between the ANS and the alveolar process
5-13	Pog	Pogonion	The most anterior point of the mandibular symphysis
5-14	J	Jugale	Point of the solid apex on the posterior edge of the zygomatic process in the zygomatic bone; the intersection of the outline of the maxillary tuberosity and zygomatic buttress
5-15	UI 11	Upper incisor 11	Midpoint of the incisal edge of tooth 11 (maxillary right central incisor)
5-16	UI 21	Upper incisor 21	Midpoint of the incisal edge of tooth 21 (maxillary left central incisor)
5-17	Mol	Molar point	Midpoint in vertical direction in the interocclusal relationship of the permanent first molars
5-18	Chin	Chin	The most lateral point of the mandibular symphysis
5-19	UIM	Upper incisal midpoint	Interincisal midpoint between UI 11 and UI 21
5-20	Co	Condylion	Most superior and central condylar point

In the first cephalometric analyses, the landmarks were defined for skeletal tissues. Burstone,[6,7] Downs,[8] Subtelny,[9] and Holdaway[10] incorporated soft tissue parameters in cephalometric analyses, adding landmarks for skin tissues. The anthropometric assessment of the skull and of the other body regions was first introduced thanks to Farkas' research.[11] The anthropologist was the first to define landmarks for the skull and gathered an enormous database of "norms" for craniofacial measures.

With the development of 3D radiography, conventionally used definitions of landmarks had to be reviewed and redefined on the three planes of space. Swennen's cephalometry atlas[12] has served as a guide to detect the exact the position of the landmarks used in the present analysis (see chapter 6, 3D Analysis of Soft Tissues). Landmarks in hard and soft tissues (Table 5-1 and 5-2) are presented in axial, sagittal, and coronal sections and on 3D renderings in the following sections.

Table 5-2 Landmarks: Soft tissues[5,13]

Figure	Abbreviation	Landmark	Definition
5-21	G'	Soft tissue glabella	Most anterior midpoint of the prominence above frontonasal suture between the eyebrows
5-22	N'	Soft tissue nasion	Cutaneous midpoint at the level of the frontonasal suture
5-23	Se'	Selion	Most posterior cutaneous midpoint at the root of the nose (nasofrontal concavity)
5-24	En'	Endocanthion	Cutaneous point located at the internal commissure of the palpebral fissure
5-25	Ex'	Exocanthion	Cutaneous point located at the external commissure of the palpebral fissure
5-26	Or'	Soft tissue orbitale	Cutaneous point underlying the right and left orbital fossae
5-27	Os'	Orbitale superius	Cutaneous point above the orbital fossa; viewed in 3D rendering, point above the right and left eyebrows
5-28	Zy'	Soft tissue zygion	Most lateral cutaneous point on the left and right zygomatic arches at the level of the zygion
5-29	Pn	Pronasale	Most anterior cutaneous midpoint of the nose tip
5-30	Sn	Subnasale	Midpoint where the columella and the upper lip meet
5-31	Sls	Subspinale (superior labial sulcus)	Most hollow midpoint of the superior labial philtrum
5-32	Ls	Labiale superius	Most anteriorly projecting midpoint of the superior labial vermilion
5-33	Li	Labiale inferius	Most anteriorly projecting midpoint of the inferior labial vermilion
5-34	Ils	Sublabiale (inferior labial sulcus)	Most hollow point of the labiomental sulcus
5-35	Pog'	Soft tissue pogonion	Most anteriorly projecting midpoint of the mandibular symphysis
5-36	Me'	Soft tissue menton	Soft tissue point corresponding to the menton
5-37	Go'	Soft tissue gonion	Most lateral cutaneous point of the right/left gonial angle at the level of the gonion
5-38	Ala	Alare	Most lateral point of each nostril
5-39	C	Columella	Constructed midpoint located at the center of the columella where the nostrils meet
5-40	Ch	Cheilion	Right and left labial commissure points
5-41	Sto	Stomion	Cutaneous midpoint of the labial fissure
5-42	Chin'	Soft tissue chin	Most lateral chin point at the level of the osseous chin

The aim of this chapter is to explain the correct interpretation of anatomical structures seen in sagittal, coronal, and axial views and the accurate location of the landmarks that are necessary to process 3D cephalometry (Fig 5-1).

Definition of the External Reference System

The external reference system (Table 5-3) is defined by:

- The sagittal plane of reference
- The axial plane of reference
- The coronal plane of reference

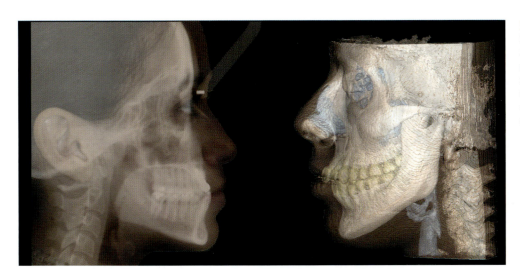

Fig 5-1 The transformation from diagnosis using 2D records (photographs and lateral cephalometric radiographs) to 3D images that include all tissues of the patient (skeletal, soft tissues, airways).

Table 5-3 Planes of reference[12]

Abbreviation	Plane of reference	Definition
Sag	External sagittal (x)	Plane defined between the SAG1, SAG2, and SAG3 points inserted manually into the sagittal window; first "0" image obtained from CT data.
Ax	External axial (z)	Plane defined between the AX1, AX2, and AX3 points manually into the sagittal window; first "0" image obtained from CT data.
Cor	External coronal (y)	Plane defined between the COR1, COR2, and COR3 points inserted manually into the sagittal window; first "0" image obtained from CT data

Figs 5-2a and 5-2b Volumetric reconstruction of the face using axial, coronal, and sagittal reference planes. The midsagittal construction plane, the maxillary plane, the mental plane, and the superior facial plane are also highlighted.

The use of an external 3D reference system (Fig 5-2a) is simple and avoids errors due to distortion in the presence of craniofacial asymmetries. It is nevertheless very important that the skull is placed in natural head position during the exam.[11]

Definition of Construction Planes

Construction planes are planes used in 3D cephalometric analysis (Fig 5-2b and Table 5-4). They can pass through:

- Two cutaneous points and one reference plane (axial, sagittal, or coronal)
- One cutaneous point and two reference planes (axial, sagittal, or coronal)

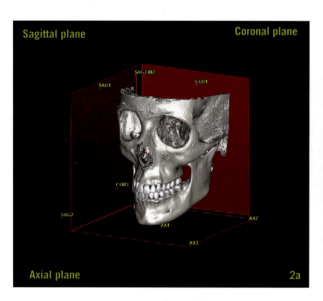

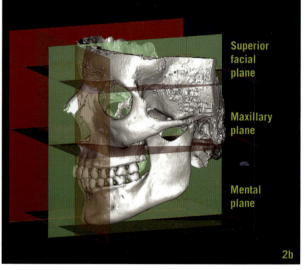

Table 5-4 Construction planes		
Abbreviation	Construction plane	Definition
SFP	Superior facial plane	Plane passing through nasion (N) perpendicular to the coronal (y) and sagittal (x) planes
ANSPl	Maxillary plane	Plane passing through the anterior nasal spine (ANS) parallel to the axial plane (z)
MePl	Mental plane	Plane passing through menton parallel to the subnasal plane

Atlas of Skeletal Landmarks

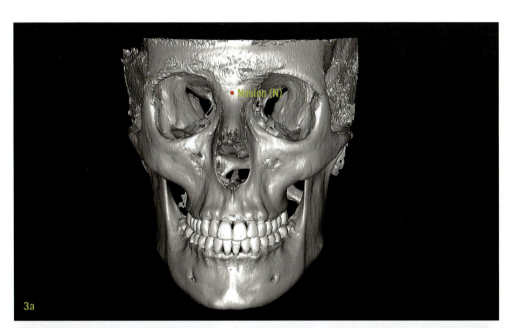

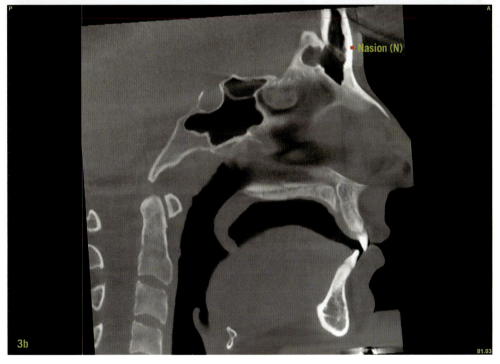

Figs 5-3a and 5-3b NASION (N): point of intersection between the frontal and the nasal bones (a) 3D view. (b) Sagittal view.

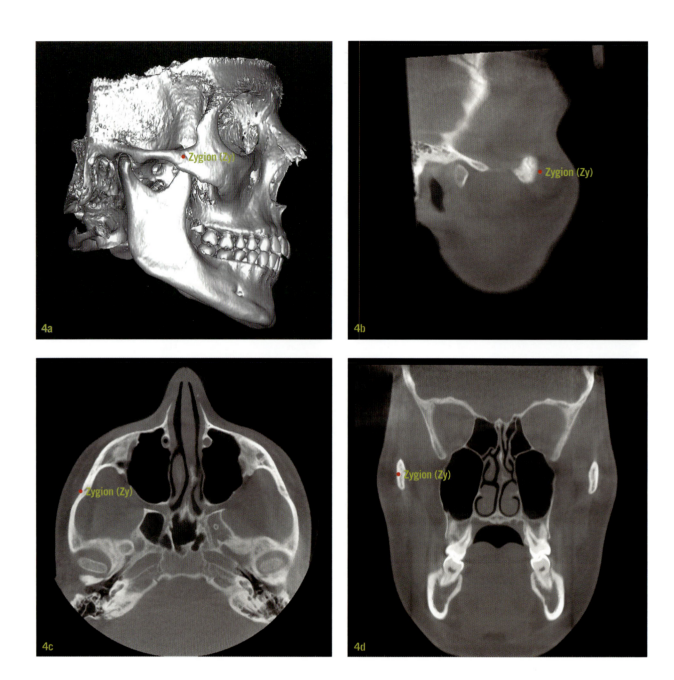

Figs 5-4a to 5-4d ZYGION (Zy): point of transition of the zygomaticotemporal suture corresponding to the maximum lateral prominence of the zygomatic arch. *(a)* 3D view. *(b)* Sagittal view. *(c)* Axial view. *(d)* Coronal view.

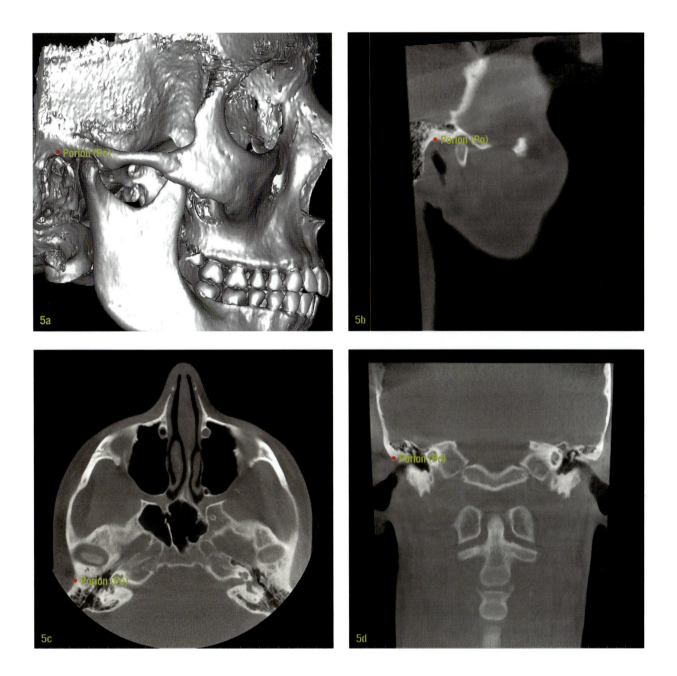

Figs 5-5a to 5-5d PORION (Po): highest point on the superior edge of the bony external auditory canal. *(a)* 3D view. *(b)* Sagittal view. *(c)* Axial view. *(d)* Coronal view.

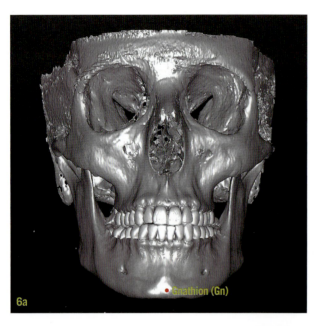
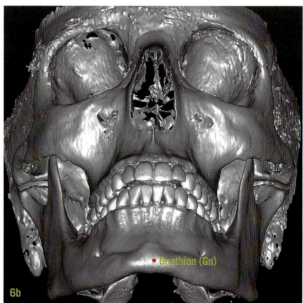
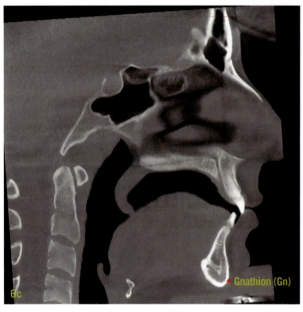

Figs 5-6a to 5-6c GNATHION (Gn): point at the intersection of the anterior edge of the mandibular symphysis and the bisector of the angle formed by two straight lines, one passing through N-Pog and one passing through Me, tangent to the inferior edge of the mandibular body. *(a and b)* 3D view. *(c)* Sagittal view.

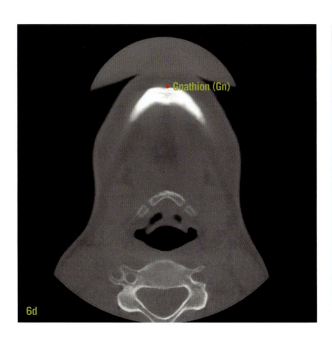 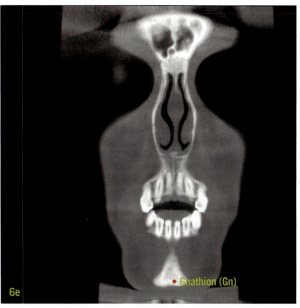

Figs 5-6d and 5-6e GNATHION (Gn). *(d)* Axial view. *(e)* Coronal view.

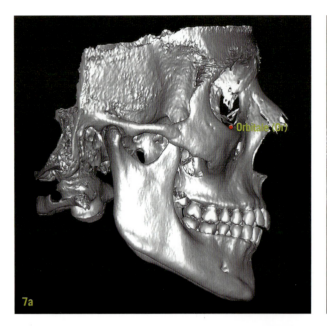
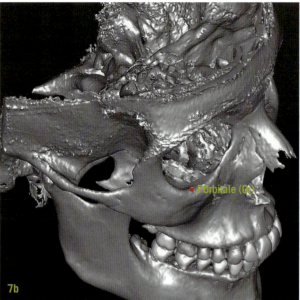
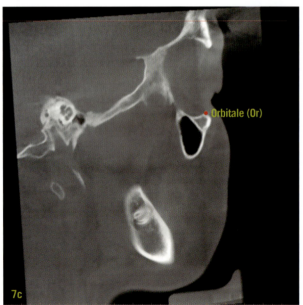

Figs 5-7a to 5-7c ORBITALE (Or): the lowest point of the infraorbital profile. *(a and b)* 3D view. *(c)* Sagittal view.

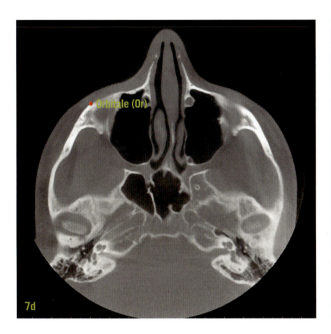
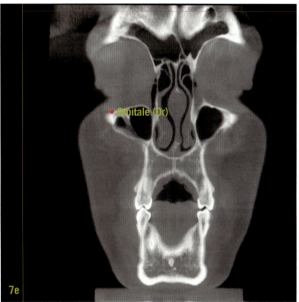

Figs 5-7d and 5-7e ORBITALE (Or). *(d)* Axial view. *(e)* Coronal view.

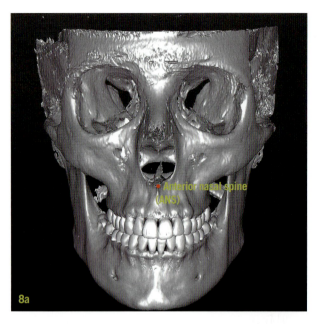
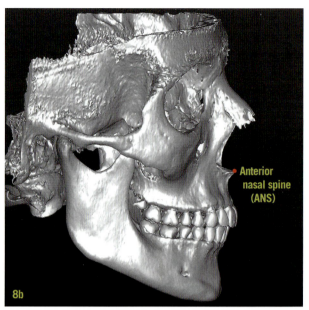
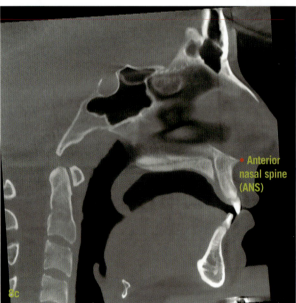

Figs 5-8a to 5-8c ANTERIOR NASAL SPINE (ANS): most anterior point of the maxillary profile at the level of the median palatal suture. *(a and b)* 3D view. *(c)* Sagittal view.

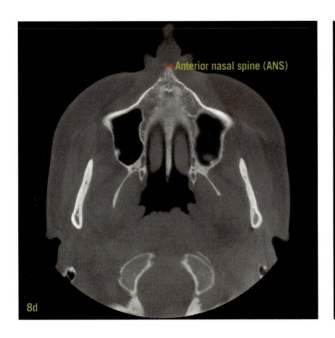 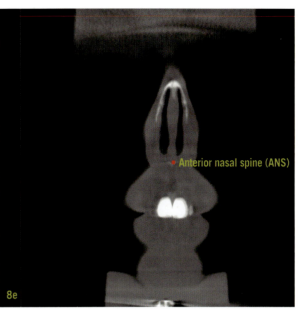

Figs 5-8d and 5-8e ANTERIOR NASAL SPINE (ANS). *(d)* Axial view. *(e)* Coronal view.

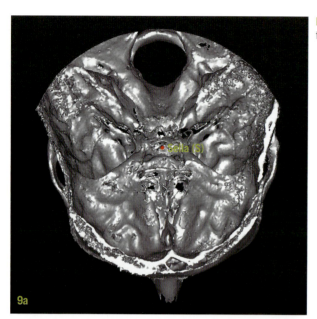

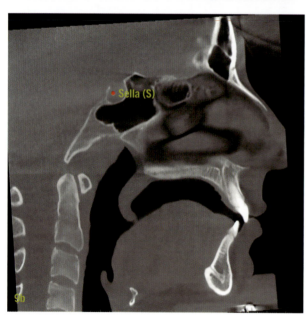

Figs 5-9a and 5-9b SELLA (S): arithmetically central point of sella turcica. *(a)* 3D view. *(b)* Sagittal view.

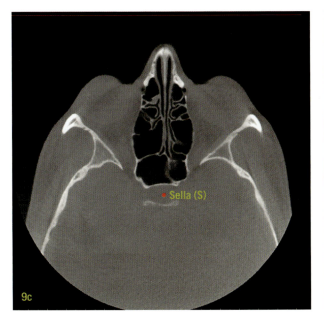
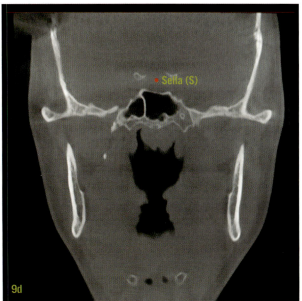

Figs 5-9c and 5-9d SELLA (S). *(c)* Axial view. *(d)* Coronal view.

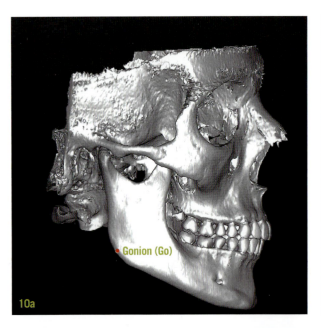
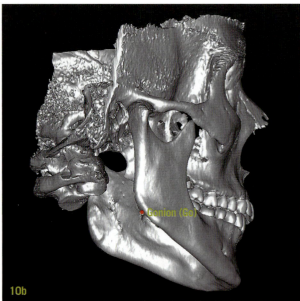
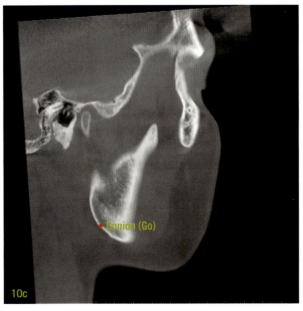

Figs 5-10a to 5-10c GONION (Go): most posterior inferior point on angle of mandible; located at the bisector of the angle formed by two straight lines, one along the posterior of the ramus and one along the inferior edge of the mandibular body. *(a and b)* 3D view. *(c)* Sagittal view.

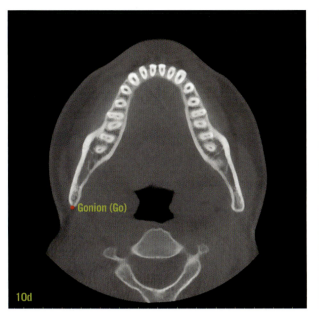
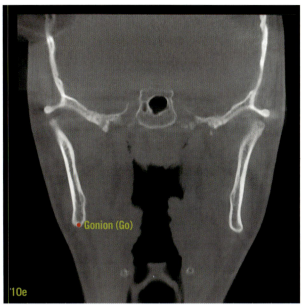

Figs 5-10d and 5-10e GONION (Go). *(d)* Axial view. *(e)* Coronal view.

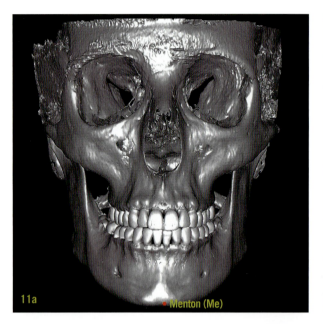
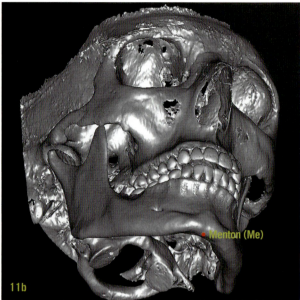
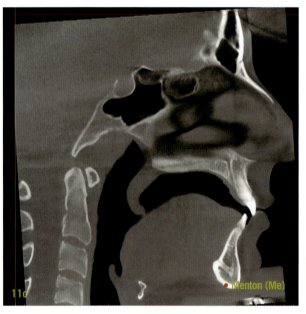

Figs 5-11a to 5-11c MENTON (Me): most recessed point, on the horizontal plane, of the inferior edge of the mandible at the level of the symphysis. It is the most inferior point of the chin at the level of the midline. *(a and b)* 3D views. *(c)* Sagittal view.

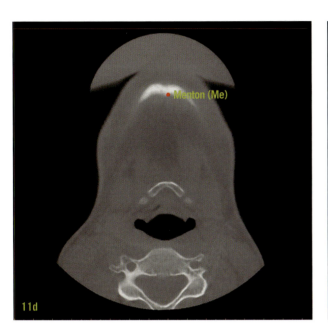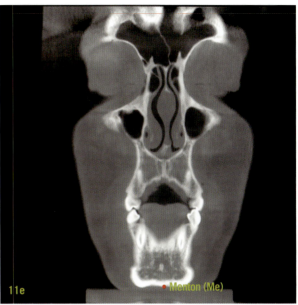

Figs 5-11d and 5-11e MENTON (Me). *(d)* Axial view. *(e)* Coronal view.

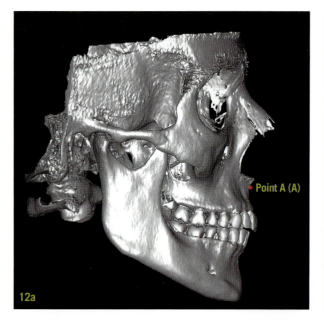
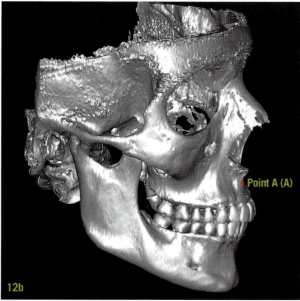
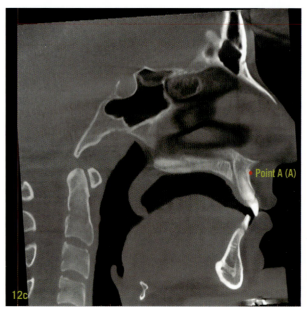

Figs 5-12a to 5-12c POINT A (A): most posterior point on the midline of the maxilla between ANS and the alveolar process. *(a and b)* 3D view. *(c)* Sagittal view.

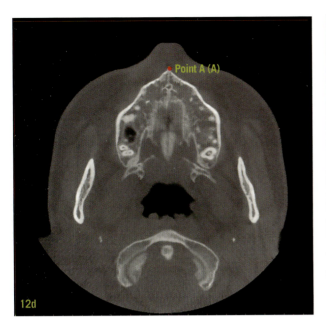
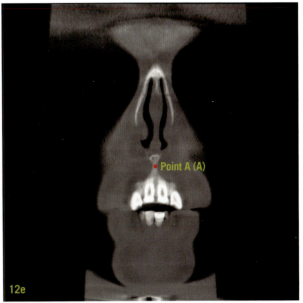

Figs 5-12d and 5-12e POINT A (A). *(d)* Axial view. *(e)* Coronal view.

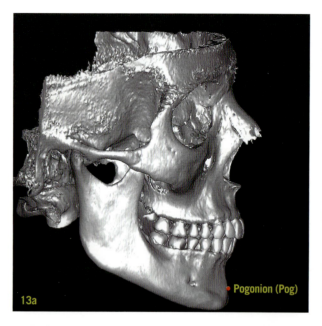
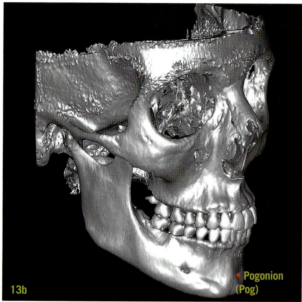
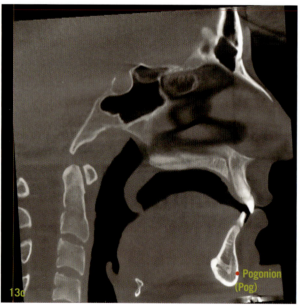

Figs 5-13a to 5-13c POGONION (Pog): most anteriorly projecting point of the mandibular symphysis. *(a and b)* 3D views. *(c)* Sagittal view.

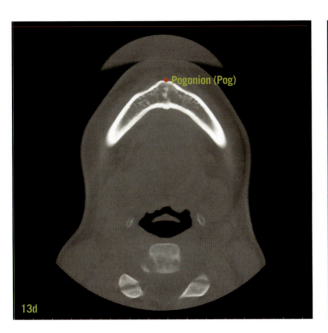 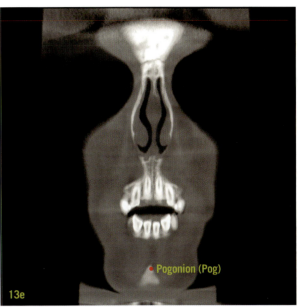

Figs 5-13d and 5-13e POGONION (Pog). *(d)* Axial view. *(e)* Coronal view.

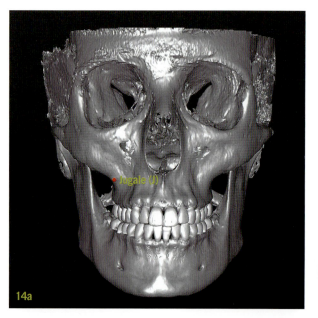
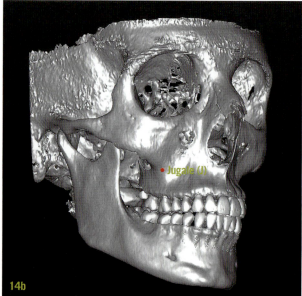
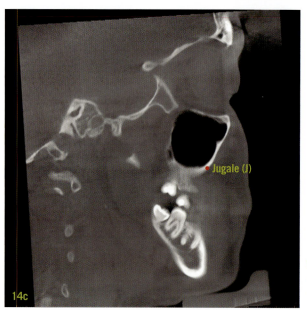

Figs 5-14a to 5-14c JUGALE (J): point of the solid apex on the posterior edge of the zygomatic process in the zygomatic bone; the intersection of the outline of the maxillary tuberosity and zygomatic buttress. *(a and b)* 3D view. *(c)* Sagittal view.

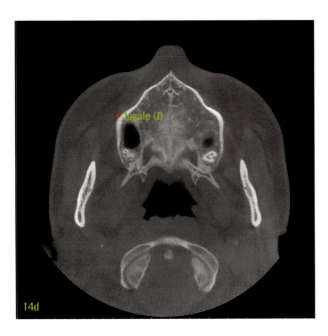
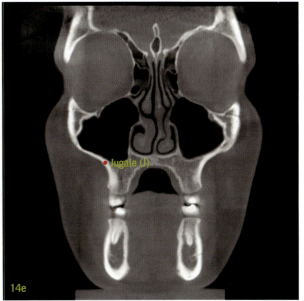

Figs 5-14d and 5-14e JUGALE (J). *(d)* Axial view. *(e)* Coronal view.

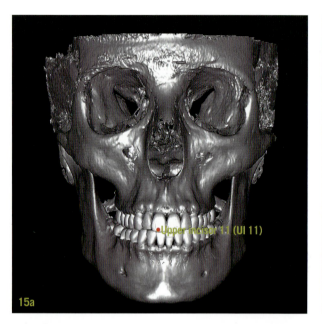
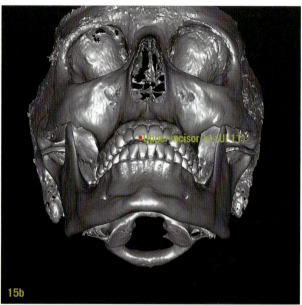
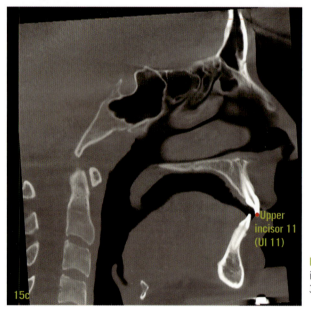

Figs 5-15a to 5-15c UPPER INCISOR 11 (UI 11): midpoint of the incisal edge of tooth 11 (maxillary right central incisor). *(a and b)* 3D view. *(c)* Sagittal view.

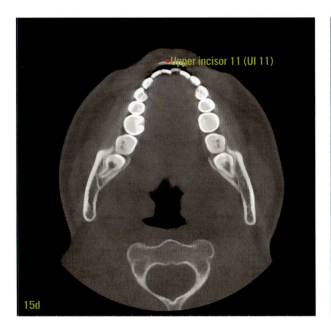
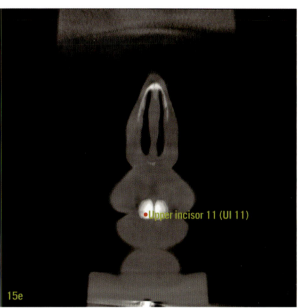

Figs 5-15d and 5-15 e UPPER INCISOR 11 (UI 11). *(d)* Axial view. *(e)* Coronal view.

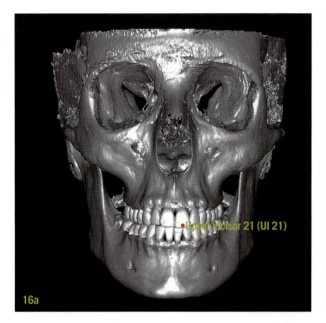
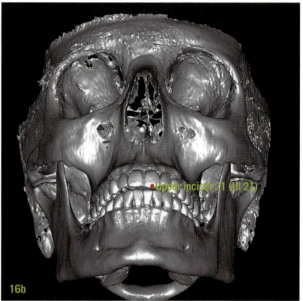
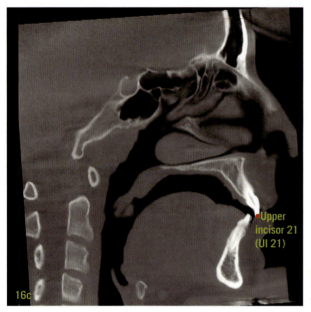

Figs 5-16a to 5-16c UPPER INCISOR 21 (UI 21): midpoint of the incisal edge of tooth 21 (maxillary left central incisor). *(a and b)* 3D view. *(c)* Sagittal view.

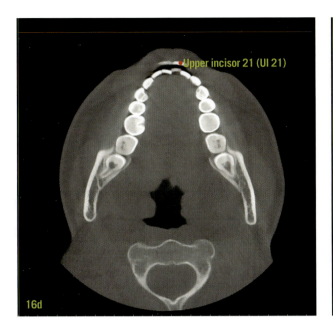
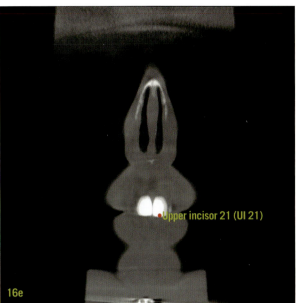

Figs 5-16d and 5-15e UPPER INCISOR 21 (UI 21): view of the landmark on the axial plane. *(d)* Axial view. *(e)* Coronal view.

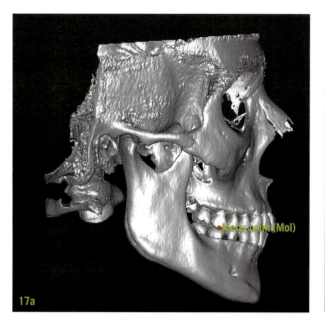
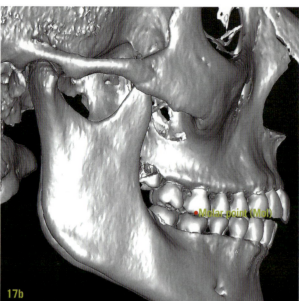
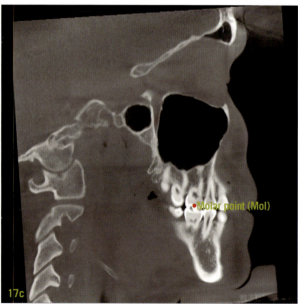

Figs 5-17a to 5-17c MOLAR POINT (Mol): midpoint in vertical direction of the interocclusal relationship between the permanent first molars. *(a and b)* 3D view. *(c)* Sagittal view.

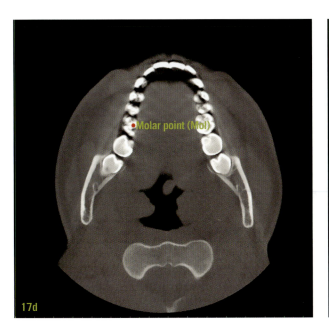 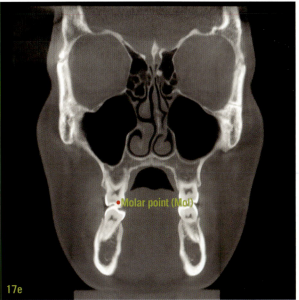

Figs 5-17d and 5-16e MOLAR POINT (Mol): view of the landmark on the sagittal plane. *(d)* Axial view. *(e)* Coronal view.

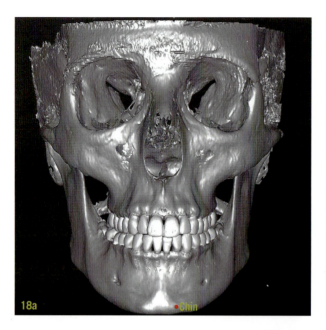
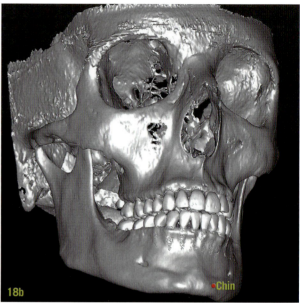
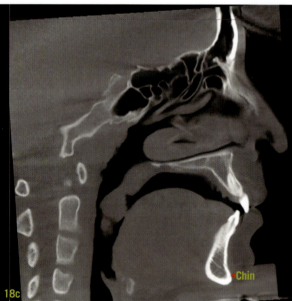

Figs 5-18a to 5-18c CHIN: most lateral point of the mandibular symphysis. *(a and b)* 3D view. *(c)* Sagittal view.

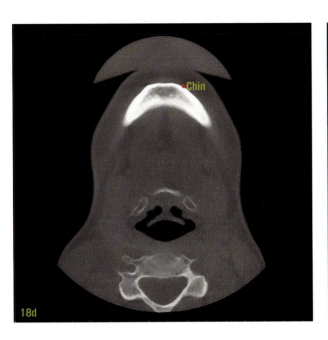
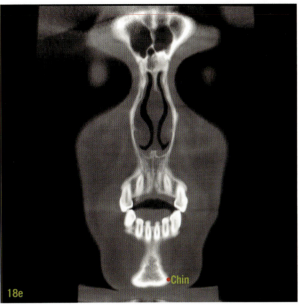

Figs 5-18d and 5-18e CHIN: *(d)* Axial view. *(e)* Coronal view.

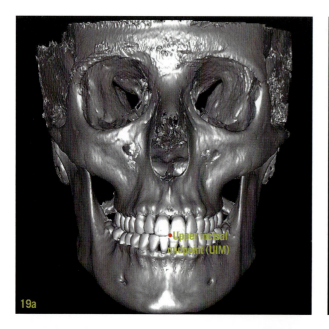
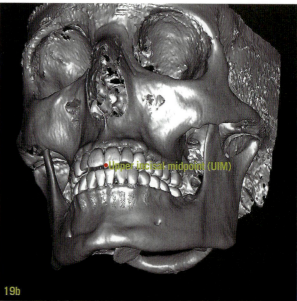
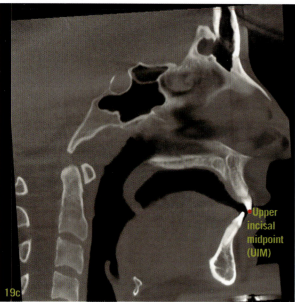

Figs 5-19a to 5-19c UPPER INCISAL MIDPOINT (UIM): interincisal midpoint between UI 11 and UI 21. *(a and b)* 3D view. *(c)* Sagittal view.

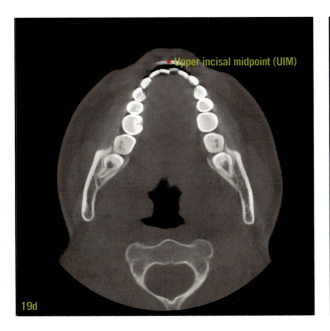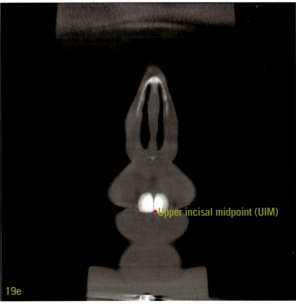

Figs 5-19d and 5-19e UPPER INCISAL MIDPOINT (UIM). *(d)* Axial view. *(e)* Coronal view.

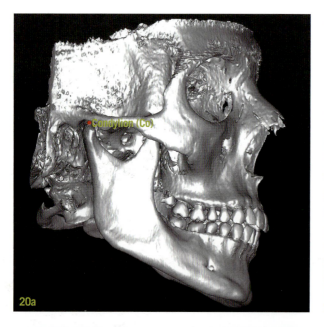
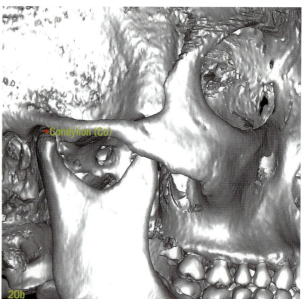
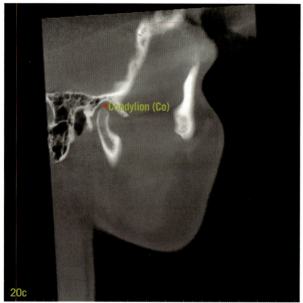

Figs 5-20a to 5-20c CONDYLION (Co): most superior and posterior point of the mandibular condyle. *(a and b)* 3D view. *(c)* Sagittal view.

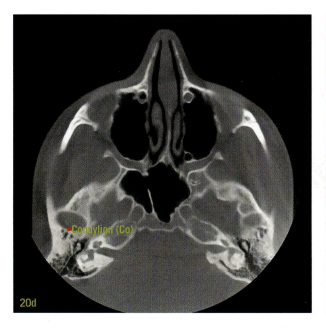
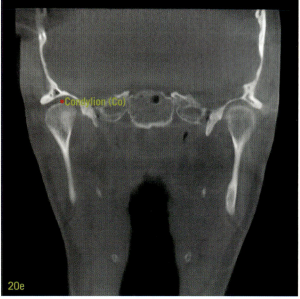

Figs 5-20d and 5-20e CONDYLION (Co). *(d)* Axial view. *(e)* Coronal view.

Atlas of Soft Tissue Landmarks

Sensitivity to perception of the anthropometric proportions of a face is limited in artists, cultivated by scholars, and the object of in-depth analysis for all those who, day by day, must contend with esthetic, maxillofacial, and orthodontic treatments. The need to measure drives the need for a system that can provide data to classify facial proportions. A 3D view of the human face through 3D rendering of facial soft tissues based on Digital Imaging and Communications in Medicine (DICOM) files of cranial scans is an ideal way to visualize facial proportions.

All anthropometric systems adopted to perform measurements require the identification of specific points at the skin level that must be recognized and codified adequately.

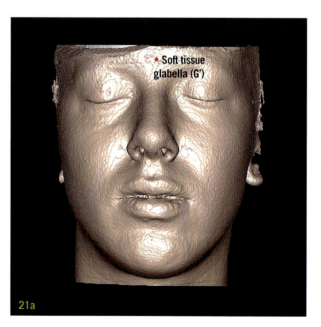
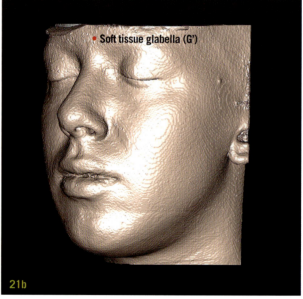

Figs 5-21a and 5-21b SOFT TISSUE GLABELLA (G'): the most anterior midpoint of the prominence above the frontonasal suture between the eyebrow arches; *(a)* 3D frontal view; *(b)* 3D ¾ view.

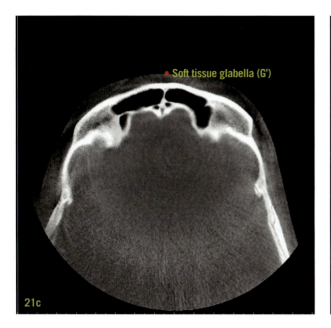

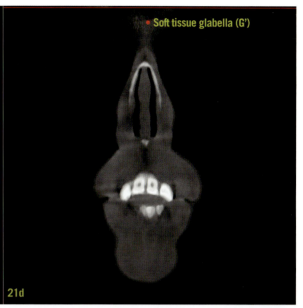

An atlas of landmarks of soft tissues in 3D images requires control of the selected point, not only in terms of volumetric rendering but also on the axial, coronal, and sagittal planes, which can be viewed by processing DICOM files.

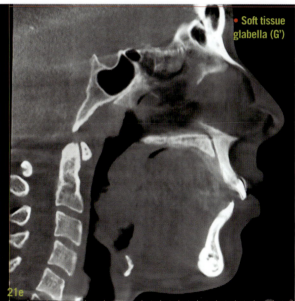

Figs 5-21c to 5-21e SOFT TISSUE GLABELLA (G'): *(c)* axial CBCT section; *(d)* frontal CBCT section; *(e)* sagittal CBCT section.

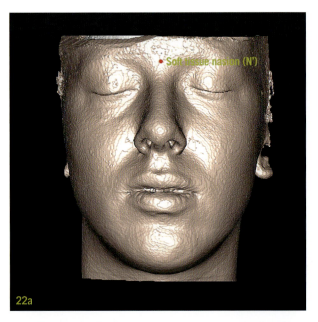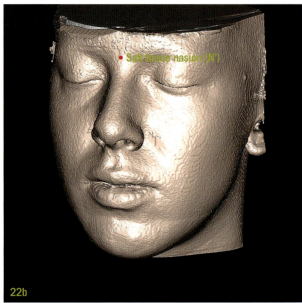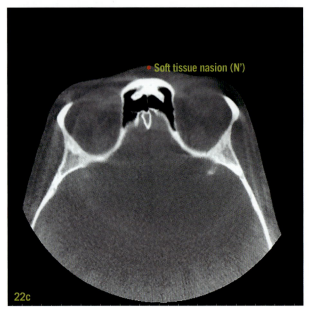

Figs 5-22a to 5-22c SOFT TISSUE NASION (N'): cutaneous midpoint at the level of the frontonasal suture; *(a)* 3D frontal view; *(b)* 3D ¾ view; *(c)* axial CBCT section.

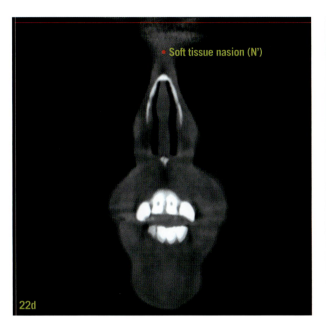
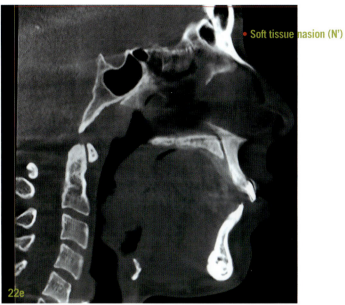

Figs 5-22d to 5-22e SOFT TISSUE NASION (N'); *(d)* CBCT frontal section; *(e)* CBCT sagittal section.

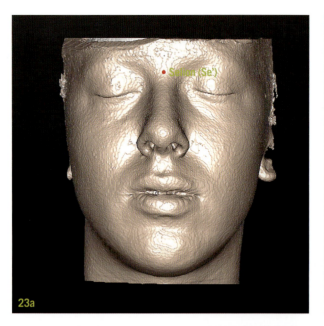
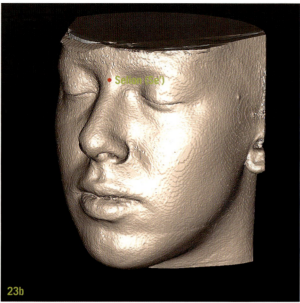
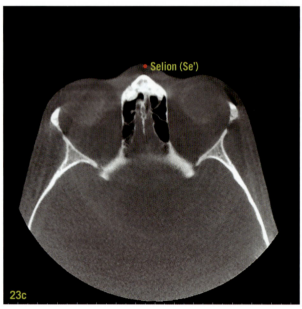

Figs 5-23a to 5-23c SELION (Se'): posterior cutaneous midpoint at the root of the nose (nasofrontal concavity); *(a)* 3D frontal view; *(b)* 3D ¾ view; *(c)* CBCT axial section.

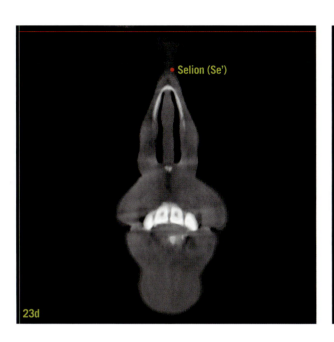
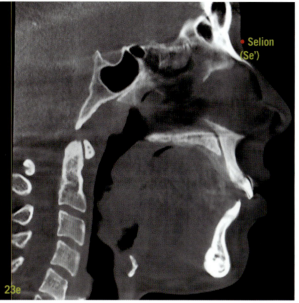

Figs 5-23d and 5-23e SELION (Se'); *(d)* CBCT frontal view; *(e)* CBCT sagittal section.

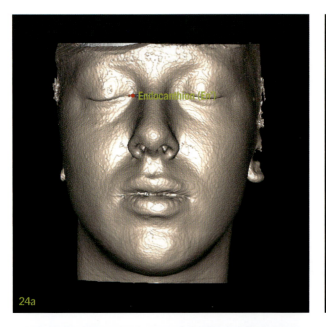
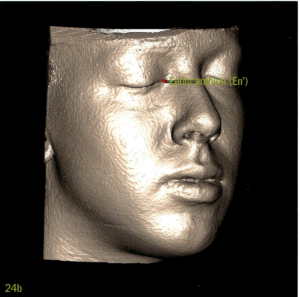
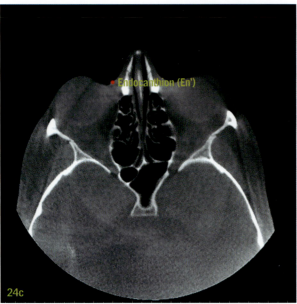

Figs 5-24a to 5-24c ENDOCANTHION (En'): cutaneous point located at the internal commissure of the palpebral fissure; *(a)* 3D frontal view; *(b)* 3D ¾ view; *(c)* axial CBCT view.

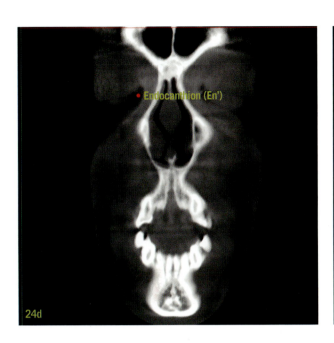 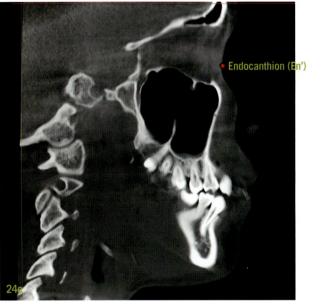

Figs 5-24d and 5-24e ENDOCANTHION (En'); *(d)* CBCT frontal section; *(e)* CBCT sagittal section.

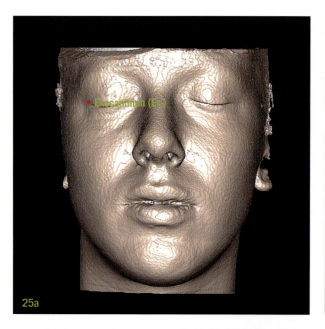
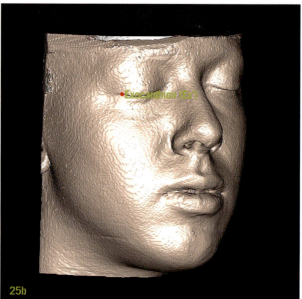
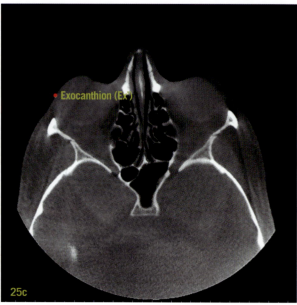

Figs 5-25a to 5-25c EXOCANTHION (Ex'): cutaneous point located at the external commissure of the palpebral fissure; *(a)* 3D frontal view; *(b)* 3D ¾ view; *(c)* axial CBCT section.

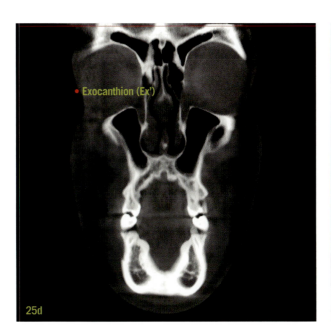
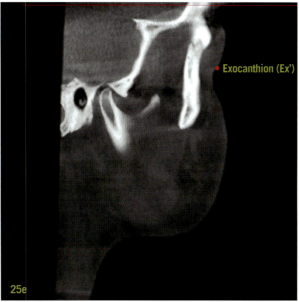

Figs 5-25d and 5-25e EXOCANTHION (Ex'); *(d)* CBCT frontal section: *(e)* CBCT sagittal view.

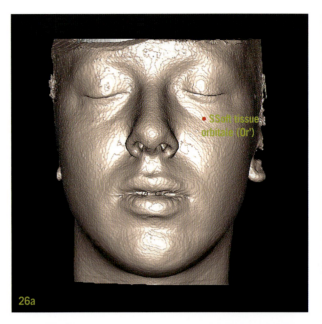

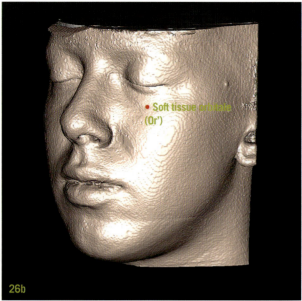

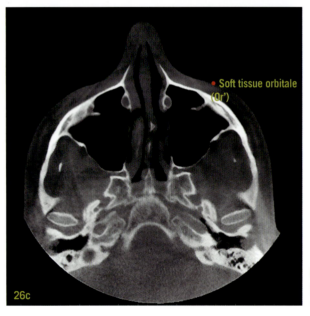

Figs 5-26a to 5-26c SOFT TISSUE ORBITALE (Or'): cutaneous point underlying the right and left orbital fossae; *(a)* 3D frontal view; *(b)* 3D ¾ view; *(c)* CBCT axial view.

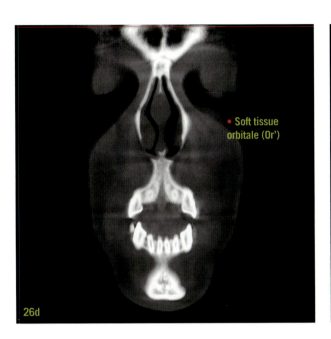
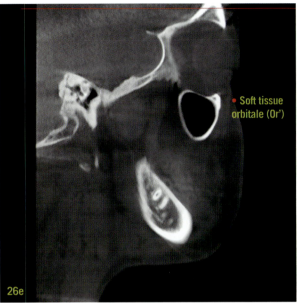

Figs 5-26d and 5-26e SOFT TISSUE ORBITALE (Or'); *(d)* CBCT frontal view; *(e)* CBCT sagittal view.

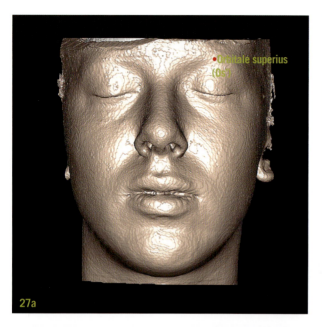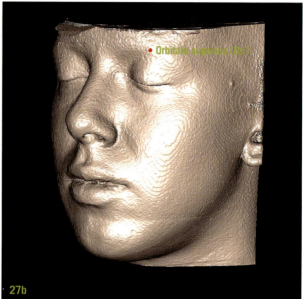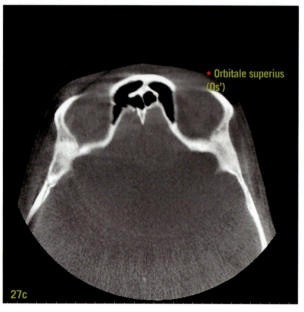

Figs 5-27a to 5-27c ORBITALE SUPERIUS (Os'): cutaneous point above the orbital fossa above the right and left eyebrows; *(a)* 3D frontal view; *(b)* 3D ¾ view; *(c)* CBCT axial view.

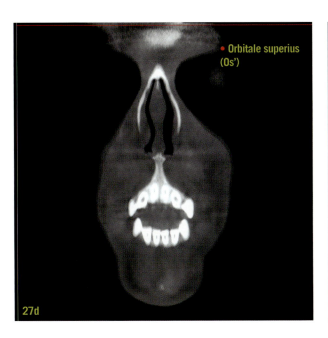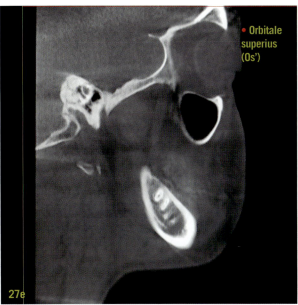

Figs 5-27d and 5-27e ORBITALE SUPERIUS (Os'); *(d)* CBCT frontal section; *(e)* CBCT sagittal section.

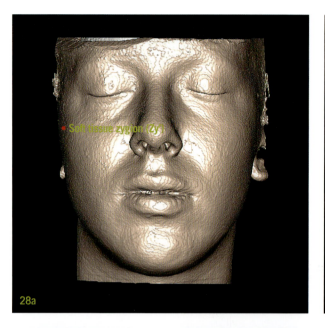
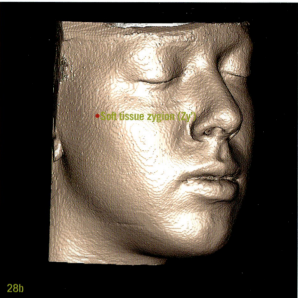
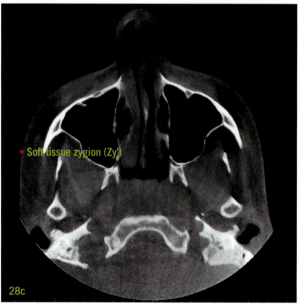

Figs 5-28a to 5-28c SOFT TISSUE ZYGION (Zy'): most lateral cutaneous point on the right/left zygomatic arch at level of the bony zygion; *(a)* 3D frontal view; *(b)* 3D ¾ view; *(c)* CBCT axial section.

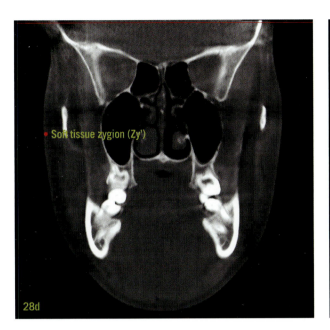 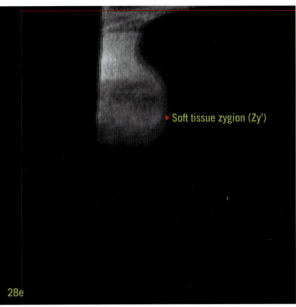

Figs 5-28d and 5-28e SOFT TISSUE ZYGION (Zy'); (d) CBCT frontal view; (e) CBCT sagittal section.

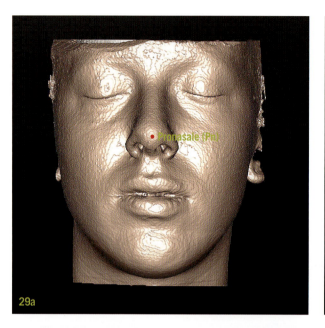
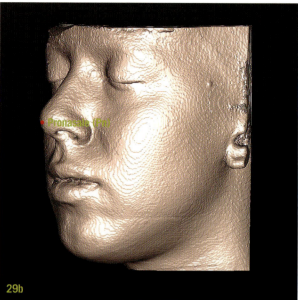
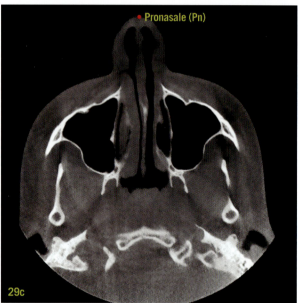

Figs 5-29a to 5-29c PRONASALE (Pn): most anterior cutaneous midpoint of the nose tip; *(a)* 3D frontal view; *(b)* 3D ¾ view; *(c)* CBCT axial section.

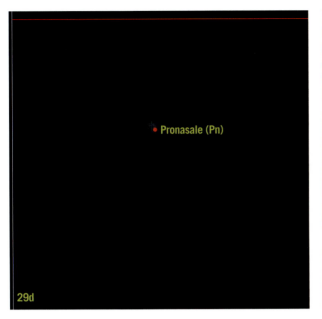
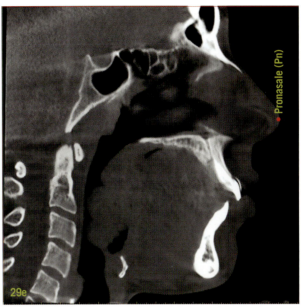

Figs 5-29d and 5-29e PRONASALE (Pn); *(d)* CBCT frontal section; *(e)* CBCT sagittal section.

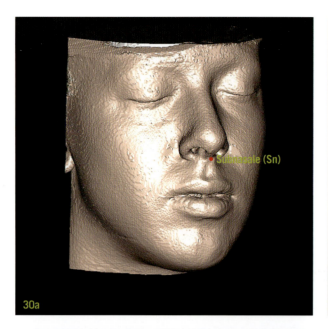
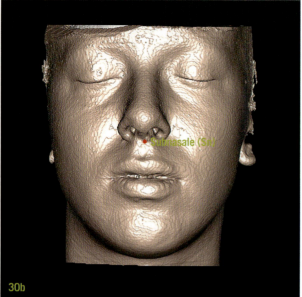
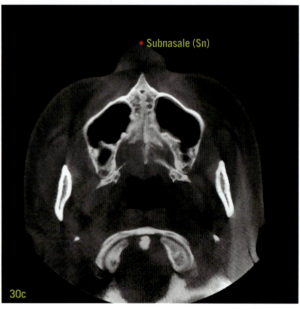

Figs 5-30a to 5-30c SUBNASALE (Sn); *(a)* 3D frontal view; *(b)* 3D ¾ view; *(c)* CBCT axial section.

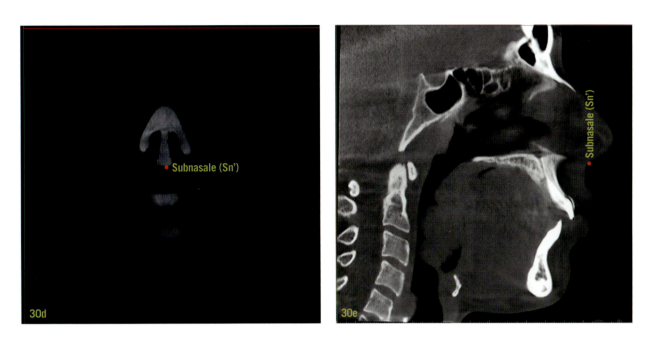

Figs 5-30d and 5-30e SUBNASALE (Sn); *(d)* CBCT frontal section; *(e)* CBCT sagittal section.

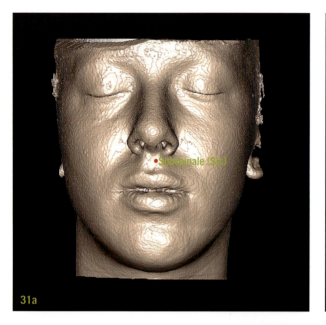
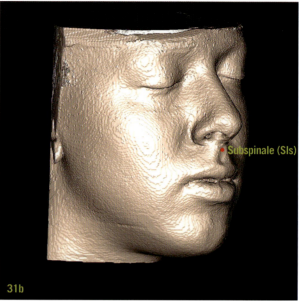
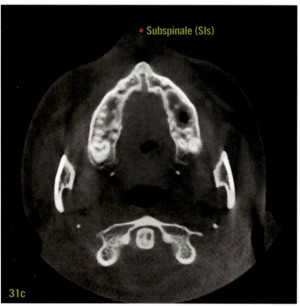

Figs 5-31a to 5-31c SUBSPINALE (SUPERIOR LABIAL SULCUS) (SIs): most hollow midpoint of the superior labial philtrum; *(a)* 3D frontal view; *(b)* 3D ¾ view; *(c)* axial CBCT view.

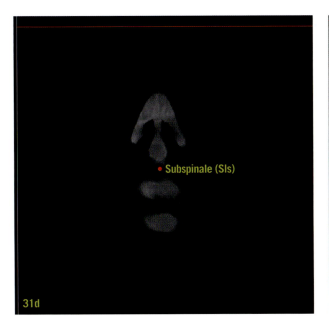
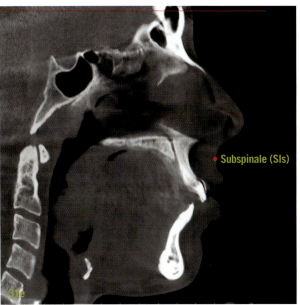

Figs 5-31d and 5-31e SUBSPINALE (SUPERIOR LABIAL SULCUS) (Sls); *(d)* CBCT frontal view; *(e)* CBCT sagittal view.

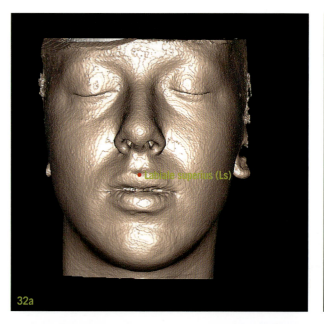
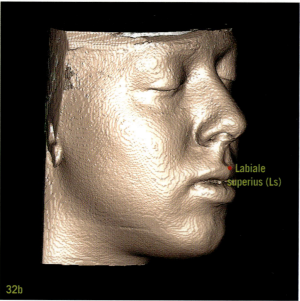
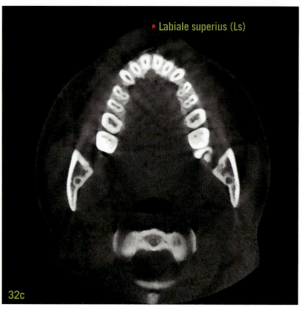

Figs 5-32a to 5-32c LABIALE SUPERIUS (Ls): most anteriorly projecting midpoint of the superior labial vermilion; *(a)* 3D frontal view; *(b)* 3D ¾ view; *(c)* CBCT axial section.

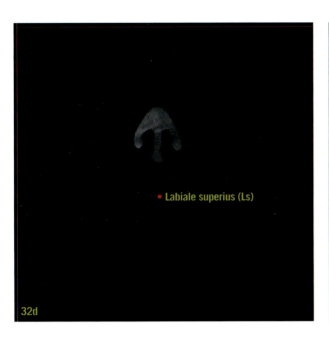 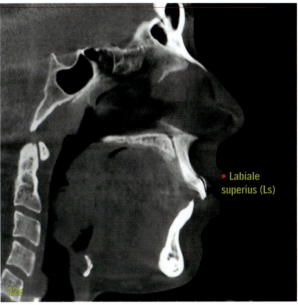

Figs 5-32d and 5-32e LABIALE SUPERIUS (Ls); *(d)* CBCT frontal view; *(e)* CBCT sagittal view.

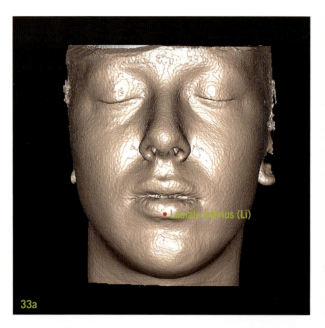
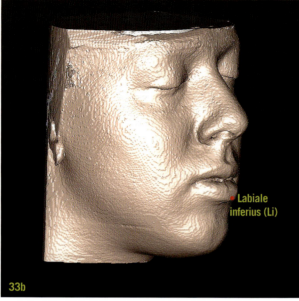
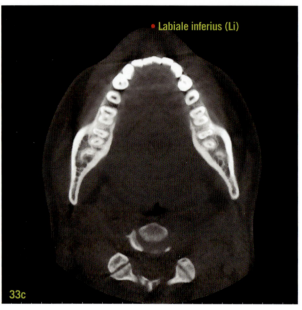

Figs 5-33a to 5-33c LABIALE INFERIUS (Li): most anteriorly projecting midpoint of the inferior labial vermilion; *(a)* 3D frontal view; *(b)* 3D ¾ view; *(c)* CBCT axial section.

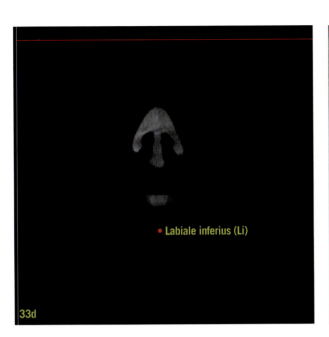
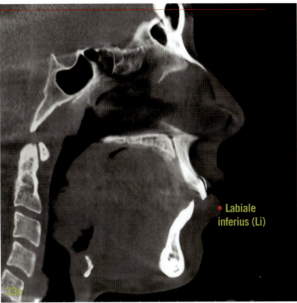

Figs 5-33d and 5-33e LABIALE INFERIUS (Li); *(d)* CBCT frontal section; *(e)* CBCT sagittal section.

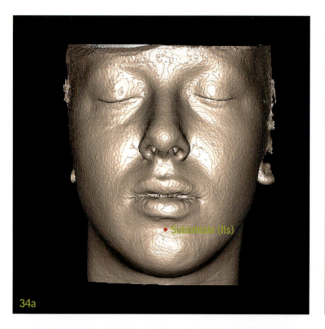
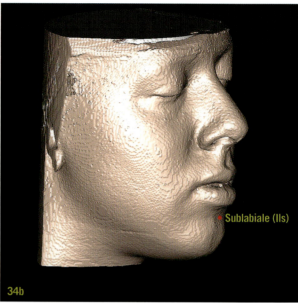
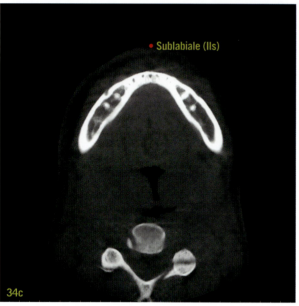

Figs 5-34a to 5-34c SUBLABIALE (INFERIOR LABIAL SULCUS) (Ils): most hollow midpoint of the labiomental sulcus; (a) 3D frontal view; (b) 3D ¾ view; (c) CBCT axial section.

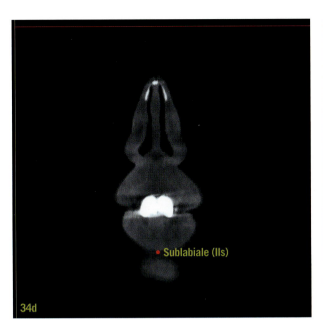
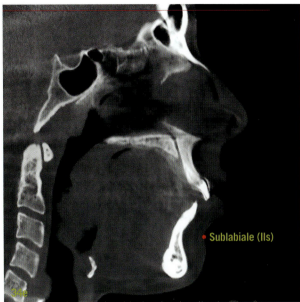

Figs 5-34d and 5-34e SUBLABIALE (INFERIOR LABIAL SULCUS) (Ils); *(d)* CBCT frontal section; *(e)* CBCT sagittal section.

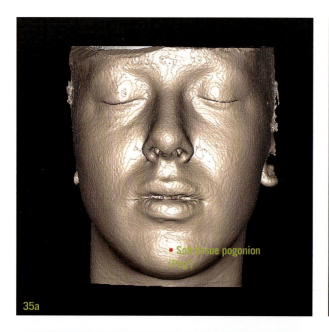
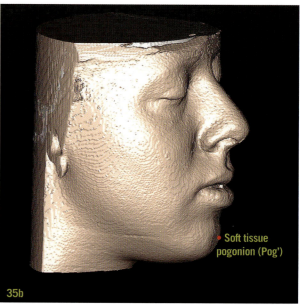
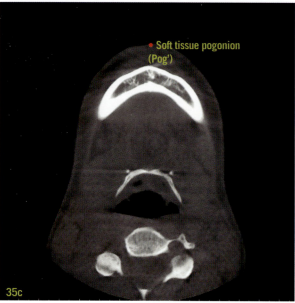

Figs 5-35a to 5-35c SOFT TISSUE POGONION (Pog'): most anteriorly projecting midpoint of the mandibular symphysis; *(a)* 3D frontal view; *(b)* 3D ¾ view; *(c)* CBCT axial view.

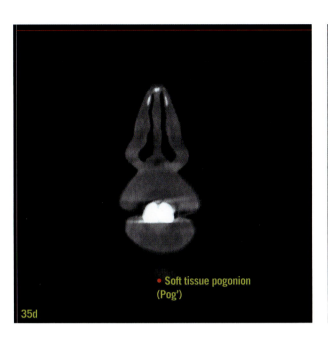 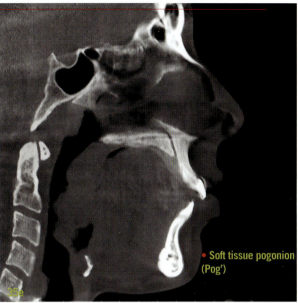

Figs 5-35d and 5-35e SOFT TISSUE POGONION (Pog'); *(d)* CBCT frontal view; *(e)* CBCT sagittal view.

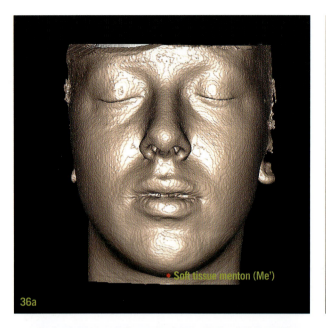
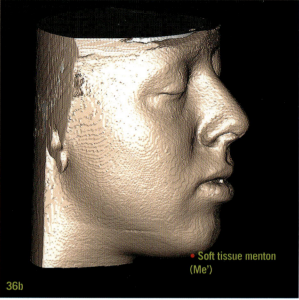
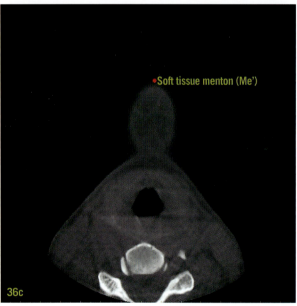

Figs 5-36a to 5-36c SOFT TISSUE MENTON (Me'): cutaneous point corresponding to bony menton; *(a)* 3D frontal view; *(b)* 3D ¾ view; *(c)* CBCT axial section.

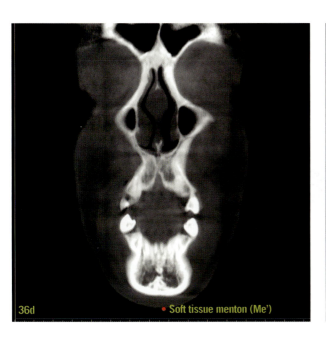 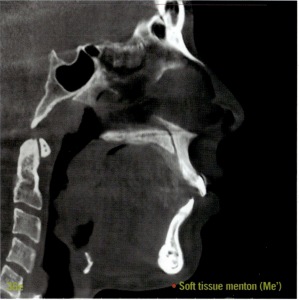

Figs 5-36d and 5-36e SOFT TISSUE MENTON (Me'); *(d)* CBCT frontal section; *(e)* CBCT sagittal view.

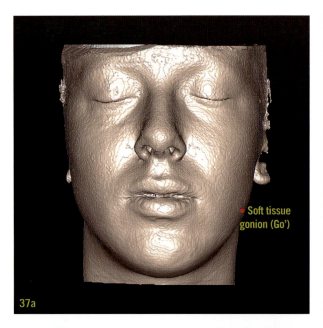
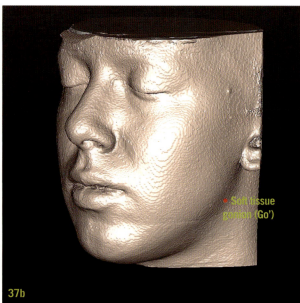
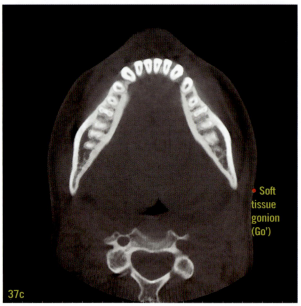

Figs 5-37a to 5-37c SOFT TISSUE GONION (Go'): most lateral cutaneous point of the right/left gonial angle at level of the bony gonion; *(a)* 3D frontal view; *(b)* 3D ¾ view; *(c)* CBCT axial section.

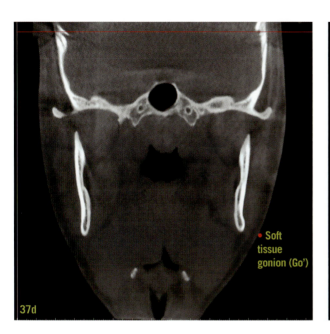
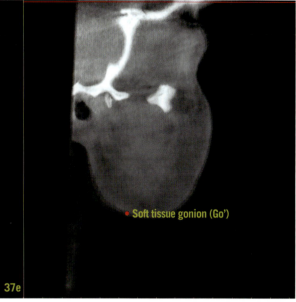

Figs 5-37d and 5-37e SOFT TISSUE GONION (Go'); *(d)* CBCT frontal view; *(e)* CBCT sagittal section.

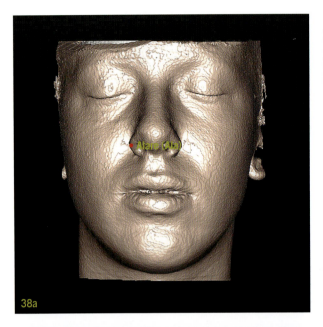
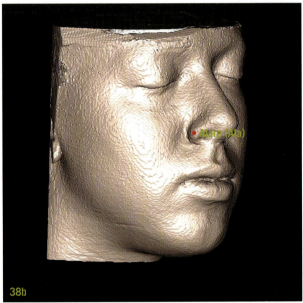
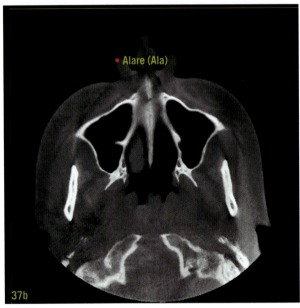

Figs 5-38a to 5-38c ALARE (Ala): most lateral point of each nostril; *(a)* 3D frontal view; *(b)* 3D ¾ view; *(c)* CBCT axial section.

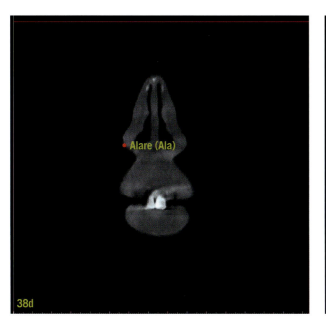
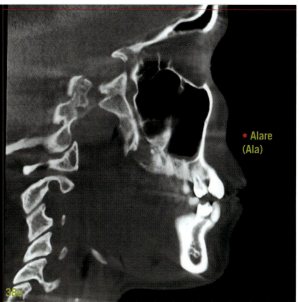

Figs 5-38d and 5-38e ALARE (Ala); *(d)* CBCT frontal view; *(e)* CBCT sagittal section.

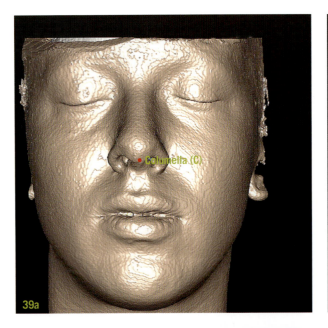
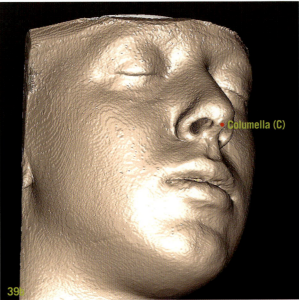
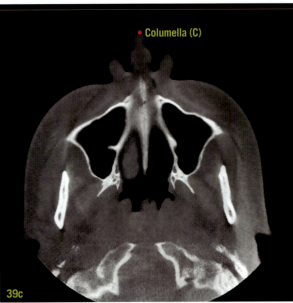

Figs 5-39a to 5-39c COLUMELLA (C): constructed midpoint located at the center of the columella at the level of the nostrils; *(a)* 3D frontal view; *(b)* 3D ¾ view; *(c)* CBCT axial section.

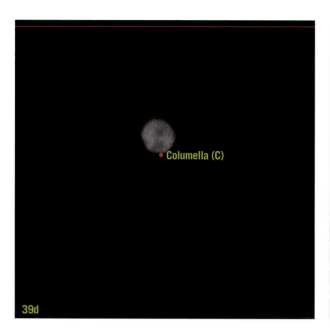 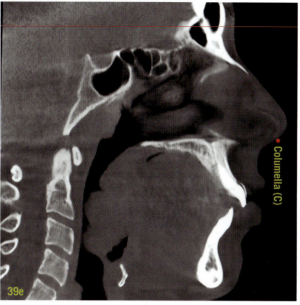

Figs 5-39d and 5-39e COLUMELLA (C); *(d)* CBCT frontal view; *(e)* CBCT sagittal section.

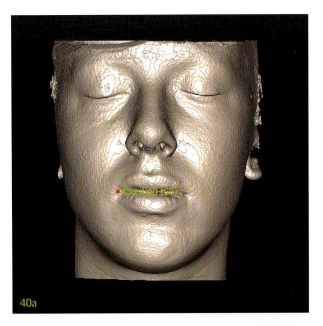
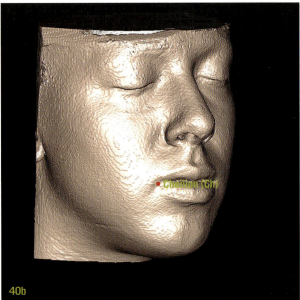
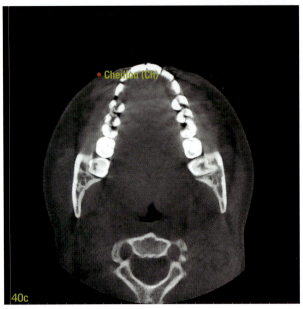

Figs 5-40a to 5-40c CHEILION (Ch): point of right and left labial commissure; *(a)* 3D frontal view; *(b)* 3D ¾ view; *(c)* CBCT axial section.

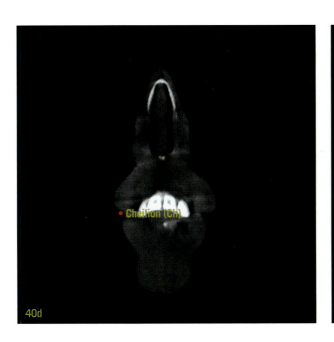 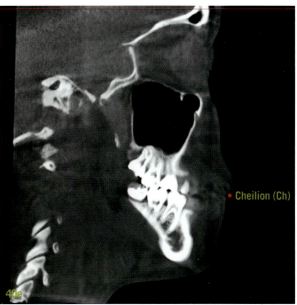

Figs 5-40d and 5-40e CHEILION (Ch); *(d)* CBCT frontal section; *(e)* CBCT sagittal section.

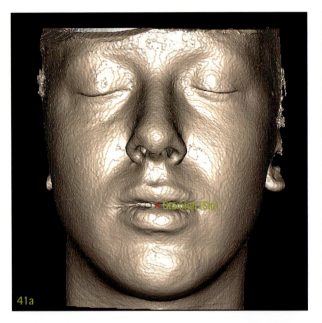
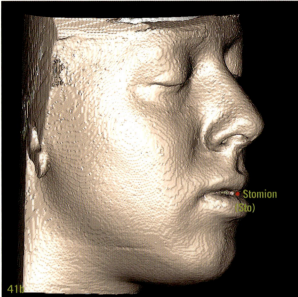
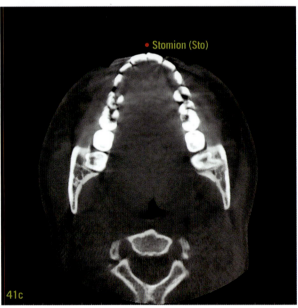

Figs 5-41a to 5-41c   STOMION (Sto): cutaneous midpoint of the labial fissure; *(a)* 3D frontal view; *(b)* 3D ¾ view; *(c)* CBCT axial section.

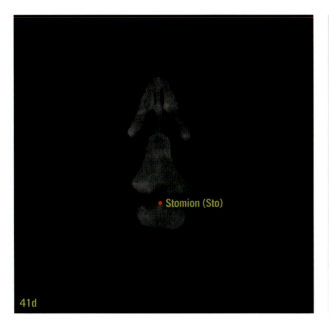
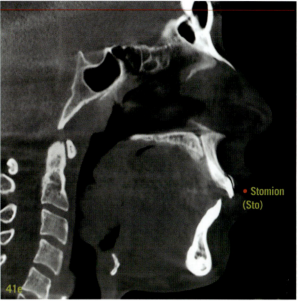

Figs 5-41d and 5-41e STOMION (Sto); *(d)* CBCT frontal view; *(e)* CBCT sagittal section.

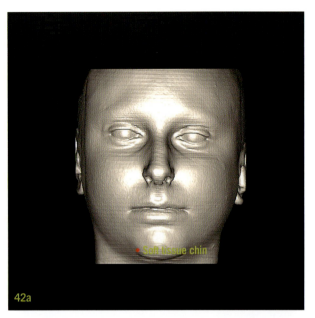
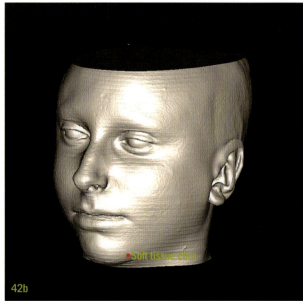
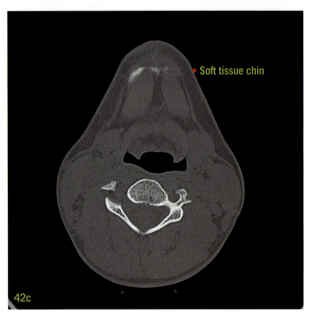

Fig 5-42a to 5-42c SOFT TISSUE CHIN: most lateral point of the chin at the level of the bony chin; *(a)* 3D frontal view; *(b)* 3D ¾ view; *(c)* CBCT axial section.

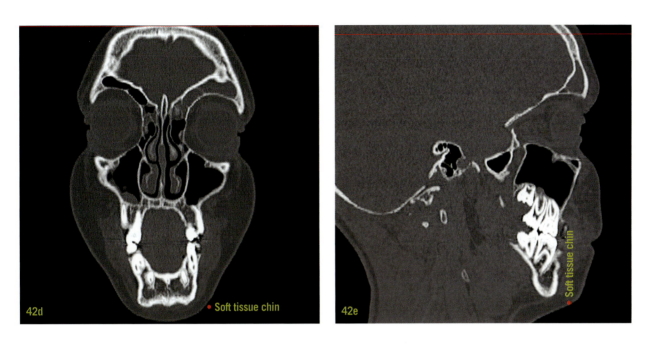

Figs 5-42d and 5-42e SOFT TISSUE CHIN; *(d)* frontal CBCT section; *(e)* CBCT sagittal section.

References

1. Houston WJ. The analysis of errors in orthodontic measurements. Am J Orthod 1983;83:382–390.
2. Richtsmeier JT, Paik CH, Elfert PC, Cole TM 3rd, Dahlman HR. Precision, repeatability, and validation of the localization of cranial landmarks using computed tomography scans. Cleft Palate Craniofac J 1995;32:217–227.
3. Olszewski R, Tanesy O, Cosnard G, Zech F, Reychler H. Reproducibility of osseous landmarks used for computed tomography based three-dimensional cephalometric analyses. J Craniomaxillofac Surg 2010;38:214–221.
4. Williams FL, Richtsmeier JT. Comparison of mandibular landmarks from computed tomography and 3D digitizer data. Clin Anat 2003;16:494–500.
5. Gateno J, Xia JJ, Teichgraeber J. A new three-dimensional cephalometric analysis for orthognathic surgery. J Oral Maxillofac Surg 2011;69:606–622.
6. Burstone CJ. The integumental profile. Am J Orthod 1958:44:1–25.
7. Burstone CJ. Lip posture and its significance in treatment planning. Am J Orthod 1967;53:262–284.
8. Downs WB. Analysis of the dentofacial profile. Angle Orthod 1956,26:191–212.
9. Subtelny JD. A longitudinal study of soft tissue facial structures and their profile characteristics, defined in relation to underlying skeletal structures. Am J Orthod 1959;45:481–507.
10. Holdaway RA. A soft tissue cephalometric analysis and its use in orthodontic treatment planning. Part I. Am J Orthod 1983;84:1–28.
11. Farkas LG. Examination. In: Farkas LG (ed). Anthropometry of the Head and Face in Medicine, ed 2. New York: Raven Press, 1994.
12. Swennen GRJ, Schutyser FAC, Hausamen J-E. Three-Dimensional Cephalometry: A Color Atlas and Manual. Berlin: Springer-Verlag, 2006.
13. Xia JJ, Gateno J, Teichgraeber JF. New clinical protocol to evaluate craniomaxillofacial deformity and plan surgical correction. J Oral Maxillofac Surg 2009;67:2093–2106.

G Perrotti
J Nowakowska

6

3D Analysis of Soft Tissues

This chapter aims to propose a three-dimensional (3D) vision of the concept of facial harmony. In the field of medicine, the concept is not beauty or greater or lesser facial appeal but rather a search for parameters to set standard values that can be used to reconstruct and remodel a human face in line with anthropometric criteria.

Normal values are not rigid rules; instead, they are standard reference values for facilitating correction of major deviations in facial proportions through orthognathic surgery or for helping orthodontists to forecast evolution of the maxillomandibular complex during growth and the resulting facial proportions.

The use of cone beam computed tomography (CBCT) in diagnostic assessment of skeletal tissues also provides the opportunity to obtain amazing 3D reconstructions of soft tissues.

The association of 3D rendering and the possibility of developing measurement systems compatible with 3D images have given immense momentum to the study of facial proportions.

3D imaging associated with a cephalometric, multiplanar system of measurement provides a new approach to the study of esthetics of the soft tissues, with major implications on virtual dental diagnostics and maxillofacial, plastic, and implant-prosthetic surgery.

Esthetic Analysis of Soft Tissues Using 3D Cephalometry

Esthetics is a sector of philosophy dealing with knowledge of the beautiful, the artistic, and the scientific, ie, an area of moral and spiritual judgment.

In medicine, esthetics is represented by a delicate balance of many somatic and physiognomic aspects, which together determine harmony. Historical and artistic examples show how human beings have always been aware of beauty and facial appearance. This now translates into an increasing demand for esthetic outcomes from patients who have become more and more demanding in relation to treatment.

Such patients go to a dental practice not just requesting better function of their stomatognathic system but also showing an increased understanding of techniques and treatments and a desire to change the form and contours of their face towards profiles that are considered to be "more appealing."

It has now been accepted for many years that social and psychologic well-being and satisfaction with one's image are greatly influenced by physical appearance.[1-3] If the esthetic outcome is therefore increasingly important, all treatments that can lead to changes in body parts affecting the esthetic appearance, like orthodontics, must also address the foreseeable consequences and alterations through treatment. Correct diagnosis is necessary to obtain a successful outcome in orthodontics, orthognathic surgery, and prosthetic rehabilitation. This is only possible by gathering information from diagnostic casts, cephalometric tracings, and facial analysis, which, nevertheless, in modern orthodontics must also consider the patient's soft tissues so as to obtain the most satisfactory results. It is important to remember that, even if symmetry and balance are clearly recognizable in nature, the perception of appeal is subjective.[4]

Standard Esthetic Analysis

Esthetic analysis of soft tissues is an easy and fast diagnostic method allowing the clinician to obtain important indications useful in developing a correct plan of treatment. Moreover, esthetic analysis provides information on the interrelations between soft tissues and underlying bone.

Conventionally, facial esthetic analysis is performed using a series of photographic images of the patient's face in predefined projections with the head always in natural head position (NHP).

The use of NHP was introduced in orthodontics in the 1950s,[5-7] defined as the position of the head when the patient is standing before starting to walk with an horizontal visual axis. In practice, individuals are asked to look at a mirror at 1.5 meters away or to stare at a distant point. NHP as a craniofacial reference system has been supported because it is easy to reproduce interindividually and is easy to record, independently from skull references (Fig 6-1).

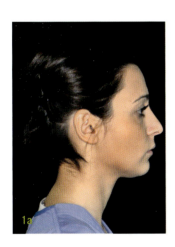 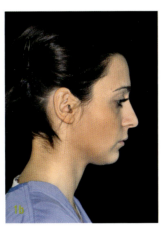 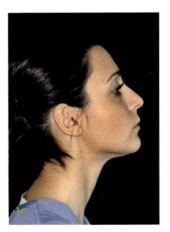

Figs 6-1a to 6-1c *(a)* The NHP is the only position that allows an objective evaluation of the facial profile. *(b)* The chin is placed too backward. *(c)* The chin is placed too forward.

Aims of the Esthetic Analysis

The facial esthetic analysis has several objectives:

- Perform a preliminary assessment of the patient to identify whether additional diagnostic (in particular, radiologic) tests are needed so as to spare patients exposure to unneeded ionizing radiation
- Assess symmetry of the face and its components
- Evaluate the parallelism between the occlusal plane and the reference lines
- Assess profile harmony
- Examine the vertical relationship between the middle and lower third of the face

2D Assessment Method

In recent years orthodontic photographs have typically been available in digital format. It is therefore common to perform a two-dimensional (2D) facial esthetic analysis using any graphic software available for personal computers. To do the analysis, it is sufficient to trace some lines and then take quick measurements. The photographic projections for this assessment of the face must be frontal and lateral.

Frontal Projection

The analysis of the face from the frontal view provides the following information:

- General facial form
- Facial symmetry
- Horizontal and vertical facial proportions
- Lips

Both horizontal and vertical reference lines are used for analysis of the frontal projection.

Horizontal Reference Lines

The bipupillary line is a straight line passing through the center of the eyes; if parallel to the horizontal plane, it represents the reference for the parallelism of the other straight lines (ie, the ophryac [eyebrow], commissural [lip], and interalar [nasal] lines). These lines can be used to analyze the inclination of the incisal and occlusal planes and the orientation of the maxillary and mandibular canines and the chin, as all straight lines should be parallel to the horizontal reference line (Figs 6-2 and 6-3).

Vertical Reference Line

The facial midline is visualized by tracing a vertical line passing through the glabella, the nose tip, the labial philtrum, and the tip of the chin (Fig 6-4). The philtrum is the most symmetric midpoint in the soft tissues, hence it is the best option to visualize the facial midline.[8]

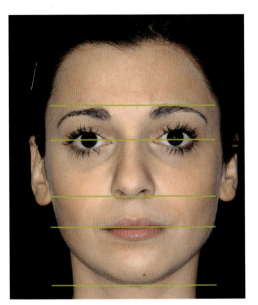

Fig 6-2 Horizontal reference lines. The ophryac (eyebrow), commissural (lip), and interalar (nasal) straight lines should be parallel to the bipupillary line passing through the center of the eyes, which is usually parallel to the horizontal plane.

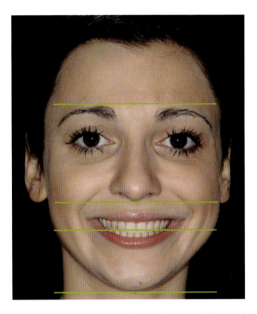

Fig 6-3 The horizontal reference lines can be used to assess the incisal plane, the maxillary and mandibular occlusal planes, and the gingival contours. The maxillary incisal plane is constructed as a line passing through the cusps of the left and right maxillary canines. The mandibular occlusal plane is defined as a line passing through the cusps of the right and left mandibular canines.

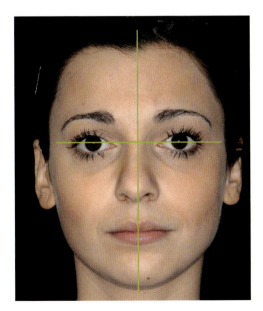

Fig 6-4 The midline divides the face into two hemifaces.

Lateral Projection

In the analysis of the lateral position, the patient's profile should be assessed with the head in standing position and the eyes staring at the horizon (NHP), in centric relation with relaxed arms. The patient is examined first on the right side, then in front, and then the left side to assess symmetry between the sides.

The analysis of the facial image in side view provides the following information:

- The different facial areas
- The angle of the facial profile
- The nasolabial angle

The assessment of the profile and of the reference lines to be traced in lateral view is discussed below (see Total Face Approach), in which a comparison is made between the conventional (2D) cephalometric analysis of soft tissues and the 3D approach.

3D Esthetic Analysis

The esthetic evaluation of soft tissues is one of the fundamental steps for correct diagnosis and preparation of an orthodontic, orthodontic-surgical, or implant-prosthetic treatment plan. Interpretation of soft tissue morphology and position through 3D analysis provides all information pertaining to esthetic facial analysis. Compared with the 2D facial analysis, the 3D assessment provides further essential information:

- Visualizes and analyzes the position of underlying hard tissues
- Increases endlessly the number of potential projections for facial analysis
- Foresees the esthetic-functional outcomes of the treatment plan
- Provides maxillofacial surgeons with additional useful information for surgical procedures

Recent advancements in technology and 3D imaging have allowed development of 3D reconstruction methods with significant diagnostic benefits compared with any 2D technique. Patients can be assessed while visualizing simultaneously the three planes of space and eliminating any distortion deriving from the use of 2D images.

Techniques of 3D Analysis of Soft Tissues

The ideal method for quantitative assessment of patients should have the following features:

- It should be noninvasive.
- It should require inexpensive equipment.
- It should allow quick execution and collection of 3D data and allow their permanent recording.
- It should allow comparison with standards for populations of the same sex, age, and ethnic group.
- It should enable use of computer-imaging, treatment simulation, and treatment selection techniques.

There are three commonly used techniques in esthetic analysis of soft tissues:

- Conventional anthropometry
- Computed anthropometry:
  - Optical devices not requiring direct contact with patients: lasers, scanners, optoelectronic devices, stereophotogrammetry, Moirè topography
  - Devices requiring direct contact with patients: electromagnets, ultrasonic probes
- 3D analysis based on volumetric reconstruction from DICOM images obtained by CBCT

Conventional Anthropometry

Anthropometry (from the Greek words *anthropos*, man, and *metron*, measure) is the science dealing with measurement of the human body as a whole or of its components. Through anthropometric studies on a skeleton, it is, for instance, possible to detect age and sex Anthropometry also has clinical applications in ergonomics, industrial design, and fashion.

Although the use of anthropometry provides accurate information for assessing a face, it is not commonly used in clinical practice, the major drawback being the relatively long time it takes, the experience required from the operator, and the need for direct contact with patients. Subsequent data collection and analysis of the results are also time-consuming.

Stereophotogrammetry

In *stereophotogrammetry* a ray of light illuminates the object to be photographed, which is "captured" simultaneously by two or more cameras at different angles with very short exposure times.[9,12] After calibration, the dedicated software acquires various images and reconstructs a 3D picture. The system not only performs a stereoscopic reconstruction of the face, it also reproduces the features of surface structures very accurately (Figs 6-5 and 6-6).

The benefit of this method compared with laser scanning methods is its very fast execution (0.75 milliseconds), reducing the chance of error associated with movement, especially in children and patients who find it difficult to remain seated. According to Weinberg et al,[13] De Menezes et al,[14] and Ghoddousi et al,[10] measurements obtained by stereophotogrammetry have an accuracy of ± 0.5 mm compared with the images acquired by direct anthropometry. The presence of artifacts, critical zones, and shadings are limitations comparable with other laser scanning devices, but in stereophotogrammetry they are less marked.

To overcome problems in locating landmarks such as zygion or gonion, several authors recommend proceeding by first identifying a landmark made by directly placing a mark using ordinary cosmetic eye liner before doing the exam.

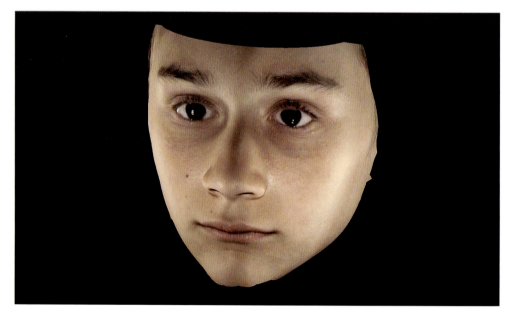

Fig 6-5 Example of 3D facial reconstruction using stereophotogrammetry.

The technique is fairly time-consuming because of data processing and creation of the 3D model after the intial photographs. Processing time depends on computing power. A major drawback is that stereophotogrammetric devices and cameras are costly, have to be calibrated before each use, and are difficult to move from place to place. It is therefore necessary to install them in a dedicated room in dental practices or clinics.

Stereophotogrammetry nevertheless provides very accurate studies of facial morphology.[15]

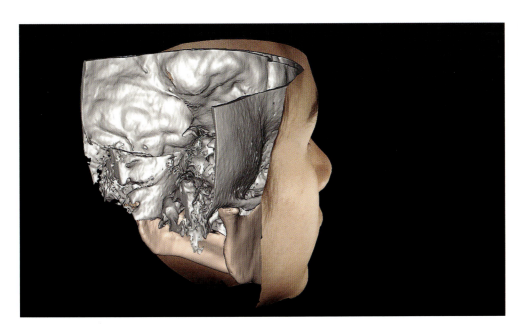

Fig 6-6 Stereophotogrammetric reconstruction in ¾ view from the posterior of the patient. Note the reconstruction of the skull base and the mandible.

Computerized 3D Esthetic Facial Analysis Using CT and CBCT Data

Digital Imaging and Communications in Medicine (DICOM) images are commonly used by most modern medical radiology units. For 3D esthetic analysis, CBCT scans are commonly used as they produce images of great quality with lower patient exposure to ionizing radiation compared with conventional techniques. DICOM images can be imported into specific software programs to collect and process the information. Axial scans are used to get a 3D reconstruction of the skull volume. Detection (segmentation) of bone structures and soft tissues is performed first, artifacts are then filtered out, and the program generates a 3D image of hard skeletal tissues and a digital reconstruction (technically, a "rendering") of soft tissues (Figs 6-7 to 6-9).

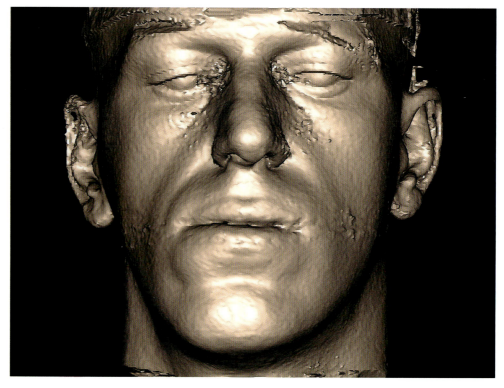

Fig 6-7 3D volumetric reconstruction of facial soft tissues obtained with software that analyzes CBCT data.

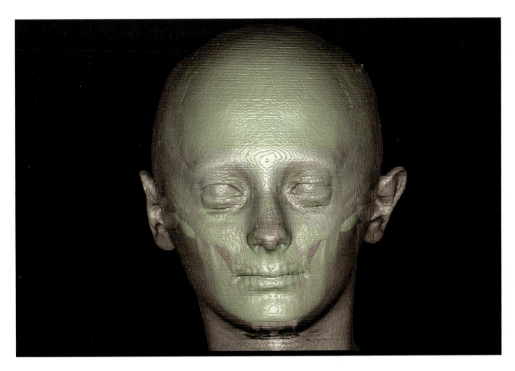

Fig 6-8 Volumetric reconstruction of hard and soft tissues obtained with a light transparence function for soft tissues.

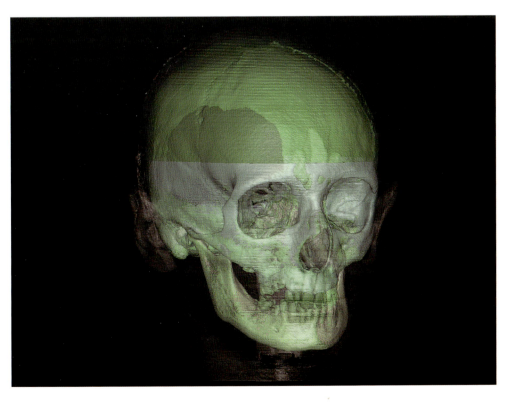

Fig 6-9 Volumetric reconstruction of soft tissues with a high transparence function: the observer can appreciate soft and underlying hard tissues.

Total Face Approach

The esthetic analysis of soft tissues can now be processed on 3D images using the selected software by proceeding through the following steps:

- Definition of the external reference system
- 3D cephalometric analysis

External Reference System

The external reference system (Fig 6-10) is defined by three planes:

- Sagittal reference plane
- Axial reference plane
- Coronal reference plane

The use of external 3D reference planes (Table 6-1) avoids errors associated with distortion in the presence of craniofacial asymmetries, and they are also easy to define.[16] It is nevertheless very important that the skull is in NHP during the exam.

Fig 6-10 External reference planes: sagittal, axial, and coronal.

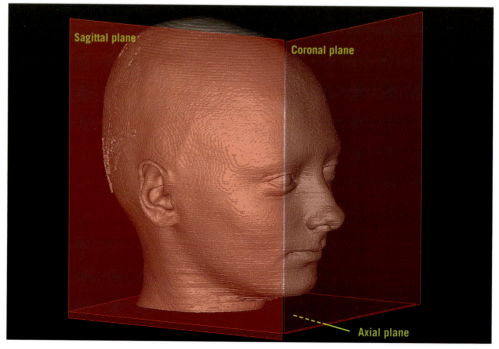

From 2D to 3D Cephalometry

Burstone,[17,18] Subtelny,[19] Schwarz,[20] and Holdaway[21] have incorporated soft tissue parameters into cephalometric analyses in orthodontics. According to Ricketts[22] the lips are contained inside the E-line, which starts from the tip of the nose and reaches the most projecting point of the chin. In relation to the E-line, the upper lip is slightly posterior to the lower lip. According to Burstone et al,[23] the anteroposterior position of the lip can be assessed with a line traced from subnasale to soft tissue pogonion, and the degree of protrusion or retrusion of the lip is measured as the linear perpendicular distance from this line to the most prominent point of both lips. In Holdaway's analysis,[21] H-line or the "harmony line" is traced tangentially to the soft tissues of the chin (soft tissue pogonion) and of the upper lip. The distance of soft tissue point A from the harmony line should not exceed 5 mm, whereas the angle between H-line and the soft tissue line traced between soft nasion and soft pogonion (H-angle) should not exceed approximately 10 degrees.

The next step, developed by RL Jacobson and A Jacobson[24] in 1994, is the 3D cephalometric analysis. Cephalometric images in 3D can be examined in any perspective. Landmarks can be correctly selected, visualizing them in an axial, sagittal, or coronal viewing window. Once each point has been defined in space through the x, y, and z coordinates, it is possible to measure the distance between points, lines, and angles. In Jacobson's analysis, four reference planes are used—anterior facial, anterior lower facial, upper facial, and midsagittal—thus allowing a detailed assessment of skull skeletal structures, soft tissues, and their relationships.[25]

The 3D cephalometric analysis proposed, the total face approach (TFA), is subdivided into four predefined modules: TFA 1, TFA 2, TFA 3, and TFA 4. Some soft tissue landmarks are identified for each part as first defined by Farkas and Munro[26] and modified by Swennen[27] so as to be precisely identified in 3D (Table 6-2). They are viewed in axial, coronal, and sagittal sections directly on CT scans and then made visible on the 3D-reconstructed skull (Fig 6-11). Measurements between points, planes, and angles to be assessed are added. Linear measures can be taken between two points, a point and a plane, or between two planes using software (Fig 6-12). It is also possible to take angular measurements.

Table 6-1 Reference and construction planes used in this study

Abbreviation	Reference planes	Definition
Sag	External sagittal (x)	Plane defined between the SAG1, SAG2, and SAG3 points inserted manually into the sagittal window. First "0" image obtained from CT data.
Ax	External axial (z)	Plane defined between the AX1, AX2, and AX3 points inserted manually into the axial window. First "0" image obtained from CT data.
Cor	External coronal (y)	Plane defined between COR1, COR2, and COR3 points inserted manually into the coronal window. First "0" image obtained from CT data.
Abbreviation	**Construction planes**	**Definition**
SFP	Superior facial plane	Plane passing through nasion (N) perpendicular to the coronal (y) and sagittal (x) planes
ANSPl	Maxillary plane	Plane passing through the anterior nasal spine (ANS) parallel to the axial plane (z)
PLs	Upper labial plane	Plane passing through labiale superius (Ls) parallel to the axial plane (z)
PLi	Lower labial plane	Plane passing through labiale inferius (Li) parallel to the axial plane (z)
MePl	Mental plane	Plane passing through menton parallel to the subnasal plane
TVP	True vertical plane	Plane passing through subnasale (Sn) parallel to the coronal plane (y)

Table 6-2 Soft tissue landmarks used in this study		
Abbreviation	Landmark	Definition
G'	Soft tissue Glabella	Skin prominence above the frontonasal suture, between the eyebrows
N'	Soft tissue nasion	Cutaneous point at the level of the frontonasal suture
Pn	Pronasale	Most prominent nasal midpoint
C	Columella	Most anterior cutaneous midpoint where the nostrils meet
Sn	Subnasale	Cutaneous midpoint where columella and upper lip meet
Sls	Subspinale (superior labial sulcus)	Most concave midpoint of the superior labial philtrum
Ls	Labiale superius	Most anteriorly projecting midpoint of the superior lip vermilion
Sto	Stomion	Cutaneous midpoint of the labial fissure
Li	Labiale inferius	Most anteriorly projecting midpoint of the inferior lip vermilion
Ils	Sublabiale (inferior labial sulcus)	Most concave midpoint of the labiomental sulcus
Pog'	Soft tissue pogonion	Anteriorly most projecting midpoint of the mandibular symphysis
Me'	Soft tissue menton	Point corresponding to bony menton in soft tissue
ZyR'/ZyL'	Soft tissue zygion right/left	Most lateral skin points in the right/left zygomatic arch at the level of bony zygion
GoR'/GoL'	Soft tissue gonion right/left	Most lateral skin points of the right/left gonial angle at the level of the gonion
Chin'	Soft tissue chin	Most lateral point of the chin at the level of the osseous chin
Or'	Soft tissue orbitale	Lowest skin point of the right and left orbital fossae

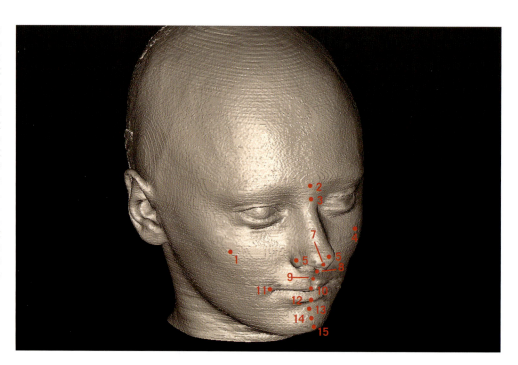

Fig 6-11 Representation of the cutaneous landmarks used in the study: 1, Soft tissue zygion right (ZyR'); 2, soft tissue glabella (G'); 3, soft tissue nasion (N'); 4, soft tissue zygion left (ZyL'); 5, right alare (AlaR); 6, pronasale (Pn); 7, cheilion right (ChR); 8, subspinale (Sls); 9, subnasale (Sn); 10, columella (C); 11, labiale superius (Ls); 12, labiale inferius (Li); 13, sublabiale (Ils'); 14, soft tissue pogonion (Pog'); 15, soft tissue gnathion (Gn'); 16, soft tissue menton (Me').

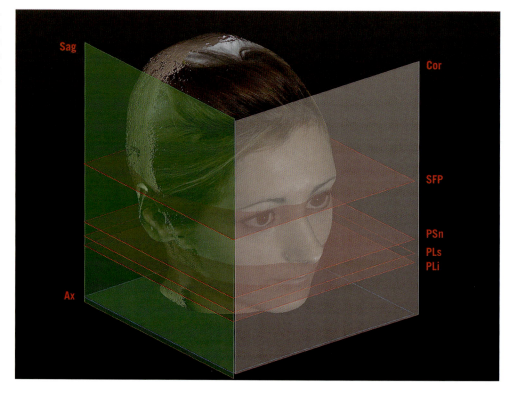

Fig 6-12 Representation of the reference and construction planes passing through the landmarks described in the text. PSn, maxillary plane.

The construction planes can pass through:

- Two cutaneous points and one reference plane
- One cutaneous point and two reference planes (axial, sagittal, or coronal)

TFA 1

The TFA 1 module is a standard profilometric analysis based on an angular value. The angle of the profile is constructed by connecting three reference points on the face: soft tissue glabella (G'), subnasale (Sn), and soft tissue pogonion (Pog'). The G', Sn, and Pog' landmarks have been determined on the sagittal, coronal, and axial DICOM sections and not on the 3D reconstruction.

Angle of the Profile

This angle is formed by soft tissue glabella (G') to subnasale (Sn) and Sn to soft tissue pogonion (Pog') (Figs 6-13 to 6-15). The profile assessment has been done by measuring this angle, which usually ranges between 165 and 175 degrees.[17] Values less than 165 degrees or greater than 175 degrees indicate skeletal discrepancies in the anteroposterior direction between the skeletal bases.

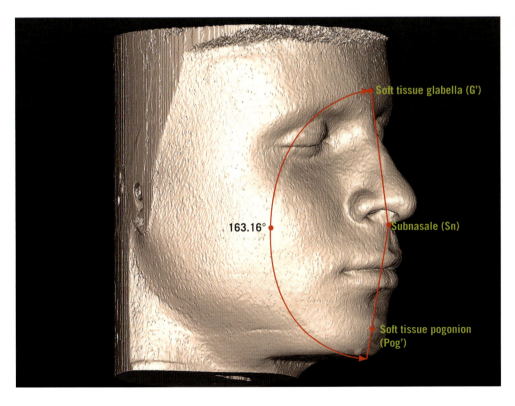

Fig 6-13 Skeletal Class I.

Convex Profile

The width of the angle is reduced, determining a posterior divergence associated with retroposition of pogonion, vertical excess of the maxilla, and, more rarely, maxillary protrusion.

Concave Profile

The value recorded when measuring the angle is greater than 180 degrees and determines an anterior divergence often associated with pogonion anteroposition, maxillary retrusion, or, less frequently, a decrease in the vertical size of the maxilla.

A concave or convex profile indicates presence of skeletal Class II or III, respectively, without indicating which of the two jaws is retruded or protruded. Marked differences in facial profiles exist among different races.[28]

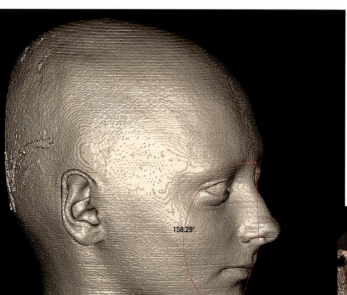

Fig 6-14 Convex profile.

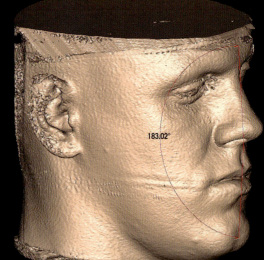

Fig 6-15 Concave profile.

TFA 2

The TFA 2 module is constructed and modified for 3D analysis starting from the cephalometric assessment of soft tissues developed by Arnett.[29-31] Arnett's cephalometric analysis is performed on 2D photographs in lateral projection, and it provides information on the areas comprising the face. The structures are analyzed with reference to the true vertical line (TVL). This line is constructed passing through subnasale, and it is perpendicular to NHP (Fig 6-16). Differently, the 3D analysis is performed by dividing the face, reconstructed in 3D, using construction planes passing through landmarks in the mandibular and maxillary area (as described in Table 6-1). The structures are then analyzed with reference to the true vertical plane (TVP) (Fig 6-17) passing through subnasale parallel to the coronal plane (y). The distances of cutaneous points are assessed with reference to the TVP (as opposed to the TVL in 2D analysis) and reflect the relationships in an anteroposterior direction between soft tissues (upper and lower lip; nose projection) and the underlying hard tissues supporting them, thus allowing assessment of the same landmarks both in skeletal and soft tissues. The second analysis uses linear measures of the mandibular and maxillary area and the nasolabial angle (an angular measure). The upper facial segment is then observed in terms of defect or excess of prominence.

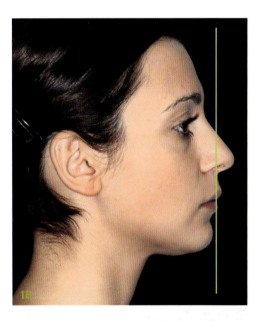

Fig 6-16 Patient's face in profile in lateral view, analyzed with reference to the TVL.

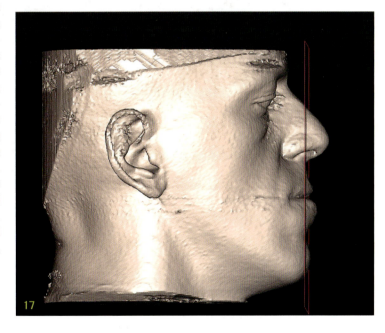

Fig 6-17 TVP passing through subnasale perpendicular to NHP.

The profile, according to Arnett,[31] can be divided into three segments or facial areas (Fig 6-18):

1. Upper middle third
2. Maxillary area
3. Mandibular area

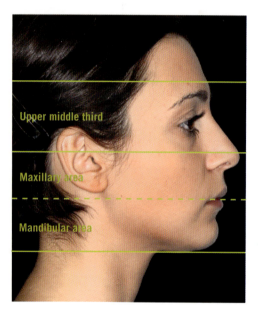

Fig 6-18 Facial division into three parts.[31]

The analysis of these segments is illustrated to readers both in 2D on photographs and on 3D-reconstructed skulls.

Upper Middle Third

The assessment of this area includes: soft tissue glabella, orbital margin, and zygomatic contour. These can be flat, normal, or prominent.

SOFT TISSUE GLABELLA

Usually, soft tissue glabella (G') is about 2 mm anterior to soft tissue nasion (N') (Figs 6-19 and 6-20). The definitions of the G' and N' landmarks are found in Table 6-2.

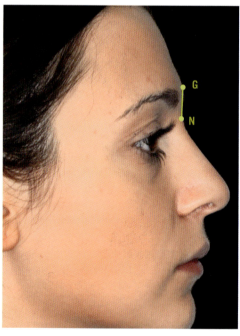

Fig 6-19 Soft tissue nasion and glabella landmarks as represented on a 2D photograph.

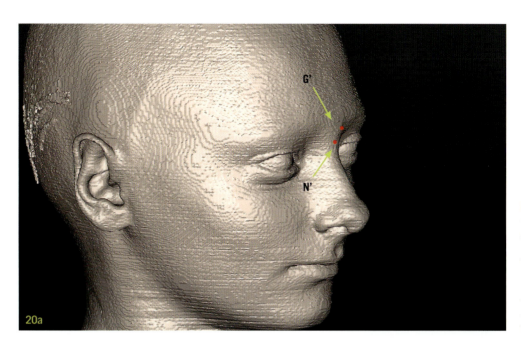

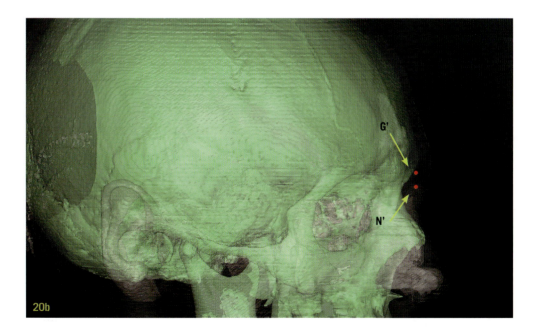

Figs 6-20a and 6-20b Soft tissue midpoints glabella (G') and nasion (N'): *(a)* Representation of the landmarks in 3D reconstruction. *(b)* Representation of the landmarks in 3D reconstruction using the transparence function.

ORBITAL MARGIN

The orbital margin landmark, or soft tissue orbitale (Or'), is the intersection between a vertical line passing through the pupil (from frontal observation) and the infraorbital margin. In assessing the profile, the orbital margin can be defined as flat, moderate, normal, or prominent (Fig 6-21).

For a definition of soft tissue orbitale, see Table 6-2.

Figs 6-21a and 6-21b Representation of the orbitale landmark and of the orbital margin: *(a)* 3D facial reconstruction. *(b)* 3D facial reconstruction in transparence.

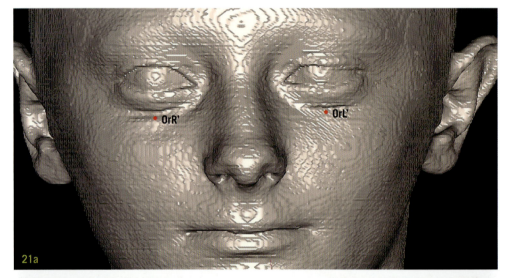

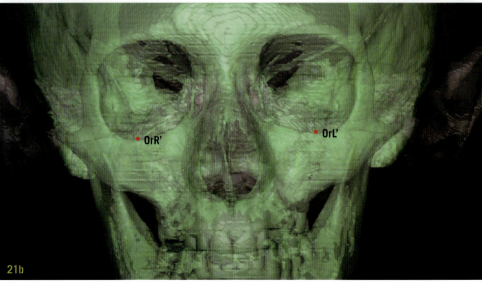

ZYGOMATIC CONTOUR

The zygomatic contour is a curved line that begins anterior to the ear, runs anteriorly through the highest point in the zygomatic contour and the subpupillary point, and ends at level of the nasal base. Ideally, it is a curved, soft, and continuous line (Figs 6-22 and 6-23).

Figure 6-24 is a ¾ view of the patient, whereas Fig 6-25 shows how a facial reconstruction can be rotated to perform assessments in various projections (aside from conventional frontal, lateral, and ¾ views).

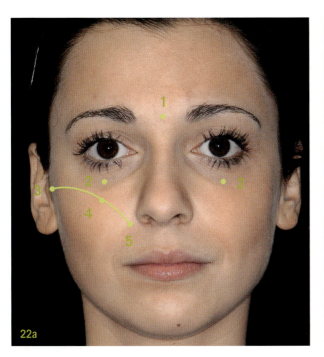
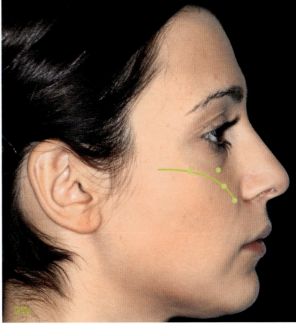

Figs 6-22a and 6-22b Zygomatic area: *(a)* frontal view; *(b)* lateral view; 1, soft tissue glabella; 2, orbital margin; 3, soft tissue zygion; 4, subpupillary point; 5, nasal base.

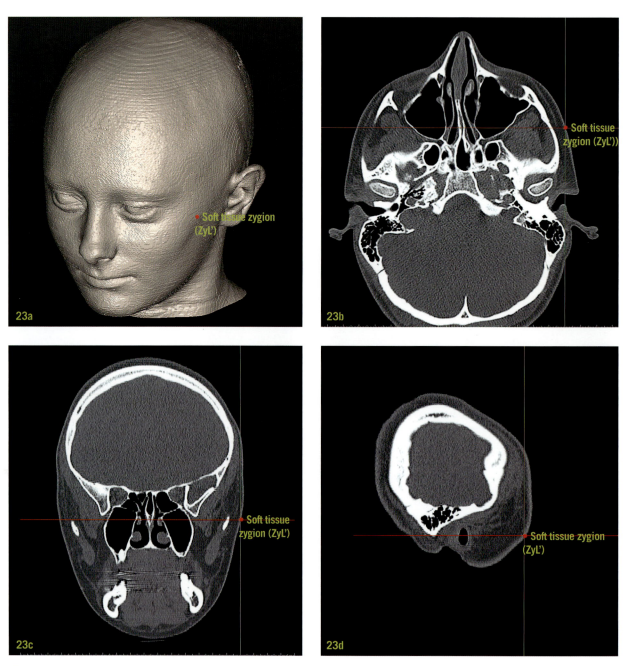

Figs 6-23a to 6-23d Soft tissue zygion: *(a)* visualization of the landmark on the 3D model; *(b)* zygion in axial view; *(c)* zygion in frontal section; *(d)* zygion in sagittal section.

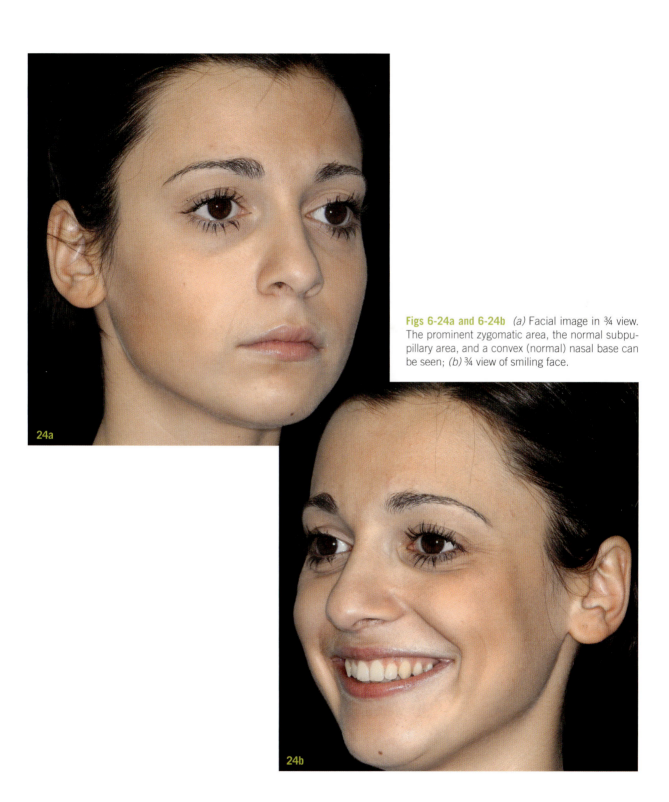

Figs 6-24a and 6-24b *(a)* Facial image in ¾ view. The prominent zygomatic area, the normal subpupillary area, and a convex (normal) nasal base can be seen; *(b)* ¾ view of smiling face.

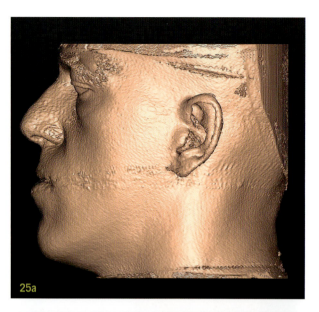
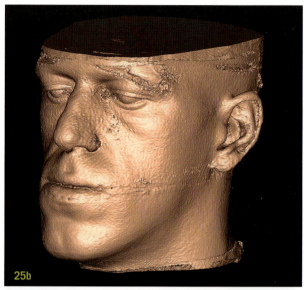
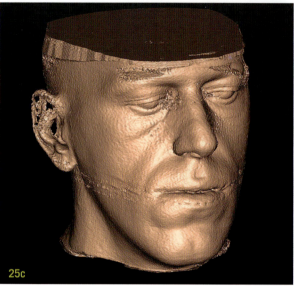
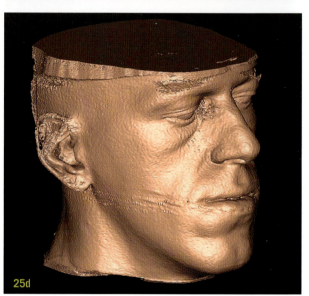

Figs 6-25a to 6-25h 3D reconstruction of photo in sequence of rotating to various views.

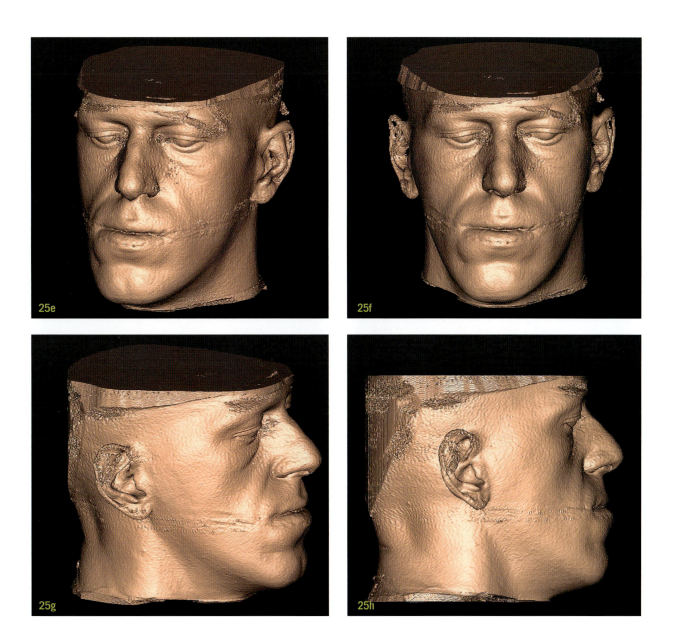

The definition of the zygion landmark can be found in Table 6-2. In the 3D analysis, the model can be rotated with reference to the x, y, and z axes. This function allows the analysis to be performed using views in addition to the conventional frontal, lateral, and ¾ projections.

Maxillary Area

In the maxillary area four soft tissue zones can be described: nasal base, prominence of the upper lip, support to the upper lip, and nose projection[32] (Figs 6-26 and 6-27). To perform the analysis, linear measures have been selected in the maxillary area: nasal projection (Pn vs TVP), the prominence of the upper lip (Ls vs TVP), and the length of the upper lip.

NASAL PROJECTION (PN VS TVP)

The nose can be described as long, normal, or short, the tip of the nose as pointing upward or downward, and the bridge of the nose as curved or sagging.

PROMINENCE OF THE UPPER LIP (LS VS TVP)

The upper lip can be defined as retruded, normal, or protruded. With reference to the TVL, the upper lip in females is usually 2.5 to 4.9 mm anterior, whereas in males it is typically 1.6 to 4 mm anterior.

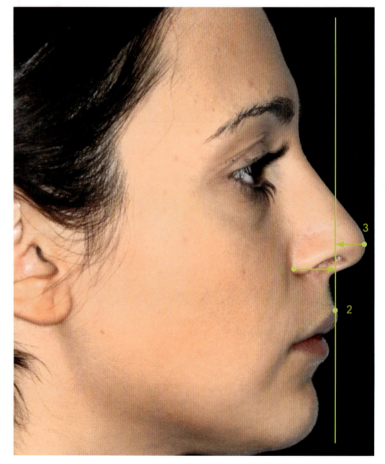

Fig 6-26 Representation of the maxillary area on a 2D photograph in lateral projection. 1, nasal base; 2, prominence of the upper lip; 3, nose projection.

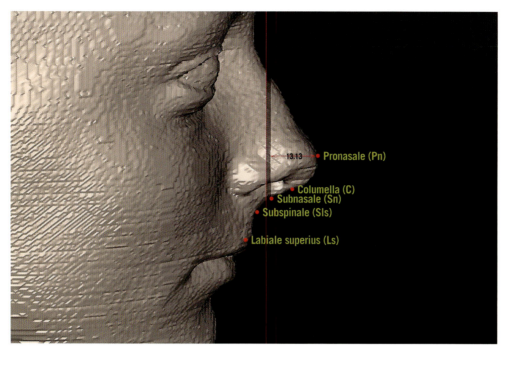

Fig 6-27 3D-reconstructed maxillary area, showing the distance of landmarks from the TVP.

Fig 6-28 Representation on 2D image: length of the upper lip, length of the lower lip and chin, and interlabial distance.

LENGTH OF THE UPPER LIP

Measured from subnasale to stomion (Sn–Sto). The interlabial distance is measured from the labiale superius to the labiale inferius (Ls–Li). The standard length of the upper lip is 19 to 22 mm; the length of the lower lip to the soft tissue chin is 42 to 48 mm, and it occupies the lower two-thirds of this space. The interlabial distance is about 1.5 mm, and it is greater in women than in men because of the greater length of lips (Figs 6-28 and 6-29).

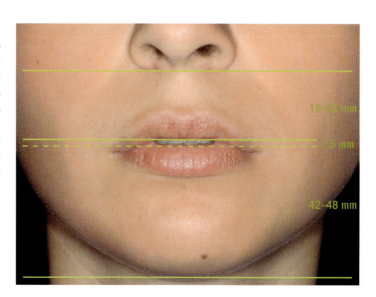

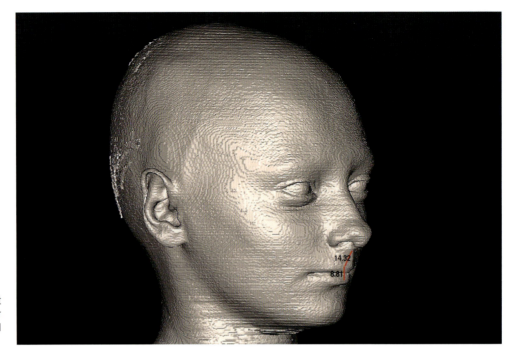

Fig 6-29 Measurement of the length of the upper lip and of the interlabial distance shown in 3D.

Mandibular Area

In the mandibular area it is possible to observe three soft tissue zones[32]: the prominence of the lower lip, the prominence of the soft tissue pogonion, and the length and contour of throat (Figs 6-30 to 6-33).

In the mandibular area the following measurements have been selected: prominence of the lower lip and prominence of the soft tissue pogonion.

PROMINENCE OF THE LOWER LIP
The lower lip can be defined as retruded, normal, or protruded. In females, the prominence of the lower lip with reference to the TVL is 0.5 to 3.3 mm; in males, 1.2 to 3.2 mm. The labiomental fold can be described as accentuated, normal, or flattened.

PROMINENCE OF THE SOFT TISSUE POGONION
The soft tissue pogonion can be defined as retruded, normal, or protruded. Normal values with reference to the TVL in females are −4.5 to −0.7 mm; in males, −5.3 to −1.7 mm.

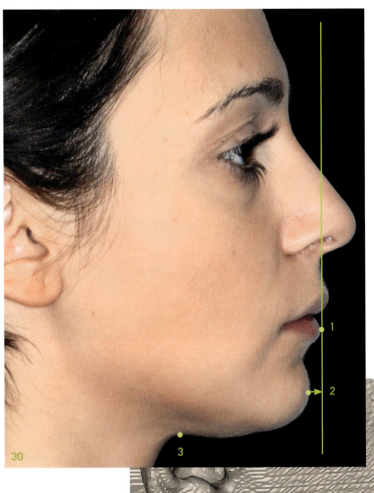

Fig 6-30 Representation of the mandibular area in 2D lateral view: 1, prominence of the lower lip; 2, soft tissue pogonion; 3, neck/throat junction.

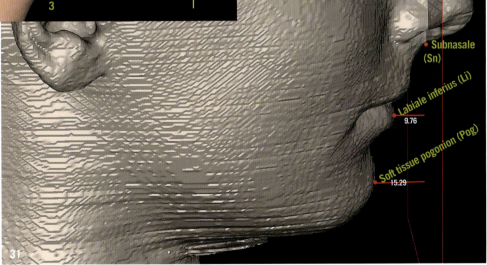

Fig 6-31 Representation of the mandibular area in 3D reconstruction. Notice the projection of the lower lip and the chin with reference to the TVP.

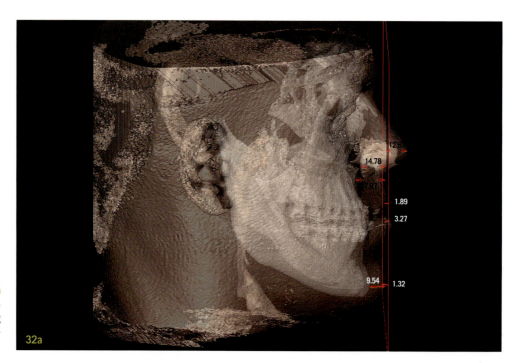

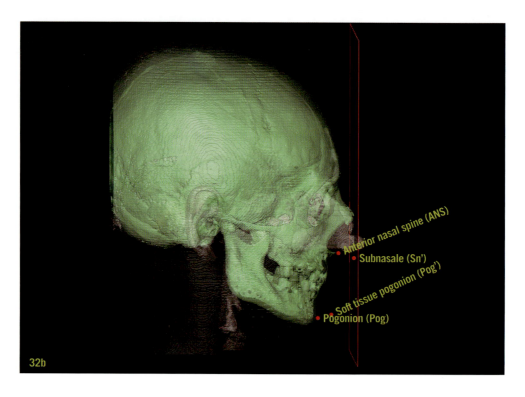

Figs 6-32a and 6-32b Projection of soft tissues and underlying hard tissues with reference to the TVP.

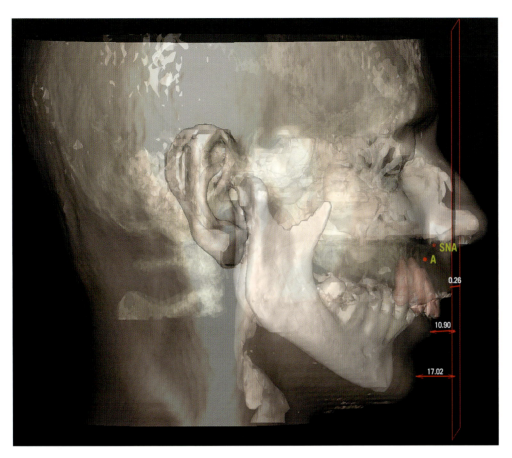

Fig 6-33 In the image it is possible to see the prominences of the upper and lower lips with reference to the TVP and, at the same time, to compare the position of soft tissues with reference to the underlying hard tissues and to assess dental support. This patient presents a very marked case of lower lip retrusion, evident retrusion of the mandible, and poor mandibular dental support. It is also possible to observe an increase in overjet and proclination of the maxillary incisors. The upper lip is short, and, as a consequence, there is an increase in the exposure of the maxillary incisors.

Nasolabial Angle

The nasolabial angle is formed by the intersection of two lines at the level of the subnasale landmark: a line tangent to the nasal base and the other to the outer edge of the upper lip (Figs 6-34 to 6-37). The mean value of this angle is about 90 to 95 degrees in men and 100 to 105 degrees in women.[31] The 3D assessment allows not only measurement of the nasolabial angle and its comparison with standard values but also analysis of the factors it depends on: nose tip, lip length, lip thickness, maxillary position, and dental support.

Fig 6-34 Slightly open labial angle (107.39 degrees).

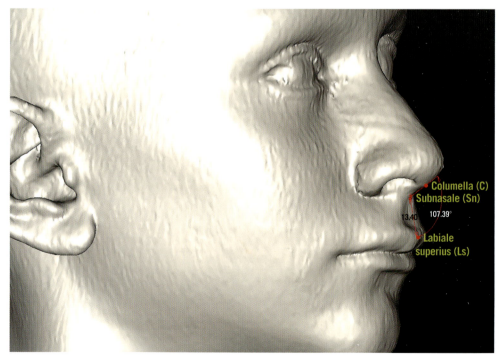

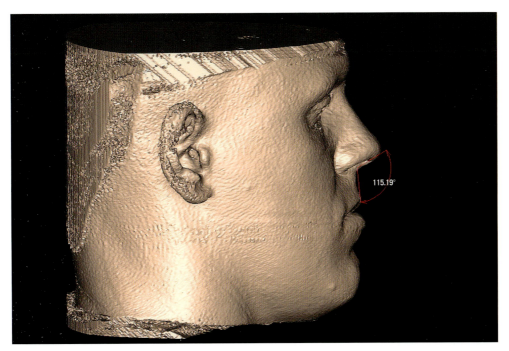

Fig 6-35 Open nasolabial angle (115.19 degrees), with significant maxillary retrusion.

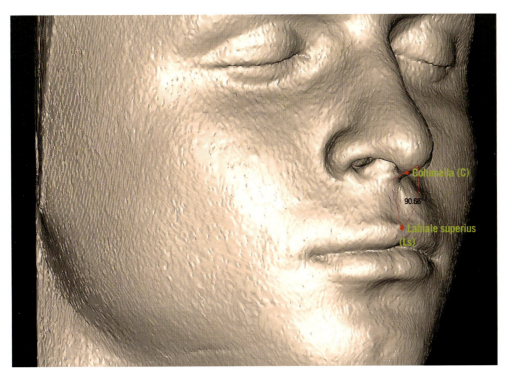

Fig 6-36 Normal nasolabial angle (91.66 degrees).

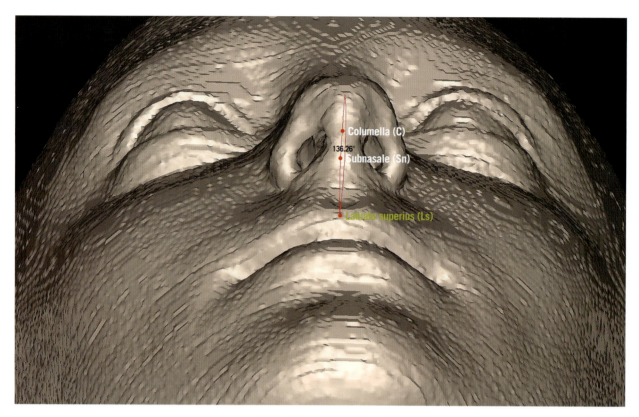

Fig 6-37 Nasolabial angle seen from below the chin.

TFA 3

Vertical Height of the Face and Lower Middle Third

The TFA 3 3D analysis is performed to assess the vertical dimensions of the face and of the lower middle third (Figs 6-38 to 6-40). Changes from the standard inevitably imply lack of harmony in the vertical dimension as measured with reference to the axial plane (z).

A decrease/increase in the lower vertical height with reference to the total facial dimension is defined respectively as short face (Fig 6-41) or long face (Fig 6-42). Furthermore, it is possible to assess an excess or defect in maxillary or chin height.

The anterior vertical dimension of the face is measured from the plane passing through the soft tisse nasion landmark to the soft tissue menton (N'–Me' distance), which should normally be 137 ± 4.7 mm, whereas the lower vertical dimension is measured from the vertical plane passing through subnasale to the plane passing through the soft tissue menton (Sn–Me'). The lower third should vary between 77 and 85 mm in men and 67 and 75 mm in women.[32]

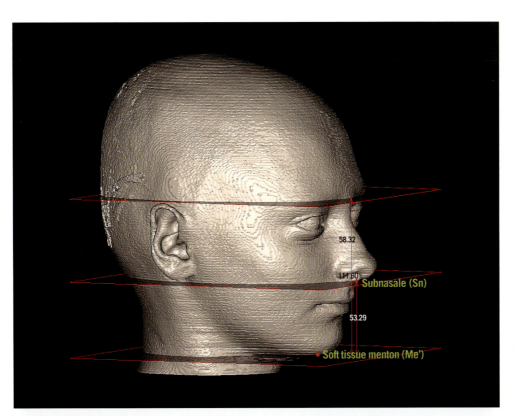

Fig 6-38 Assessment of the anterior vertical dimension of the face: total vertical (N'–Me') and lower (Sn–Me') dimensions.

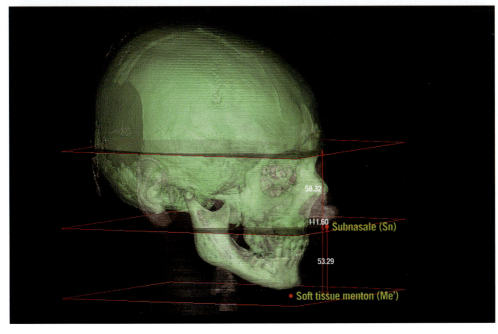

Fig 6-39 Assessment of the anterior vertical dimension of the face using the soft tissue transparence function.

Assessment of the Lower Third

The lower third of the face (see Fig 6-40) consists of the upper lip (one-third of the space) and the chin (two-thirds). The interlabial distance is measured from the lowest point of the upper lip to the highest point of the lower lip.

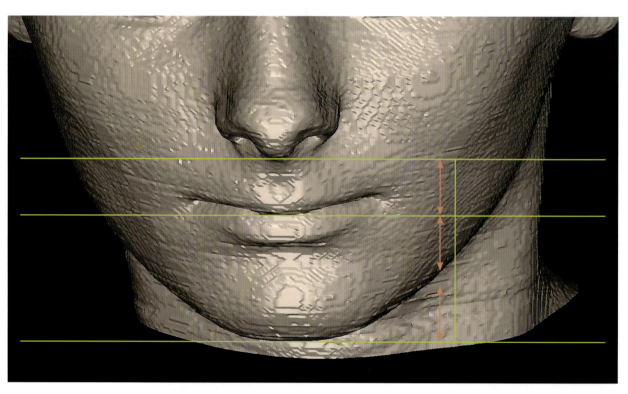

Fig 6-40 In the lower third of the face, the upper lip usually occupies one-third of the space and the lower lip with the chin, two-thirds. However, in this patient the length of the upper lip *(orange arrow)* occupies less than one-third of the space. Further investigation will be needed to detect whether the length of the upper lip is less than the standard, or whether the segment of the lower lip including the chin is too long.

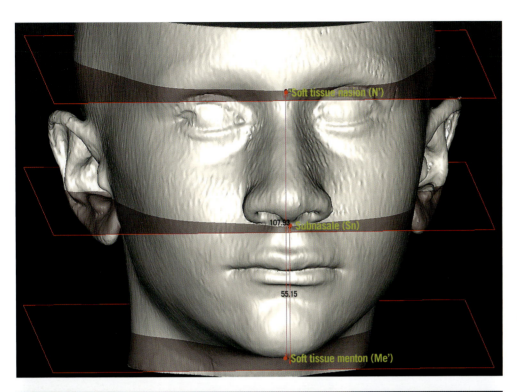

Fig 6-41 Example of face with reduced lower vertical dimension in relation to the total vertical dimension (short face).

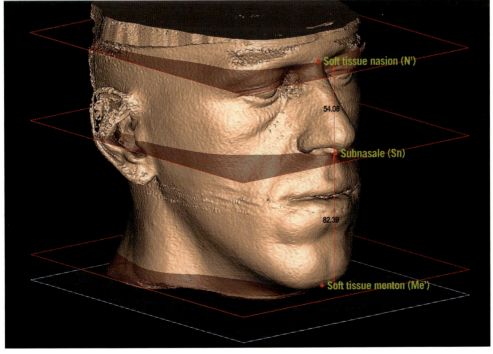

Fig 6-42 Example of long face: the lower vertical dimension is increased with reference to the total vertical dimension (long face).

Lips

The assessment of the lower third of the face includes an analysis of the lips, which can be classified according to their shape or size as thin, medium, or thick (Fig 6-43). During life, lips undergo physiologic thinning. The desire to maintain a young facial appearance with turgid lips has prompted frequent use of esthetic surgery to modify the shape and volume of the lips.

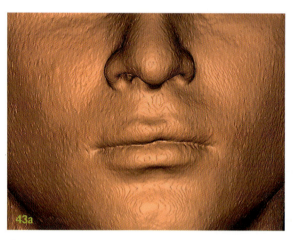
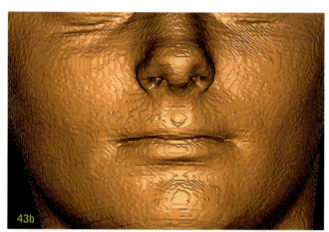
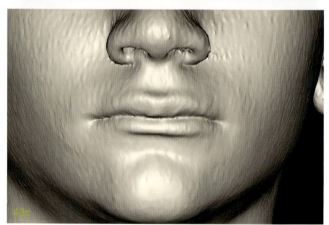

Fig 6-43a to 6-43c Various shapes and sizes of lips (3D volumetric reconstruction).

TFA 4

Analysis of Symmetry

Symmetry was conventionally analyzed on 2D photographs by drawing a midline dividing the face into two parts. The line had to be perpendicular to the bipupillary line (see Fig 6-4).

The intersection of the midline with the horizontal planes created a sort of proportionally organized network allowing analysis of symmetry between the right and left side of the face. A slight asymmetry of the face would fall into the norm, and asymmetry is only noticed by the observer if the discrepancy between right and left side exceeds 3%.[8]

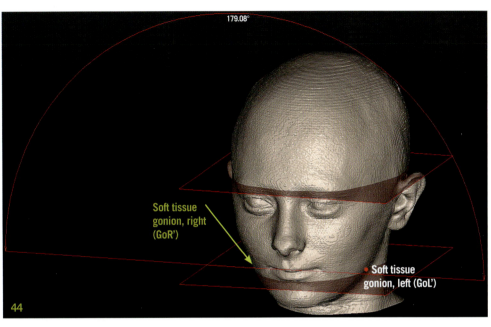

Fig 6-44 Parallelism of the plane containing the right and left soft tissue gonion, relative to the superior facial plane (SFP).

Fig 6-45 Parallelism of the plane containing the right and left soft tissue endocanthion relative to the SFP.

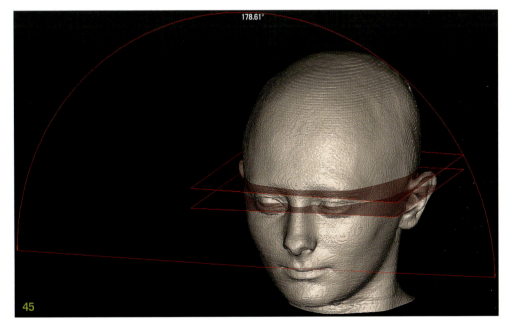

The 3D symmetry analysis, as opposed to that done in 2D, is performed by measuring the parallelism between planes and reference planes (superior facial plane and mental plane) (Fig 6-44 to 6-47; also see Table 6-1). Alternatively, the same analysis can be performed by measuring the distance of landmarks to the reference planes (Figs 6-48 and 6-49). In symmetric patients, the planes passing through the right and left landmarks should be parallel to the reference planes. A slight tilt (about 3 degrees) does not indicate asymmetry as this still falls into the range. A greater tilt, on the contrary, can indicate asymmetry.

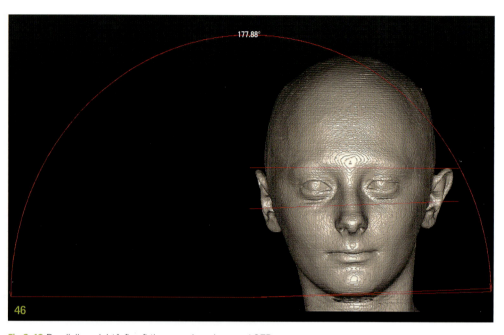

Fig 6-46 Parallelism right/left soft tissue zygion plane and SFP.

Fig 6-47 The patient presents marked mandibular asymmetry as seen from the right/left soft tissue zygion plane with reference to the SFP (175.3 degrees).

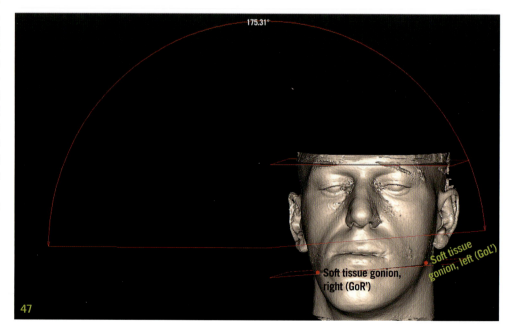

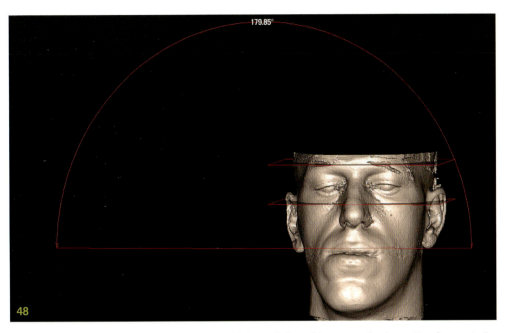

Fig 6-48 Assessment of symmetry of the median third: parallelism of the zygomatic plane with reference to the SFP (179.85 degrees). There is no symmetry of the middle third.

Fig 6-49 The asymmetry of the chin can be measured as the distance of the landmark to the plane: the distance of the right and left soft tissue chin to the SFP is shown (difference, 2.2 mm).

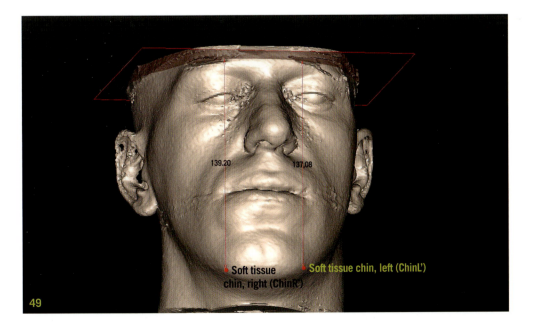

Diagnostic 3D AnalyDiagnostic Work-up: 3D Analysis of Soft Tissues with Mutiplanar Cephalometric Analysis: Clinical Cases

CLINICAL CASE 1
Female patient MM, aged 20 years
Skeletal diagnosis:
Skeletal Class II, hypodivergent skeletal pattern, reduced vertical dimension
Dental diagnosis:
Deep bite, multiple tooth agenesis: maxillary right lateral incisor, canine, first and second premolars and second molar; maxillary left lateral incisor, canine, second premolar and second molar; mandibular right second molar; mandibular left second premolar and second molar

Patient medical history: hypothyroidism treated with levothyroxine.
At initial visit: skeletal Class II, dental Class II, short face, deep bite; multiple agenesis of teeth as noted (see box at left).
Diagnostic steps: diagnostic set-up and CBCT imaging; orthodontic and implant-surgical treatment planning; esthetic and skeletal assessment (Figs 6-50 to 6-56).
Treatment plan:

- Oral rehabilitation after extracting primary (primary maxillary left second molar and maxillary right canine and molars) and permanent teeth (maxillary right and left lateral incisors and maxillary left first premolar)
- Guided bone regeneration
- Provisional prosthesis
- Implant placement: maxillary right and left lateral incisors, canines, and second premolars
- Final prosthesis

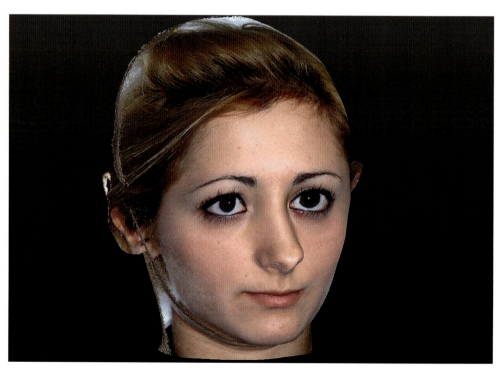

Fig 6-50 3D photograph of the patient.

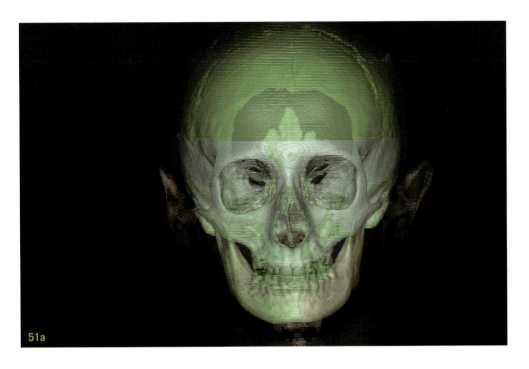

Fig 6-51 3D volumetric reconstruction of soft tissues and hard tissues using the transparence function.

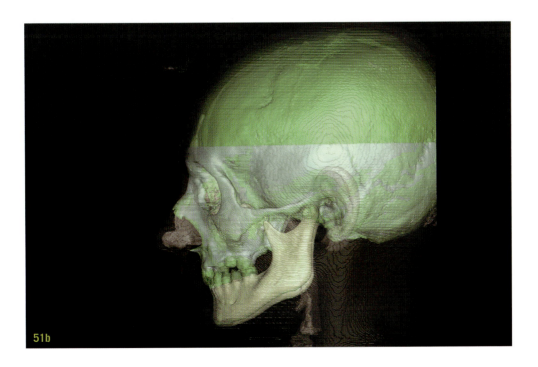

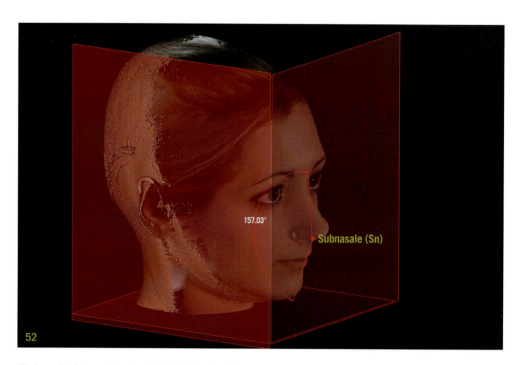

Fig 6-52 Profile angle typical of skeletal Class II.

Fig 6-53 The profile is convex, showing retrusion of the mandible and of the lips with reference to the TVP.

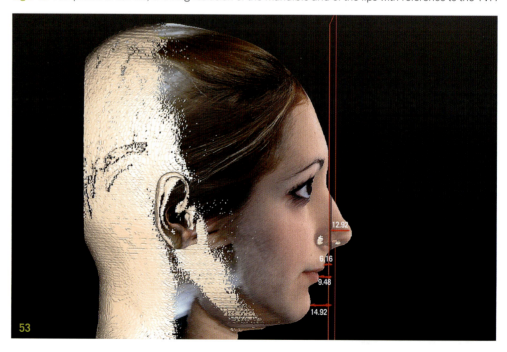

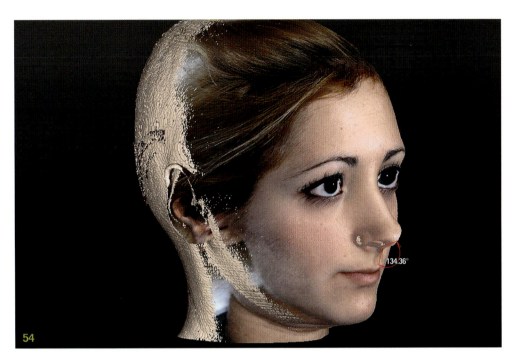

Fig 6-54 Open nasolabial angle.

Fig 6-55 Total vertical dimension.

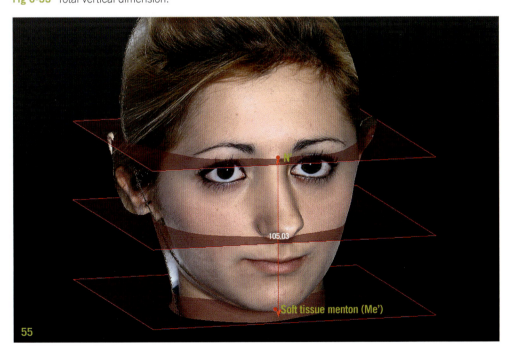

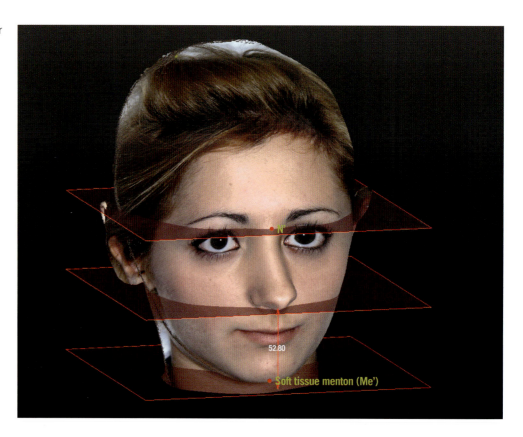

Fig 6-56 Reduced lower vertical dimension.

Orthognatic surgery with pre- and postsurgical orthodontic treatment.
Patient medical history: noncontributory.
Initial patient visit, 15 years of age: skeletal Class III, maxillary deficiency, mandibular prognathism, hyperdivergent skeletal pattern; lateral deviation to the right; periodic follow-up visits planned to monitor residual growth: no TMJ condition.
17 years of age: presence of acute left TMJ condition with mild symptoms, clicking when opening the mouth, and a tendency toward right lateral deviation; periodic follow-up visits to monitor residual growth, stabilization plate.
19 years of age: beginning of the fixed orthodontic treatment with maxillary and mandibular bands, CBCT imaging and 3D facial photographs (Proface, PlanMeca), and planning of orthognathic surgery (Figs 6-57 to 6-65). Patient skeletal Class III, maxillary retrusion, mandibular protrusion, chin asymmetry.
20.5 years of age: orthognathic surgery.
21 years of age: removal of orthodontic appliance; splinting of mandibular canine to canine; maxillary removable retainer; after 6 months, follow-up CBCT scan and 3D Proface photographs for postsurgery esthetic assessment (Figs 6-66 to 6-73).

CLINICAL CASE 2
Orthognathic surgery
Male patient TD, aged 21 years
Skeletal diagnosis:
Skeletal Class III, maxillary deficiency, mandibular prognathism, hyperdivergent skeletal pattern

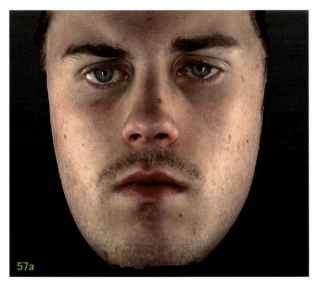
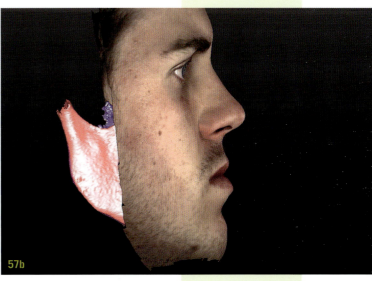

Figs 6-57a and 6-57b
3D photographs of patient in frontal and lateral views before surgery.

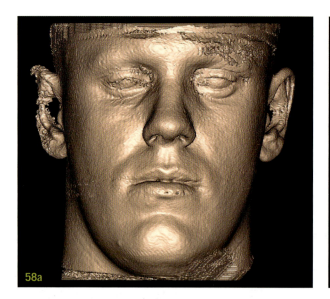
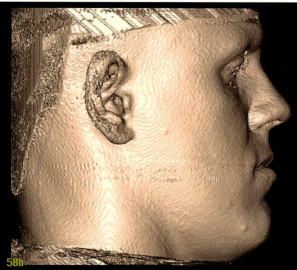

Figs 6-58a and 6-58b 3D volumetric reconstruction of the patient's face obtained with CBCT using orthodontic software (Materialise).

Fig 6-59 Angle of the profile typical for skeletal Class III.

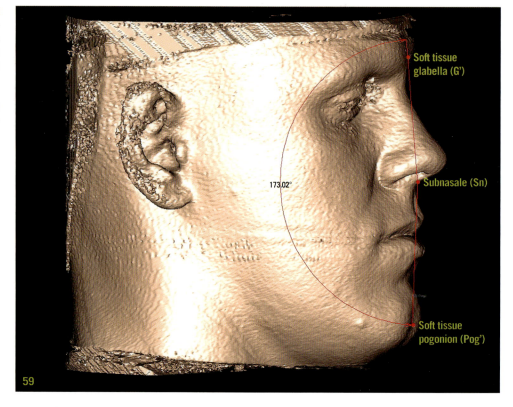

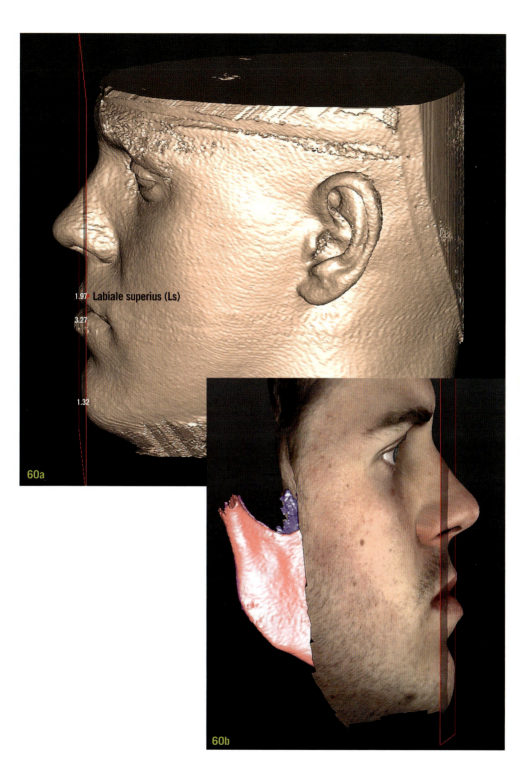

Figs 6-60a and 6-60b Profilometric analysis with reference to the TVP. The observer can notice a slight maxillary retrusion and protrusion of the mandible and the lower lip.

Fig 6-61 Measurement of the nasolabial angle, which is slightly open (standard: 90 to 95 degrees for men).

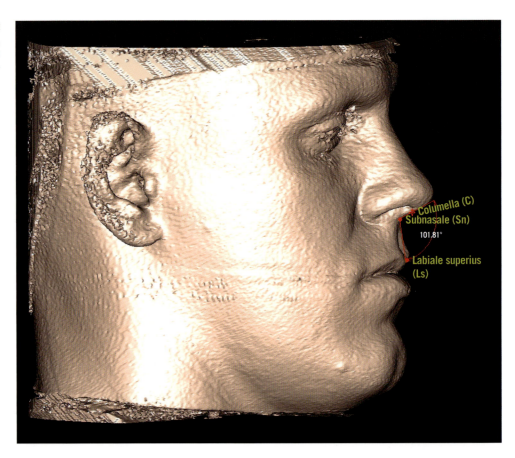

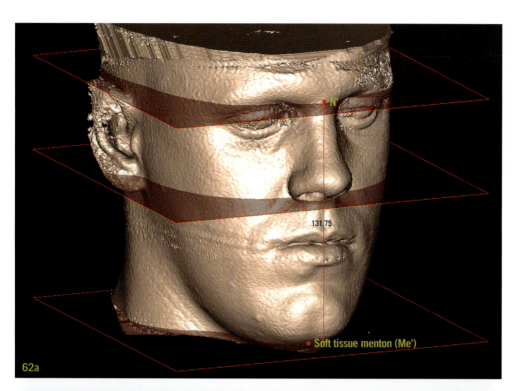

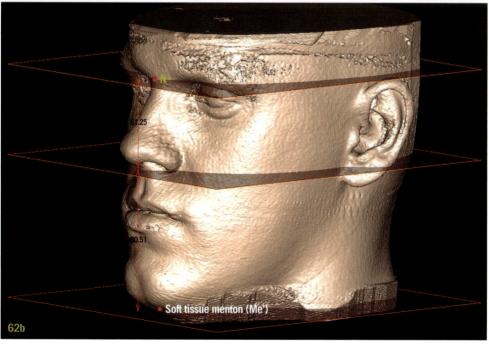

Figs 6-62a and 6-62b Measurement of the total vertical dimension (N'–Me') and of the lower vertical dimension (Sn–Me'). The total and lower vertical dimensions are within the standard (ie, N'–Me' 137.7 ± 6.5 mm, Sn–Me' 81.1 ± 4.7 mm in men).[32]

Fig 6-63 Comparison of measurements for the right and left chin landmarks with reference to the SFP. Chin asymmetry is evident.

Fig 6-64 Measurement of the soft tissue gonion plane tilt with reference to the SFP. The pogonion plane is parallel.

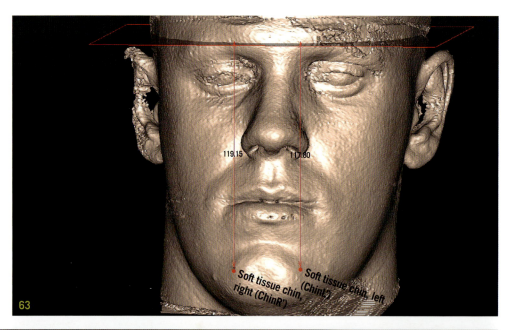

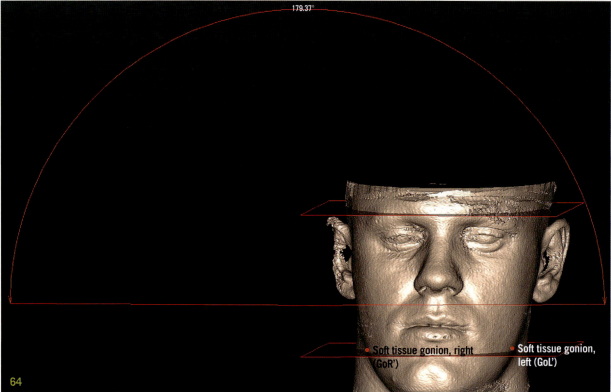

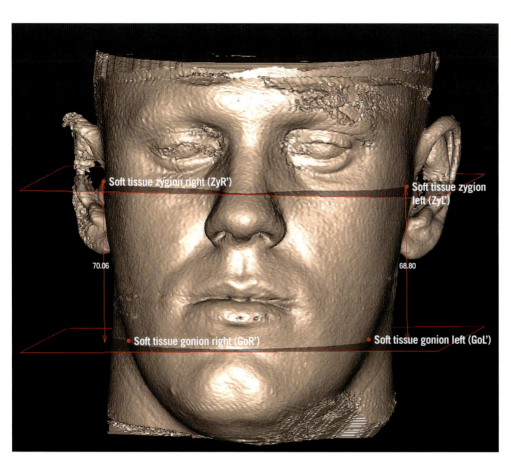

Fig 6-65 Measurement of the distance between the zygion and gonion planes at right and left. The measurement shows that the left side of the patient is about 2 mm shorter than the right.

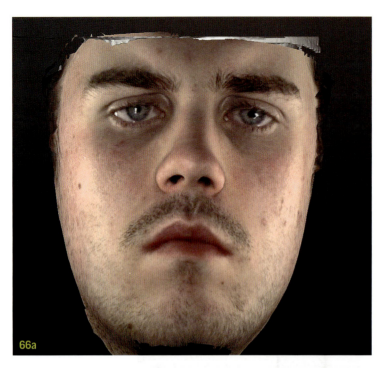

Esthetic Assessment After Orthognathic Surgery

Six months after bimaxillary orthognathic surgery, a new CBCT examination was requested, and new 3D photographs (Proface) were taken for a postsurgical esthetic analysis (Figs 6-66 to 6-73).

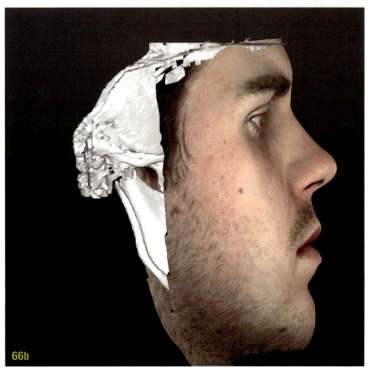

Figs 6-66a and 6-66c 3D photograph of the patient obtained with CBCT and stereophotogrammetry (Proface) after orthognathic surgery.

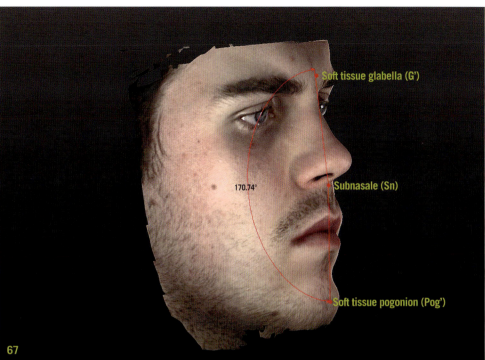

Fig 6-67 Profilometric analysis: angle of the profile. The observer can note that the value of the profile angle has decreased from about 173 degrees to about 170 degrees after surgery (see Fig 6-59).

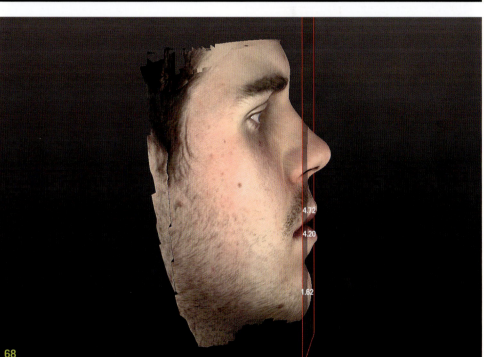

Fig 6-68 Profilometric analysis performed with reference to the TVP. It is possible to observe the improvement in profile after surgery through correction of maxillary retrusion and mandibular protrusion.

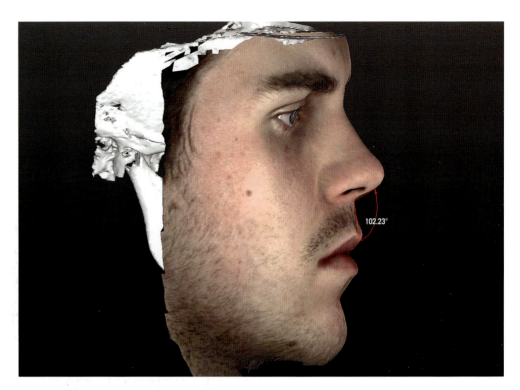

Fig 6-69 Measurement of the nasolabial angle, which has not changed from the presurgical value (see Fig 6-61).

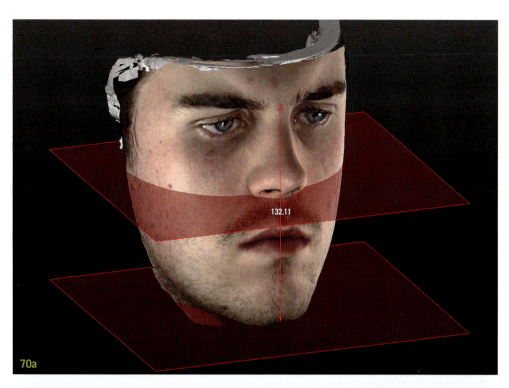

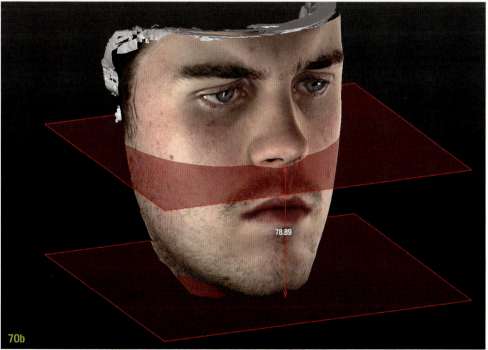

Figs 6-70a and 6-70b The total (N'–Me') and lower (Sn–Me') vertical dimensions have not changed after surgery.

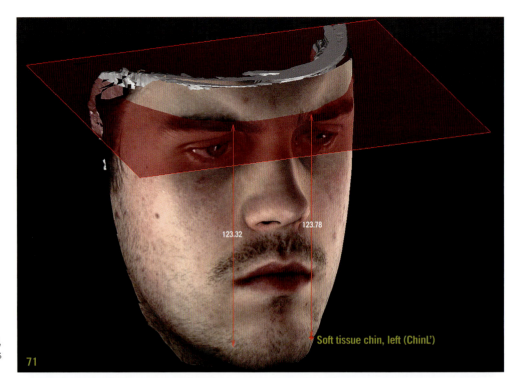

Fig 6-71 After surgery, chin asymmetry has been corrected.

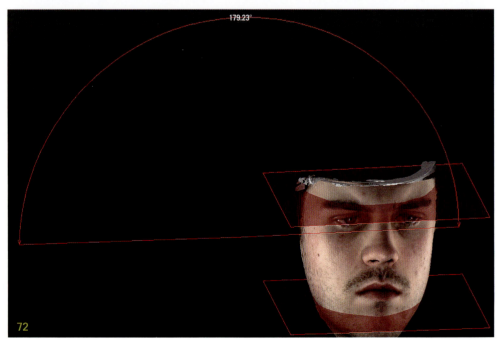

Fig 6-72 The parallelism of the gonion plane with reference to the SFP has not changed after surgery.

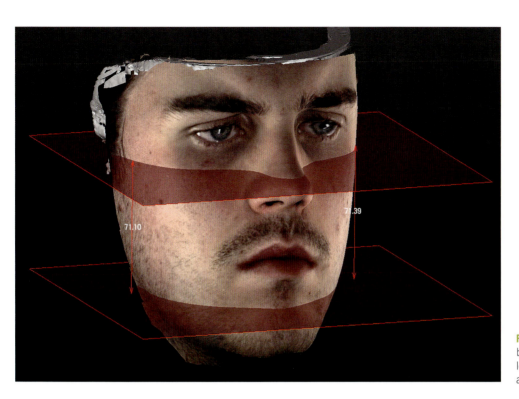

Fig 6-73 The distances between the right and left soft tissue pogonion and zygion are identical.

The 3D analysis allows the clinician to perform several tasks:

- Assess the relationship of the various facial components
- Check the symmetry of the facial segments in relation to the SFP
- Measure total facial height and the height of the various segments
- Assess the anteroposterior relationships of soft tissues and underlying hard tissues with reference to the TVP

Therefore, 3D analysis allows the clinician to do a precise and accurate assessment and diagnosis, and it also guides the clinician in facial evaluation when preparing oral rehabilitation or planning corrective surgery.

We nevertheless recommend the use of numeric values as an indication of facial harmony or disharmony. According to Tessier, "harmony and disharmony do not depend on angles, distances, lines, surfaces or volumes; they stem from proportions."[33]

References

1. Varela M, Garcià Camba JE. Impact on the psychologic profile of adult patients: A prospective study. Am J Orthod Dentofacial Orthop 1995;108:142–148.
2. Kitay D, BeGole EA, Eans CA, Giddon DB. Computer-animated comparison of self-perception with actual profiles of orthodontic and nonorthodontic subjects. Int J Adult Orthodon Orthognath Surg 1999;14:125–134.
3. Knight H, Keith O. Ranking facial attractiveness. Eur J Orthod 2005;27:340–348.
4. Jung D. Schwarze CW, Tsutsumi S. Profile and skeletal analyses—A comparison of different assessment procedures [in German]. Fortschr Kieferorthop 1984;45,304–323.
5. Downs WB. Analysis of the dentofacial profile. Angle Orthod 1956;26:191–212.
6. Moorrees CF, Gron AM. Principles of orthodontic diagnosis. Angle Orthod 1966;36:258–262.
7. Moorrees C, Kean MR. Natural Head Position: A basic consideration in the interpretation of cephalometric radiographs. Am J Phys Anthropol 1958;16:213–234.
8. Fradeani M. Esthetic Rehabilitationn in Fixed Prosthodontics, vol 1. London: Quintessence, 2004.
9. Majid Z, Chong CA, Ahmad A, Setan H, Setan H, Samsudin AR. Photogrammetry and 3D laser scanning as spatial data capture techniques for a national craniofacial database. Photogramm Rec 2005;20:48–68.
10. Ghoddousi H, Edler R, Haers P, Wertheim D, Greenhill D. Comparison of three methods of facial measurement. Int J Oral Maxillofac Surg 2007;36:250–258.
11. Sawyer AR, See M, Nduka C. 3D stereophotogrammetry quantitative lip analysis. Aesthetic Plast Surg 2009;33:497–504.
12. Wong JY, Oh AK, Ohta E, et al. Validity and reliability of craniofacial anthropometric measurement of 3D digital photogrammetric images. Cleft Palate Craniofac J 2008;45:232–239.
13. Weinberg SM, Scott NM, Neiswanger K, Brandon CA, Marazita ML. Digital three-dimensional photogrammetry: Evaluation of anthropometric precision and accuracy using a Genex 3D camera system. Cleft Palate Craniofac J 2004;41:507–518.
14. De Menezes M, Rosati R, Ferrario VF, Sforza C. Accuracy and reproducibility of a 3-dimensional stereophotogrammetric imaging system. J Oral Maxillofac Surg 2010;68:2129–2135.
15. Hennessy RJ, McLearie S, Kinsella A, Waddington JL. Facial shape and asymmetry by three-dimensional laser surface scanning covary with cognition in a sexually dimorphic manner. J Neuropsychiatry Clin Neurosci 2006;18:73–80.
16. Gateno J, Xia JJ, Teichgraeber JF. A new three-dimensional cephalometric analysis for orthognathic surgery. J Oral Maxillofac Surg 2011;69:606–622.
17. Burstone CJ. The integumental profile. Am J Orthod 1958;44:1–25.
18. Burstone CJ. Lip posture and its significance in treatment planning. Am J Orthod 1967;53:262–284.
19. Subtelny JD. A longitudinal study of soft tissue facial structures and their profile characteristics, defined in relation to underlying skeletal structures. Am J Orthod 1959;45:481–507.
20. Schwarz AM. Roentgenostatics: A practical evaluation of the x-ray headplate. Am J Orthod 1961;47:561–585.
21. Holdaway RA. A soft tissue cephalometric analysis and its use in orthodontic treatment planning. Part I. Am J Orthod 1983;84:1–28.
22. Ricketts RM. Cephalometric analysis and synthesis. Angle Orthod 1961;31:141–156.
23. Burstone CJ, James RB, Legan H, Murphy GA, Norton LA. Cephalometrics for orthognathic surgery. J Oral Surg 1978;36:269–277.
24. Jacobson RL. Facial analysis in two and three dimensions. In: Jacobson A (ed). Radiographic Cephalometry: From Basics to Videoimaging. Chicago: Quintessence, 1994:273–294.
25. Jacobson RL. Three dimensional cephalometry. In: Jacobson A, Jacobson RL (eds). Radiographic Cephalometry: From Basics to 3D imaging, ed 2. Chicago: Quintessence, 2006: 249–253.
26. Farkas LG, Munro IR. Anthropometric Facial Proportions in Medicine. Springfield: Charles C Thomas, 1987.

27. Swennen GRJ. 3-D cephalometric soft tissue landmarks. In: Swennen GRJ, Schutyser F, Hausamen JE (eds). Three-Dimensional Cephalometry: A Color Atlas and Manual. Berlin: Springer, 2005: 186–226.
28. Owens EG, Goodacre CJ, Loh PL, et al. A multicenter interracial study of facial appearance. Part 1: A comparison of extraoral parameters. Int J Prosthodont 2002;15:273–282.
29. Arnett GW, Bergman RT. Facial keys to orthodontic diagnosis and treatment planning. Part I. Am J Orthod Dentofacial Orthop 1993;103:299–312.
30. Arnett GW, Bergman RT. Facial keys to orthodontic diagnosis and treatment planning. Part II. Am J Orthod Dentofacial Orthop 1993;103:395–411.
31. Arnett GW, Jelic JS, Kim J. Soft tissue cephalometric analysis: Diagnosis and treatment planning of dentofacial deformity. Am J Orthod Dentofac Orthop 1999;116:239–253.
32. Arnett GW, McLaughlin RP. Pianificazione Estetica e Programmazione Ortodontica in Chirurgia Ortognatica. Milan: Elsevier Masson, 2006:65–75.
33. Tessier P. Anatomical classification of facial, craniofacial and lateral facial clefts. J Oral Maxillofac Surg 1976;4:69–92.

G Perrotti

7

3D Analysis of the Temporomandibular Joint

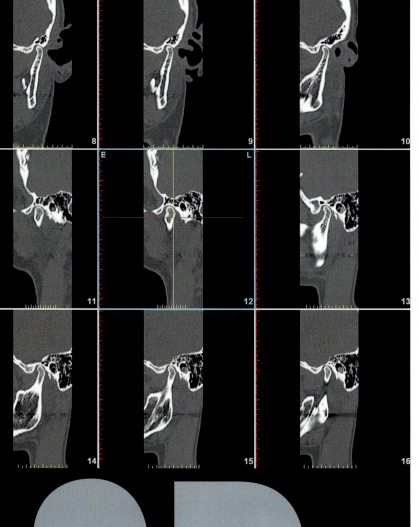

Study of the degenerative/erosive processes of articular condyles has been performed for years using conventional 2D images such as magnetic resonance imaging (MRI) and, in severe cases, with multislice spiral computed tomography (MSCT).

Currently, cone beaam CT (CBCT), if the radiation exposure is properly controlled, allows a nosologic, careful, and detailed classification of joint degenerations and, therefore, an accurate diagnosis.

While CBCT is not the examination of choice for chronic dysfunctional conditions, it is now more common to use CBCT than CT in condylar fractures and for a detailed analysis of degenerative processes in the condylar head.

Anatomy and Pathology of the TMJ

Good knowledge of the anatomy of the TMJ and its muscles and ligaments is the first requisite for proper treatment of pathologies affecting this joint (Fig 7-1).

Temporomandibular Joint

The TMJ is a bilateral and complete diarthrosis.[1] It consists of two articular surfaces, the mandibular condyle and the glenoid or articular fossa of the temporal bone, with the articular disk in the middle.
Each joint consists of four distinct anatomical components:

- Mandibular condyle
- Articular surface with the squamous portion of the temporal bone
- Articular disk
- Articular capsule

The condyle is part of the mandibular condylar process that extends superiorly, posteriorly, and medially.

- Its shape is variable and usually ovoid; its mediolateral diameter is about 20 mm, and its anteroposterior diameter is about 10 mm.
- The long axes of the paired condyles converge posteriorly, forming an obtuse angle

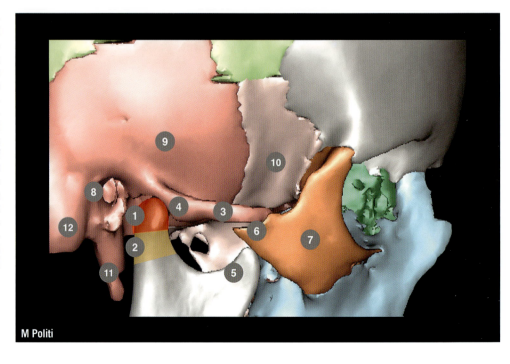

Fig 7-1 3D reconstruction of the relevant cranial bones and TMJ structures: (1) condylar head; (2) condylar neck; (3) zygomatic process of the temporal bone; (4) articular eminence of the temporal bone; (5) coronoid process of the mandible; (6) temporal process of the zygomatic bone; (7) zygomatic bone; (8) internal acoustic meatus; (9) temporal bone; (10) sphenoid bone; (11) styloid process of the temporal bone; (12) mastoid process of the temporal bone.

of about 170 degrees that opens anteriorly. The zygomatic process is part of the temporal bone, and it includes the articular fossa and the articular eminence.

The fossa is concave anteroposteriorly and mediolaterally, and its roof is in close relation with the middle cranial fossa.

The articular eminence is a bony ridge continuing laterally in the root of the zygomatic arch. It is convex anteroposteriorly and slightly concave mediolaterally.

The articular disk is made of fibrous connective tissue and has a biconcave shape, thin at the center and thicker in its anterior and posterior parts. This part of the disk continues posteriorly as retrodiscal tissue, which consists of highly vascularized loose connective tissue. The articular disk has several distinguishing features:

- It divides the joint into two separate compartments, the superior and the inferior articular compartments.
- It is made of dense connective tissue, and it is affixed to the articular ligament.
- Its profile corresponds to the temporal articular surface in its superior part and to the condylar surface in its inferior part.
- The central part is biconcave and thin; the posterior part is in continuity with a pad of highly vascularized and highly innervated loose connective tissue (Fig 7-2).

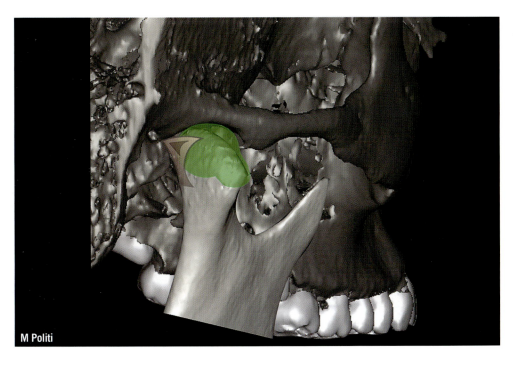

Fig 7-2 3D image of the mandible and the splanchnocranium or facial skeleton. The articular disk connected to the posterior lamina is highlighted in green.

The joint is covered by an articular capsule with an outer layer of fibrous connective tissue in continuity with the ligament and with the collagen fibers of the disk, and it contains the synovial fluid.

- It surrounds the joint, and it is fixed superiorly to the peripheral articular eminence of the temporal bone and inferiorly to the neck of the condylar process.
- It is well developed laterally and medially, while anteriorly and posteriorly it is in continuity with the loose adjacent tissue.

Its lateral thickening constitutes a stand-alone anatomical component, the temporomandibular ligament.

The synovial fluid secreted by the cells of the synovial tissue that fills the synovial cavities plays an important mechanical function; it lubricates and protects the articular tissues, and it also delivers nutrients to the structural elements of the nonvascularized parts. Under normal conditions, the fluid is a dialyzed byproduct of plasma, rich in proteoglycans and hyaluronic acid with few phagocytes, monocytes, and lymphocytes. The number of these cells increases noticeably when there is an inflammatory process.

Temporomandibular Ligament

The temporomandibular ligament consists of two distinct parts (Fig 7-3):

- An outer part with oblique fibers from the articular tubercle to the neck of the condyle.
- An inner part with nearly horizontal fibers from the articular tubercle to the condylar neck and to the posterior part of the disc.

Overview of TMJ Pathology

Pain in the orofacial region of nondental origin is the most common symptom in temporomandibular diseases. Pain can affect masticatory muscles and the preauricular area.
The American Academy of Orofacial Pain categorizes temporomandibular disorders as muscular, articular, and masticatory.[2]

TMJ pathologies can be classified as:

- Myofascial syndrome
- Craniocervical mandibular dysfunction
- Muscular tension migraine
- Fibromyalgia
- Arthritic degeneration of the TMJ, which is subdivided into:
  - Degenerative arthritis with low inflammatory index: osteoarthritis (a degenerative articular condition)
  - Degenerative arthritis with high inflammatory index: *(1)* infective arthritis, *(2)* rheumatoid arthritis in the young and in the adult, *(3)* metabolic arthritis (gout, psoriatic arthritis, lupus erhythematosus, ankylosing spondylitis, Reiter syndrome, arthritis associated with ulcerative colitis)

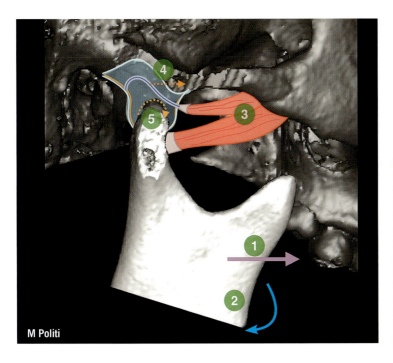

Fig 7-3 3D image of a mandible during opening of the mouth, with visualization of the structures involved in motion: (1) protrusion; (2) downward movement; (3) lateral pterygoid muscle; (4) forward movement of the disk and of the superior articular compartment; (5) rotating movement of the inferior articular compartment.

These diagnostic classifications are based on symptoms reported by patients and on their clinical examination; however, clinical examination alone is not sufficient to fully appreciate the bony tissue components and soft tissues of the TMJ. Radiologic exams are therefore performed to complete the diagnostic work-up.

Over the last 30 years, advancements in imaging have contributed to improved diagnosis of temporomandibular pathologies.

Radiologic Examinations of the TMJ

Various imaging modalities are used to assess the TMJ:

- Panoramic radiograph, the first-llevel exam[3]
- CT to assess bony components[4]
- MRI to assess all soft tissues in the joint[5]

The exam of choice to assess the TMJ is MRI, which allows the clinician to view both hard and soft tissues. MRI is performed

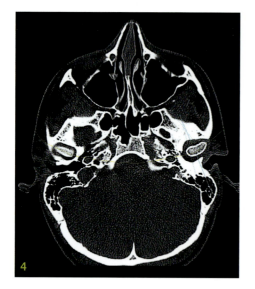
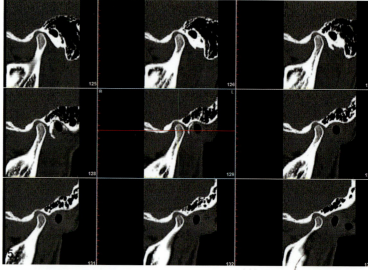

Fig 7-4 Axial view of normal condyles with the panoramic curve passing through the long axis of the condyles; this curve allows visualization of cross-sectional views.

Fig 7-5 Cross-sectional images of normal condyles.

Fig 7-6 3D rendering of facial bones in which the reconstruction of the condyles and their relationship with the glenoid fossa are well defined.

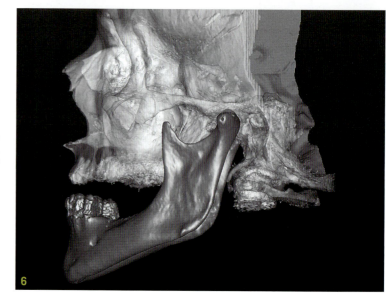

with both an open and a closed mouth, which is not desirable in CBCT because this will double the radiation exposure.

The radiographic examination is an essential part of the diagnosis and management of TMJ disorders. The aim of TMJ radiographic analysis is to assess the cortical and trabecular bony structures and their integrity, to measure the severity of lesions, to monitor progression in bone changes, and to evaluate response to treatment.[4]

An accurate TMJ assessment using conventional 2D radiographs may be insufficient due to overlapping of anatomical structures.

Panoramic radiography is useful as a preliminary screening tool to assess articular bone pathologies. Although it is a simple technique, it has several limitations that reduce its value in TMJ assessment. The structures are often distorted, and there is frequent overlapping of the zygomatic processes.[3] Panoramic radiography is not very reliable or sensitive in detecting bone changes, and its value in radiographic TMJ assessment is therefore limited.

With CT, sensitivity in detecting bone changes ranges from 53% to 90%, and specificity from 73% to 95%. CT provides excellent viewing of a broad spectrum of bone changes such as osteophytes (bone spurs), condylar erosion, fractures, dislocations, ankyloses, and abnormal growth such as condylar hyperplasia. Studies on cadaver samples have shown that CT has a sensitivity of 75% and a specificity of 100% in detecting bone changes with a positive predictive value of 100% and a negative predictive value of 78%.[5] Nevertheless, the high cost and the relatively high dose of radiation have limited the use of CT in TMJ assessment.

With the introduction of CBCT, it is now possible to obtain 3D images of bony structures in the facial skeleton with a much lower impact in terms of exposure to ionizing radiation. CBCT imaging is by far quicker, and it provides an image of both joints in a single scan during a 360-degree rotation around the patient's head.

Better access to CBCT equipment offers several benefits compared with multislice CT scans. With CBCT, the radiation dose is much lower than with CT; CBCT image resolution is typically higher than in CT protocols for TMJ imaging. Accuracy in detecting changes in bone surfaces and intraoperator reliability are comparable[6] for CBCT and multislice CT, with CBCT outperforming panoramic radiographs in that regard.

Recent guidelines recommend CT as the first-line examination of TMJ bone changes.[7] Because of the lower radiation dose and the increasing availability of CBCT equipment, it is now becoming the exam of choice in assessing TMJ bony components (Figs 7-4 to 7-6).

There are some parameters that influence image quality in CBCT. Crucial factors are the x-ray beam, the size of the FOV, the kind of detector, and the size of voxels reconstructed. These parameters change depending on the CBCT scanner used, but most units allow these parameters to be selected.

Therefore, when a specific TMJ assessment is performed by CBCT, it is important for clinicians to set up these parameters so as to obtain ideal images in this diagnostic task.[7]

In regard to the field of view (FOV), simpler units can be used with a collimated FOV of 4 cm × 4 cm × 4 cm and image capture with a voxel size of 78 µm or larger.

These scans with small FOVs can provide sufficient anatomical coverage including the condylar head, the glenoid fossa, and the articular TMJ eminence. A complete chin-apex FOV can be required. This can also be used in TMJ analysis. With these units, the size of the collimated image can vary from 10 to 20 cm (it is usually 15 cm) and the range of voxels from 200 to 400 μm. Of course, a complete FOV produces an image volume including both TMJs. Depending on the diagnostic task, it may be necessary to request an FOV for the entire maxillofacial skeleton to allow assessment of craniofacial asymmetry.[7]

Indications for CBCT Analysis of the TMJ

With CBCT it is possible to analyze the mandibular condyle, its position in the glenoid fossa, and the underlying cortical and trabecular bone structures. The following changes in TMJ bone components require prescription of a CBCT[8]:

- Osteoarthritis
- Rheumatoid arthritis
- Malignant tumors
- Condylar fractures
- Morphological changes of the condyle as a consequence of orthognathic surgery
- Condylar remodeling areas
- Idiopathic bone resorption

The criteria for classifying structural condylar changes according to Koyama et al[9,10] are (Figs 7-7 to 7-17):

1. Normal condyle: no increase in thickness or change in condylar surface from physiological conditions
2. Flattened condyle: flattened contour of the anteroposterior or posterosuperior portion of the condyle
3. Eroded condyle: modification towards superficial cell proliferation or erosion with change towards a hypodense bony structure, with or without roughening of the outer condylar surface
4. Deformed condyle: formation of osteophytic spurs without proliferation or hypodense tissue
5. Deformed condyle with osteophytes
6. Deformed and eroded condyle

Structural changes of condyles in osteoarthritic processes can appear in form of subchondral cysts, subchondral sclerosis, formation of osteophytes, condylar erosion, and remodeling.

The glenoid fossa is considered as positive when there is flattening, erosion, and/or sclerosis and as negative when the fossa appears to be normal.

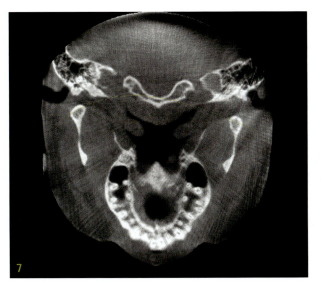

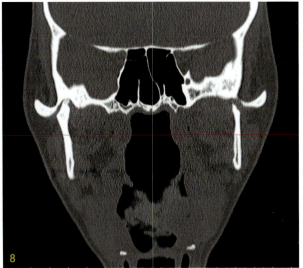

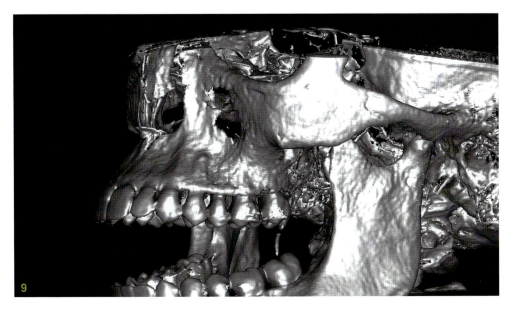

Fig 7-7 Axial image of the panoramic curve.

Fig 7-8 Coronal view showing the stage of erosion of the left condyle.

Fig 7-9 3D rendering of the patient in Fig 7-5.

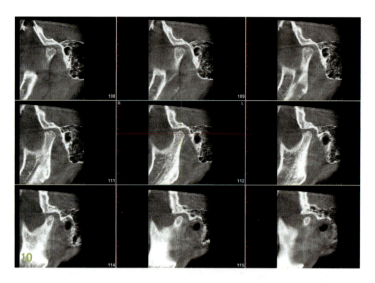
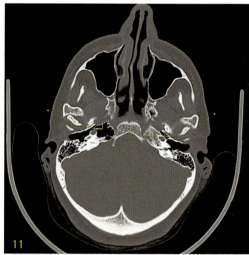

Fig 7-10 Cross-sectional image showing condylar erosion.
Fig 7-11 Panoramic curve.
Fig 7-12 Cross-sectional images showing severe erosion with condylar remodeling.

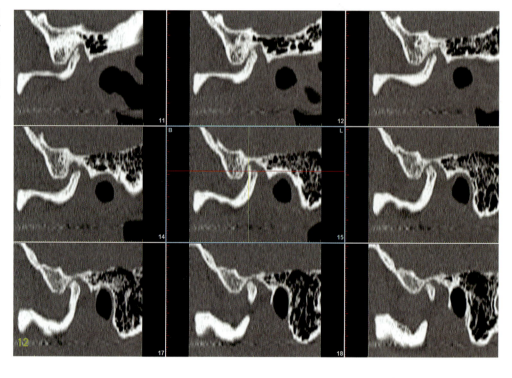

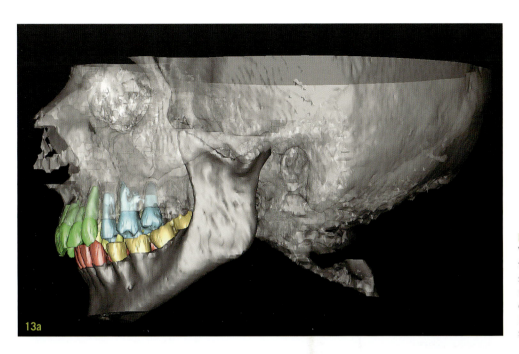

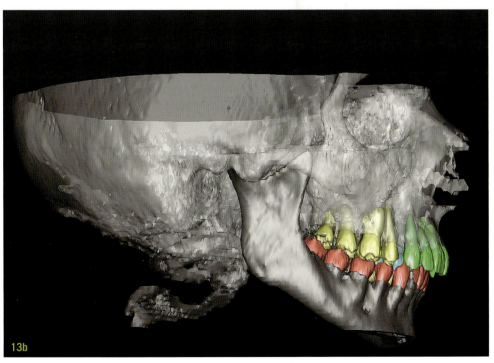

Figs 7-13a and 7-13b Volumetric reconstruction of the face. Observe the condylar remodeling and the large coronoid process on both the right and left sides.

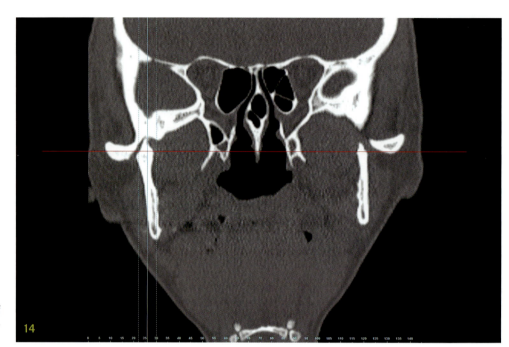

Fig 7-14 Coronal view of idiopathic bilateral condylar resorption.

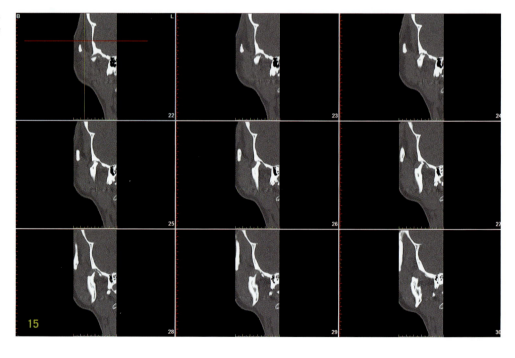

Fig 7-15 Cross-sectional view of severely eroded condyles.

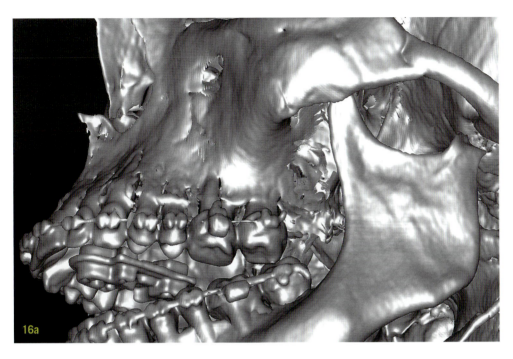
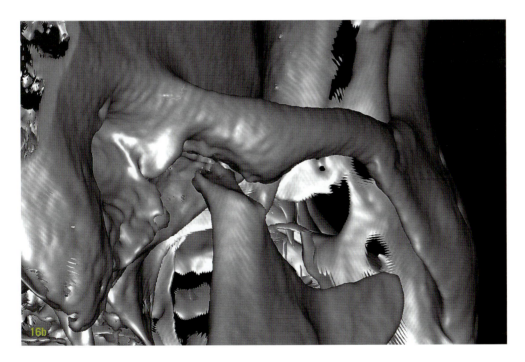

Figs 7-16a and 7-16b 3D views of condylar resorption.

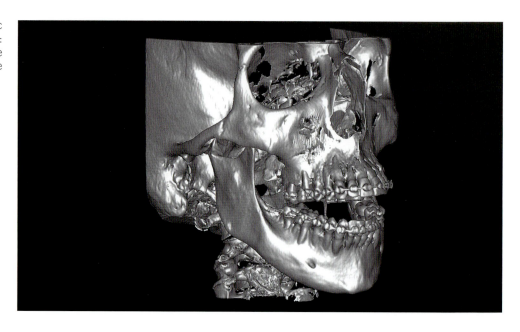

Fig 7-17 Volumetric rendering of the face: observe the open bite caused by progressive condylar erosion.

Optimal Imaging of Condylar Morphology

CBCT of the TMJ produces a set of scans whose thickness ranges from 0.3 to 1 mm.[11] Individual scans can be taken on the axial, coronal, or sagittal planes, and it is possible to obtain a 3D volumetric reconstruction. The specific study of condylar morphology also includes processing of paraxial sections (cross sections).[11]

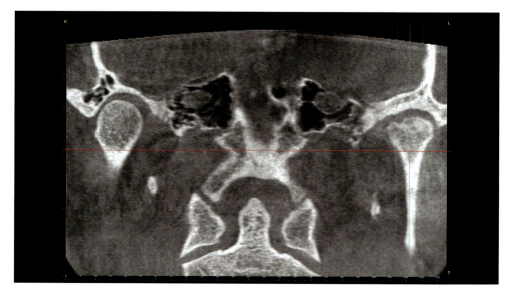

Fig 7-18 Coronal section of a girl aged 14 years: the left condyle appears eroded, although there is still adequate articular space. Erosion has appeared after widespread inflammatory processes affecting various joints and the presence of joint hyperlaxity. Acute pain has been the first pathognomonic sign associated with condylar degeneration.

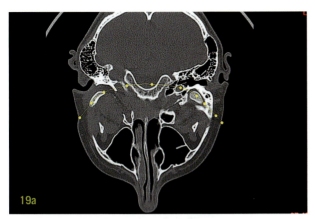

Fig 7-19a Axial view of the panoramic curve passing through the long condylar axis.

Fig 7-19b Coronal view of the sequelae of a condylar fracture in a 12-year-old patient not treated surgically. The fracture had occurred at the age of 8 years.

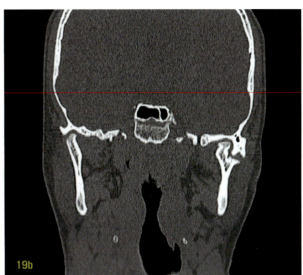

This view can be obtained with computer processing of paraxial sections of the coronal and lateral images of the perpendicular axis of the condyle. This is without question the most specific method for studying degeneration of the condylar head (Figs 7-18 and 7-19).

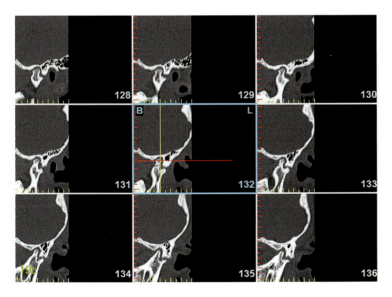

Fig 7-19c Cross-sectional view of the fractured condyle 4 years posttrauma.

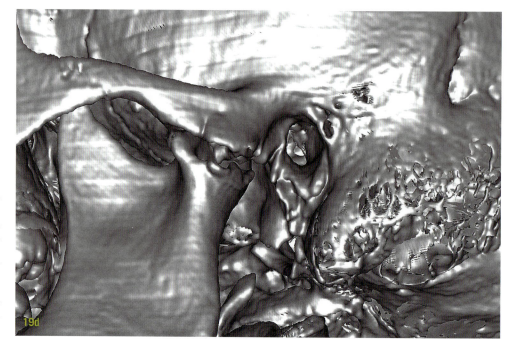

Fig 7-19d 3D reconstruction of the fractured condyle: observe the extensive bone remodeling and the structural changes in the articular bone component, and likewise in the glenoid fossa. No clinical signs of articular hypofunction or symptoms were present.

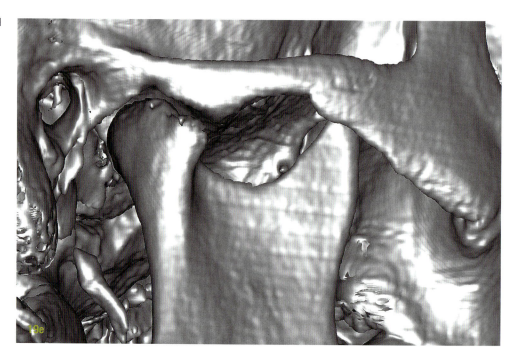

Fig 7-19e Contralateral healthy condyle.

References

1. DuBrul LE. Anatomia Orale di Sicher, ed 2. Milano: Edi Ermes, 1988.
2. de Leeuw R, ed. American Academy of Orofacial Pain. Orofacial Pain: Guidelines for Assessment, Diagnosis, and Management, ed 4. Chicago: Quintessence, 2008.
3. Barghan S, Merrill R, Tetradis S. Cone beam computed tomography imaging in the evaluation of the temporomandibular joint. Tex Dent J 2012;129:289–302.
4. Crow HC, Parks E, Campbell JH, Stucki DS, Daggy J. The utility of panoramic radiography in temporo-mandibular joint assessment. Dentomaxillofac Radiol 2005;34:91–95.
5. Alkhader M, Ohbayashi N, Tetsumura A, et al. Diagnostic performance of magnetic resonance imaging for detecting osseous abnormalities of the temporomandibular joint and its correlation with cone beam computed tomography. Dentomaxillofac Radiol 2010;39:270–276.
6. Zain-Alabdeen EH, Alsadhan RI. A comparative study of accuracy of detection of surface osseous changes in the temporomandibular joint using multidetector CT and cone beam CT. Dentomaxillofac Radiol 2012;41:185–191.
7. Kapila S, Conley RS, Harrell WE Jr. The current status of cone beam computed tomography imaging in orthodontics. Dentomaxillofac Radiol 2011;40:24–34.
8. Tanaka E, Detamore MS, Mercuri LG. Degenerative disorders of the TMJ: Etiology diagnosis and treatment. J Dent Res 2008;87:296–307.
9. Hussain AM, Packota G, Major PW, Flores-Mir C. Role of different imaging modalities in assessment of temporo-mandibular joint erosions and osteophytes: A systematic review. Dentomaxillofac Radiol 2008;37:63–71.
10. Koyama J, Nishiyama H, Hayashi T. Follow-up study of condylar bony changes using helical computed tomography in patients with temporomandibular disorder. Dentomaxillofac Radiol 2007;36:472–477.
11. Tsiklakis K, Syriopoulos K, Stamatakis HC. Radiographic examination of the temporomandibular joint using cone beam computed tomography. Dentomaxillofac Radiol 2004;33:196–201.

M Politi

8

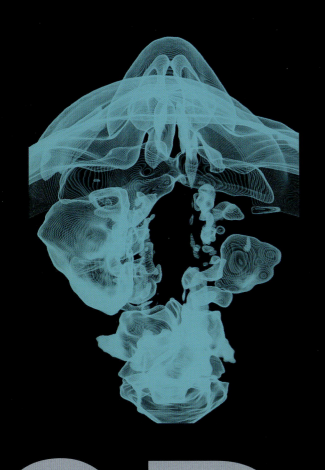

The three-dimensional (3D) virtual reconstruction of the airways through processing of CBCT images depends on the skeletal structure, the soft tissues, and the expandability and collapsibility of mucosal tissues covering the airways.

A 3D reconstruction of the airways is a good indicator of a patient's actual and potential risk of incurring obstructive respiratory conditions. It is clear that an indication of reduced airway spaces is not the only diagnostic tool required, but it can be a primary screening method to be completed with further in-depth investigation as required.

Like many other disciplines, dentistry is increasingly integrated with general medicine, and it can no longer be considered separately. Both in diagnosis and in treatment, the best approach is step-by-step teamwork.

Therefore, dentists should be able to acknowledge potential dyspnea presentations through a correct reading of the airway images, and, as a consequence, to refer their patients to specialists.

3D Analysis
Airway Spaces

Obtructive Sleep Apnea

Obstructive sleep apnea (OSA) is a collapse of the upper airways that can be partial (hypopnea) or total (apnea). It occurs during sleep, interrupting it and causing nighttime hypoxemia.[1]

More frequently, the occlusion affects the velopharyngeal sphincter, although it can also occur in other areas of the upper airways (nasopharynx, oropharynx, hypopharynx).

If the disorder persists, anoxia can cause major complications of the heart with arrhythmia or right cardiac failure, with the development of arterial hypertension likely exacerbated by deprivation of restful sleep.

OSA affects about 12% of the population aged 65 and older, 10% of middle-aged men, and 5% of women.

There is a central form of sleep apnea in which apneic episodes are secondary to transient loss of the nerve stimulus to breathing muscles during sleep; however, the more common, peripheral form, OSA, is caused by the occlusion of the upper airways.

Etiology of OSA

The mechanism whereby obstructive sleep apnea starts is not fully understood, but it is certainly caused by a combination of factors. During sleep, hypotonia of the oropharynge muscles and an increase in negative pressure induced by the diaphragm and intercostal muscles induce a physiologic decrease in the patency of the airways at the base of the tongue and on the walls of the pharynx. This reduction becomes pathologic when it is associated with anatomical abnormalities and structural defects in these areas.

Risk Factors for Obstruction of the Airways and Development of OSA

There are anatomical and nonanatomical risk factors and specific risk factors (Table 8-1).[2,3]

Anatomical Factors:
- Craniofacial abnormalities with reduction in the size of bones
  - Mandibular hypoplasia or retrognathia
  - Maxillary hypoplasia or retrognathia
- Laryngotracheomalacia
- Major deviations of the nasal septum
- Craniofacial malformation syndromes (Crouzon, Apert, and Treacher Collins syndromes, Pierre Robin sequence, achondroplasia, velocardiofacial syndrome)

- Increase in soft tissue volume
  - Fat deposition in the airways (eg, in obesity)
  - Adenotonsillar hypertrophy (especially in children)
  - Soft palate hypertrophy
  - Macroglossia with hypertrophy of the tongue base
  - Increase in the thickness of the lateral esophageal walls
  - Inflammation or edema of the nasopharyngeal space (often caused by snoring)

Nonanatomical Factors:
- Reduced dilatory activity of the pharynx muscles, weakening of the mechanoreceptive sensitivity
  - Weakening of the neuromuscular reflexes of the airways
  - Weakening of the strength and resistance of the muscles dilating the pharynx
- Reduction in lung volume
- Increase in surface tension
- Hormonal factors:
  - Presence of testosterone (male patients or testosterone intake)
  - Absence of progesterone (menopause)
  - Endocrine disorders (hypothyroidism or acromegaly)
- Genetic factors (familiarity, ethnic group, Down syndrome, Marfan syndrome)

Specific Risk Factors:
- Obesity
- Gender (male)
- Advanced age
- Intake of antidepressants or hypnotic drugs
- Intake of drugs or alcohol

Table 8-1 OSA signs and symptoms

OSA symptoms	OSA signs
Excessive daytime sleepiness	Obesity (BMI > 29 kg/m^2)
Sleep interruption (microawakenings)	Increased neck circumference (male > 43 cm; female > 41 cm)
Snoring	Increased waist circumference
Reported apnea	Retrognathia
Restless sleep	Maxillary hypoplasia
Insomnia	Overjet or malocclusion
In advanced stages:	Adenotonsillar hypertrophy
Morning migraine	Macroglossia
Irritability and depression	Edema and erythema of the soft palate
Impaired concentration	Oropharyngeal stricture (Mallampati scale)
Behavioral and cognitive disorders	Hypertension
Day and night enuresis	Cardiovascular disorders
Asphyxia-anoxia crises during sleep	Diabetes
Impotence	Thyroid disorders
Esophageal reflux	

OSA Diagnosis

Although clinical assessment is usually not enough to diagnose OSA, careful taking of the patient's history using a specific questionnaire[2] associated with thorough clinical examination to detect a combination of symptoms and risk factors can increase the diagnostic accuracy and intercept the pathology (Table 8-2).

If outpatient screening gives clear indication of a sleep disorder, it will be necessary to perform an in-depth investigation with an ear, nose, and throat examination and a referral to a center for sleep disorders where highly specific exams can be done to deliver a reliable diagnosis and provide treatment indications.

The diagnosis necessarily involves laboratory evaluation over a whole night.

Table 8-2 Epworth Sleepiness Scale[2]

How likely are you to doze off or fall asleep (not just to feel tired) under the following circumstances?

_____ Sitting, reading a book or a magazine
_____ Watching TV
_____ Sitting inactive in a public place (eg, at the theatre or in a meeting)
_____ Sitting in a car as a passenger for an hour without a break
_____ Lying down to rest in the afternoon when possible
_____ Sitting and talking to someone
_____ Sitting quietly after a meal (without drinking alcohol)
_____ In a car, while stopped for a few minutes in traffic

0 = not likely at all
1 = not very likely
2 = quite likely
3 = very likely

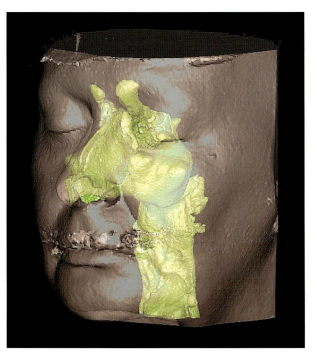

Fig 8-1 3D rendering *(in transparence)* of soft tissues and of the underlying airways *(yellow)* of a patient who has undergone a CBCT examination.

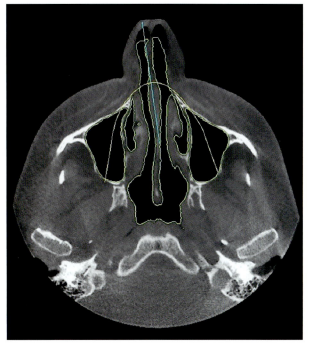

Fig 8-2 Axial slice with outline of the airways during segmentation (in this slice the maxillary sinuses and the nasal cavities are visible).

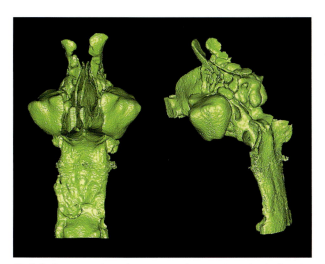

Fig 8-3 Segmentation of the upper airway volume including the paranasal sinuses, the nasal cavities, and the pharynx.

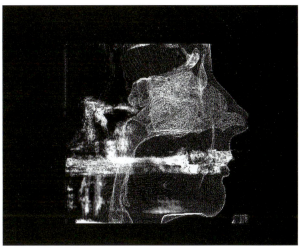

Fig 8-4 Synthesized cephalometric image utilizing a filter to highlight the airways.

OSA Diagnostic Work-up

These items indicate risk of OSA:
- Patient history and identification of risk factors (using questionnaires)
- A general clinical examination[4]
- Assessment of cardiorespiratory function
- Assessment of severity of daytime somnolence
- Body mass index (BMI)[4] > 29 kg/m^2
- Neck circumference > 43 cm (male) or > 41 cm (female)[4]
- Recurrent or persistent snoring alone or with other signs and symptoms
- Presence of at least two other symptoms in addition to recurrent and persistent snoring (breathing pauses + awakenings with shortness of breath or breathing pauses + daytime sleepiness or awakenings with shortness of breath + daytime sleepiness)
- Presence of a symptom other than recurrent snoring plus at least other two signs/symptoms
- Presence of a symptom other than recurrent and persistent snoring plus at least other one sign/symptom in individuals where snoring cannot be ascertained (ie, patients who sleep alone)
- Nighttime cardiorespiratory monitoring

Diagnostic Examinations

Laboratory polysomnography (PSG) is the most accurate exam for the diagnosis of OSA, and it must be performed by sleep experts. PSG records the frequency of apneic and hypopnic events, and it is positive if at least five or more episodes occur during 1 hour of sleep.

The severity of the pathology is measured using the apnea-hypopnea index (AHI), but other factors such as oxygen desaturation and sleep interruption recording are fundamental in staging OSA.

The greatest limitations of PSG are its high cost and the time commitment involved, which is the reason why waiting times and lists are very long.

Home sleep testing is simpler, but it measures just a few parameters. Although time and cost decrease remarkably with home sleep testing, accuracy and reliability of the results is highly variable and often limited.

Other types of OSA examinations are cephalometric images of the skull in a lateral position for the cephalometric analysis of the hypopharyngeal spaces and spiral computed tomography (CT) or cone beam CT (CBCT) of the face for the volumetric analysis of hypopharyngeal airways (Figs 8-1 to 8-4).

CT and CBCT scans required for presurgical orthognathic and implant planning are analyzed using software such as that produced by Materialise. Visualization of the upper airways and of the hypopharynx can be accomplished through 3D rendering of soft tissues by processing Digital Imaging and Communications in Medicine (DICOM) data from CT and/or CBCT scans[5] (Figs 8-5 to 8-10).

3D virtual reconstruction of the airways using software allows calculation of the volume in mm^3 of the airway space available for airflow in primary airways. This airway space depends on skeletal structures, soft

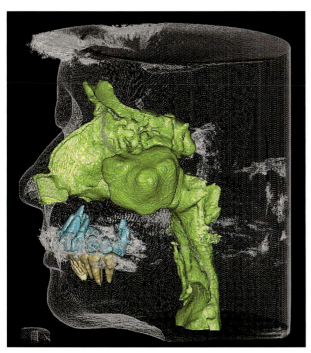

Fig 8-5 3D rendering of a patient using several kernels simultaneously; the dental arches and the airways have been reconstructed separately and highlighted in different colors, while a special kernel has been used for soft tissues to display the underlying structures.

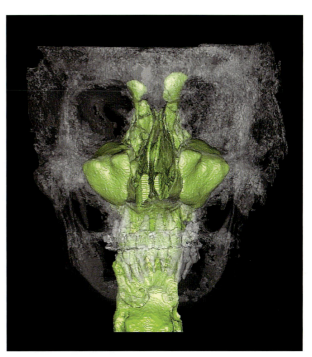

Fig 8-6 3D rendering in frontal view with bony structures reconstructed in transparence while the airways *(yellow)* have been reconstructed in opaque.

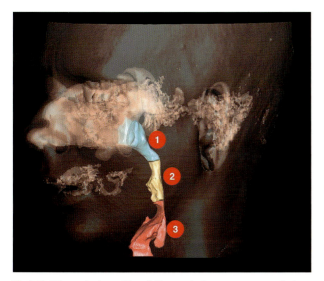

Fig 8-7 3D rendering with soft tissues in transparence and pharynx segmented into three anatomical divisions: *(1)* nasopharynx, *(2)* oropharynx; *(3)* hypopharynx.

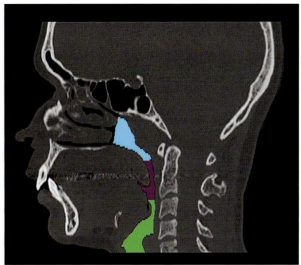

Fig 8-8 Sagittal CBCT slice with the three parts of the pharynx highlighted in different colors: nasopharynx *(blue)*, oropharynx *(purple)*, and hypopharynx *(green)*.

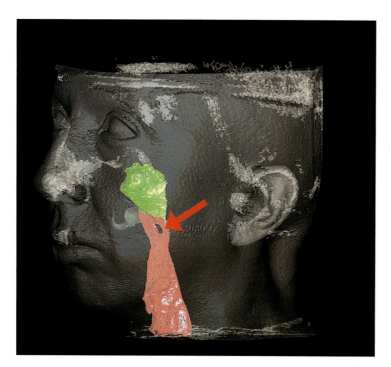

Fig 8-9 3D rendering of an OSA patient: the hypopharynx area is undergoing occlusion *(arrow)*, causing nighttime apnea.

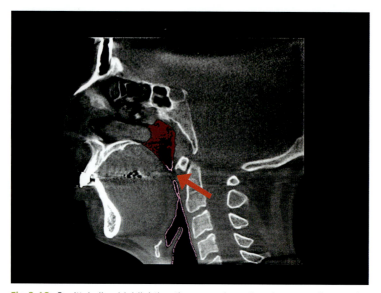

Fig 8-10 Sagittal slice highlighting the area where the pharynx collapses *(arrow)*, impairing normal patency of the airways.

tissues, and the expand ability and collapsibility of the mucous tissues covering the airways.

These calculations are not definitively indicative of airway obstruction, and it is not possible to use calculation of airway volume as a mean index of breathing volume; however, this highlights that the area of the hypopharynx can be investigated in 3D, and the results of these analyses can be correlated with other diagnostic tests done routinely for obstructive breathing pathologies. The 3D reconstruction of the airways is a good indicator of the real and potential risk for a patient to incur an obstructive breathing disorder. Therefore, clinicians who regularly take CBCT or CT scans of patients' skulls for implant placement, dental, or maxillofacial indications and who then analyze them using dedicated software for image processing and 3D reconstruction should be encouraged not to neglect the diagnostic aspect of the airways.

It is clear that the indication of reduced airway spaces is not the only diagnostic tool required, but it can be a primary screening source followed by further in-depth investigation.

In studying breathing disorders correlated with sleep, an interdisciplinary approach is necessary, and it should be always kept in mind that these patients must be followed up the rest of their lives.

Teamwork with a step-by-step methodology has established itself in diagnostics and treatment. This cooperation requires an interactive network of specialists from all disciplines of sleep medicine, including neurology, pulmonology, internal medicine, otorhinolaryngology, psychology, and others. Regular group meetings, workshops, and symposia are very important to promote constant exchange of information among disciplines for the continuous improvement of treatment quality.

References

1. Young T, Palta M, Dempsey J, Skatrud J, Weber S, Badr S. The occurrence of sleep-disordered breathing among middle-aged adults. N Engl J Med 1993;328:1230–1235.
2. Johns MW. A new method for measuring daytime sleepiness: The Epworth sleepiness scale. Sleep 1991;14:540–545.
3. Grunstein R, Wilcox I, Yang TS, Gould Y, Hedner J. Snoring and sleep apnoea in men: Association with central obesity and hypertension. Int J Obes Relat Metab Disord 1993;17:533–540.
4. Stradling JR, Crosby JH. Predictors and prevalence of obstructive sleep apnoea and snoring in 1001 middle aged men. Thorax 1991;46:85–90.
5. Stratemann S, Huang JC. Three-dimensional analysis of the airway with cone-beam computed tomography. Am J Orthod Dentofacial Orthop 2011;140:607–615.

G Perrotti
T Testori
S Ferrario
M Politi

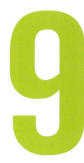

3D Analysis of Impacted Teeth

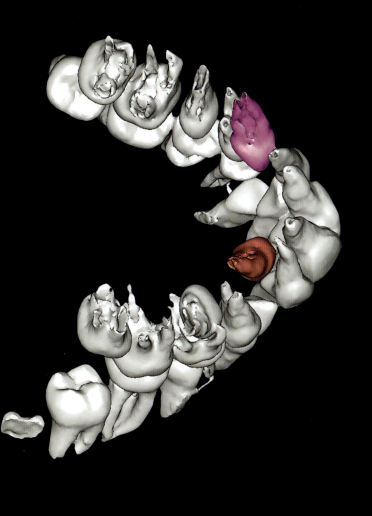

Approximately 20% of the population is likely to have one or more teeth impacted in the bone. The most commonly impacted teeth are mandibular third molars and maxillary canines, although maxillary premolar impaction is not an infrequent occurrence.

Closely related to the risk of impaction in bone of one or more teeth is the issue of correct diagnosis and indication for extraction or disimpaction aimed at the functional salvage of the tooth. A closer diagnostic examination by means of cone beam computed tomography (CBCT) is required in case of doubt and in the presence of supernumerary teeth needing extraction so as to favor the spontaneous and/or guided eruption of the impacted tooth.

If dental impaction is confirmed, the diagnostic work-up begins, which is absolutely necessary for selecting the right therapy (extraction or orthodontic salvage). This can apply, as is often the case, both to maxillary canines and to third molars that can potentially be salvaged, either in the event of loss of the second molars or as a result of an orthodontic choice when correction of the Angle class requires distalization of the first molar, extraction of the second molar, and salvage of the third molar in the position of the second molar. The operative risk connected to surgical extraction of the mandibular third molar requires accurate diagnostic analysis, and, at present, CBCT is the method of choice after panoramic radiography.

Impaction of the Permanent Maxillary Canine

Tooth Impaction

Impaction is an anomaly in dental eruption, which is defined in the literature in a number of different manners:

- Late or blocked dental eruption, accompanied by clinical and radiographic evidence that further eruption cannot be expected[1-4]
- Absence in the arch of a tooth, the root of which is completely formed, or a condition where the contralateral tooth has erupted at least 6 months earlier, and its root has fully developed[5]
- Mechanical impediment (bone or adjacent teeth) to tooth eruption, as a result of which the tooth is trapped inside the socket[6,7]
- Failure of tooth eruption into the correct position in the arch during the normal growth period[8] (Table 9-1)

Table 9-1 Differential diagnosis of the main anomalies of tooth eruption

	Dislocation	Retention	Impaction
Eruption timeline	Normal	Late	Late
Morphostructural development	Incomplete	Incomplete	Complete
Intraosseous position	Unfavorable	Usually favorable	Usually unfavorable

Permanent maxillary canine eruption disorders are common, as these teeth develop deep inside the maxillary bone and have a long path of eruption into the oral cavity.[9]

Odontogenesis

The odontogenesis of permanent maxillary canines starts at around 5 to 6 months of intrauterine life, and the first hints of calcification can be observed between 4 and 12 months. The tooth germ forms deep inside the maxillary bone, lateral to the piriform fossa, under the orbital floor and in correspondence with the anterior wall of the maxillary sinus, between the roots of the primary first molar.[10] The subsequent eruption of the primary molar creates enough space for the formation of the germ of the permanent first premolar between its roots, thus leaving the germ of the canine more cranially positioned.[11] Around the age of 4 years, the primary first molar, the germ of the first premolar, and the germ of the canine thus lie on the same vertical line[12] (Fig 9-1).

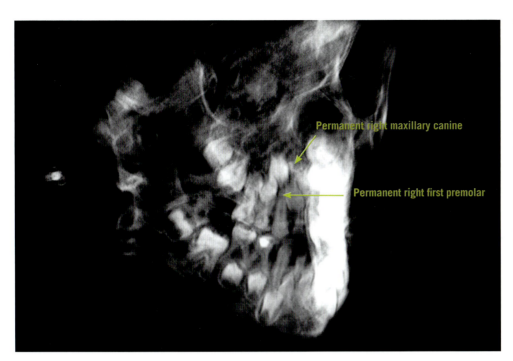

Fig 9-1 Low-radiation CBCT scan of a poorly collaborating 5-year-old female patient. This being the only radiographic image available for the patient, the decision was made to use it despite the poor quality of the 3D reconstruction. Worth noting is the intraosseous position of the germs of the canine and of the permanent first premolar; the canine is located almost apical to the premolar, and slightly palatal and mesial to it.

The enamel is fully developed around the age of 6 years, and the concurrent growth of maxillary bones provides the space for the mesiobuccal movement of permanent incisors and canines, the crowns of which are mesial to the root of the correspondent primary canines, with a vertical overlap of approximately 3 mm. The development stage between 8 and 12 years, called "the ugly duckling stage" (this being the period between the exchange of the frontal group and that of the lateroposterior sectors) (Fig 9-2), is crucial in causing canine impaction in that the crown of the canine should naturally shift from a mesiopalatal position relative to the root apex of its primary precursor to one that is mesiobuccal while, at the same time, staying distal to the root of the permanent lateral incisor; the mesial inclination of canines, which press against the apical third of the root of lateral incisors, and the narrow maxillary basal bone result in coronal distal inclination of the incisors themselves and possibly in a physiologic median diastema.[10] However, in some cases, this shift towards the palatobuccal plane does not occur, and this leads to palatal dislocation of the canine (PDC) and, potentially, to its impaction[11] (Fig 9-3).

During the eruption of the first premolar, the space freed up distally to the canine enables the premolar to slide on the disto-occlusal plane along the distal surface of the root of the lateral incisor, to fill the space between the lateral incisor and the first premolar, thus favoring correction of the "ugly duckling" dentition.[10]

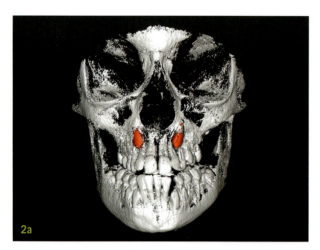

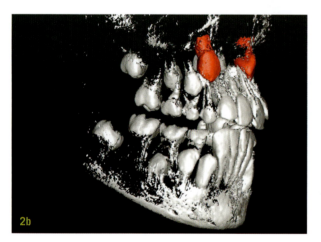
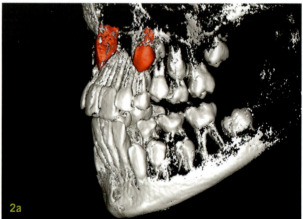

Figs 9-2a to 9-2c Physiologic development of dentition in an 8-year-old female patient. The poor quality of the 3D image is due to the low radiation dose used. The frontal view *(a)* shows the characteristic distal inclination and vestibularization of the lateral incisors and the tendency towards the formation of a physiologic median diastema. The lateral views *(b and c)* show correct root resorption of the primary canines and the distobuccal position of the crown of the permanent canines relative to the root of the lateral incisors.

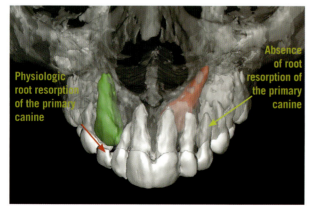

Fig 9-3 Palatal dislocation of maxillary left canine *(red)*. Worth noting is the different spatial inclination compared to the contralateral tooth *(green)*, and the absence of root resorption of the primary left canine.

Time of Eruption

Normally, maxillary canines erupt between 11 and 12 years of age, when their root is formed to the extent of three-quarters of its final length, and completely develop in the following 2 to 3 years.[12]

However, there is a broad diversity in terms of age when the canine erupts in the oral cavity:

- Coulter and Richardson (1997) report a mean age of 11.7 years for females and 12.1 years for males[11]
- Hurme (1949) deems 12.3 years for females and 13.1 years for males to be late[13]
- Thilander and Jakobsson (1968) established that 95% of canines should be present in the arch by the age of 13.9 years in females and 14.6 years in males.[2]

Differences have also been found between the eruption of canines and the biologic or dental age of the patient. In a study dating back to the year 2000, Becker and Chaushu looked for a confirmation of Newcomb's insight (1959), that, based upon his experience, he had noted a clinically significant correlation between potential impaction of permanent teeth and moderately-to-severely late tooth maturation.[14] The findings of this study showed that patients with buccal canine ectopia have a normal dental age corresponding to their actual age, whereas patients with palatal canine ectopia have a marked tendency to late tooth development. To be more precise, in approximately half of the cases, the dental age corresponds to the actual one, whereas in the remaining half the dental age is delayed. This phenomenon would suggest the existence of two different categories of canine palatal dislocation, presumably with different etiology.

The study of Baccetti et al[15] helps clinicians estimate the period of eruption of canines. Indeed, it takes the maturation of cervical vertebrae (cervical stage [CS]) as a reference to assess the degree of dentoskeletal development in growing patients (Fig 9-4). The findings confirm a broad diversity as to the real age when the canine erupts. With reference to the biologic age, permanent canines naturally erupt during the prepubertal age (CS1–CS2) in 56.6% of cases; in the remaining cases, these teeth spontaneously erupt within the year of pubertal peak, or, at the latest, the following year (CS3–CS4). In no case has spontaneous eruption of canines been observed during the postpubertal development stage (CS5–CS6). It can be concluded that the absence of the canine in the arch during the postpubertal stage of development is indicative of a late eruption of the tooth at issue (Fig 9-5).

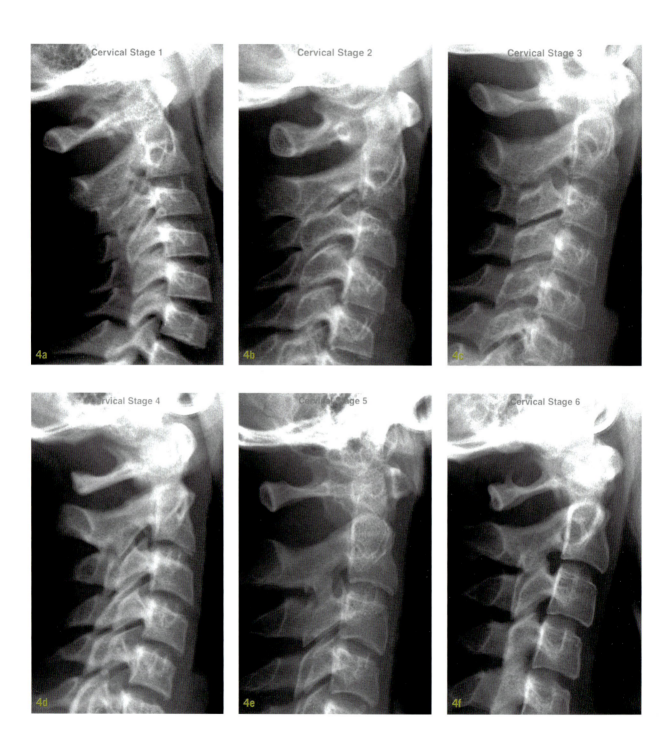

Figs 9-4a to 9-4f Representation of the six stages of cervical vertebral maturation (CVM). CS1 *(a)* and CS2 *(b)* are prepubertal stages; CS3 (c) and CS4 (d) comprise the period of peak growth; CS5 *(e)* and CS6 *(f)* are postpubertal stages.[15]

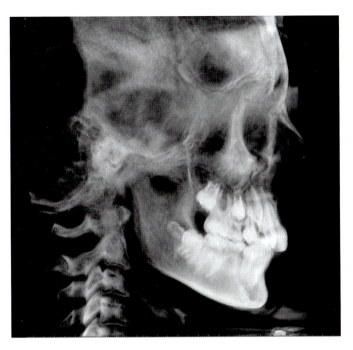

Fig 9-5 CBCT sintered lateral cephalometric image of the patient in Fig 9-3. The cervical vertebrae being in an advanced stage of maturation (CS5), further spontaneous eruption of the palatally dislocated canine cannot be expected.

Eruption Path

Several authors agree that the maxillary canine follows a longer and more tortuous eruption path compared to all other teeth.[11]

In 1997, Coulter and Richardson measured in the three dimensions of space the natural eruption path of 60 canines in the age range of 5 to 15 years using lateral and posterolateral cephalometric images taken once a year.[11]

The average distance traveled by a canine was found to be 21.99 mm, with most of the movement occurring between 9 and 12 years of age. This shift, if broken down into the three spatial planes (ie, considering the shift on every plane as the result of the algebraic sum of all shifts between 5 and 15 years of age for every tooth), is as follows:

- 11.48 mm anteroposterior, mainly between 9 and 12 years of age
- 18.56 mm apico-occlusal, mainly between 9 and 12 years of age
- 2.67 mm palatobuccal, mainly between 10 and 12 years of age

The palatobuccal shift of the tooth between 10 and 12 years of age appears to be particularly significant in that, before this period, the germ tends to move in the opposite direction, ie, towards the palate. Failure to complete this shift is believed to be involved in the palatal impaction of the canine.[16] Using the same method, in 1999 McSherry and Richardson quantified the eruption path of 20 palatally ectopic canines.[17]

- On the sagittal plane, ectopic canines show a more limited shift both anteroposteriorly (as with the study men-

tioned above, this is an apparent movement; with a traditional orientation of the radiograph, a mesial shift of malpositioned canines would be shown) and apico-occlusally, as compared to normally erupting canines.
- On the frontal plane, ectopic canines show a gradual and continuous movement towards the palate in the 10-year range analyzed, without the usual change of shift to a buccal pattern.

These findings appear to support a genetic etiology of canine palatal impaction rather than a mechanic one.

Epidemiology

Maxillary canine impaction is a frequently occurring dental anomaly.[9] After mandibular third molars, maxillary canines are the most frequently impacted teeth, followed by the maxillary third molars, the second premolars, and the maxillary central incisors.[10]

The prevalence of this disorder stands at 1% to 2% of the population[1,4,9]; however, the statistical data reported in the literature are not uniform, and the percentage varies based on the sample selected and on the type of study conducted. Bilateral impaction is more rare than unilateral impaction, and the percentage of this phenomenon ranges from 8% to 45%, considering palatal impactions alone.[9,18]

Females are more frequently affected than males, in a 2:1 ratio[1,4,9,11] or 3:1 ratio,[19] with maxillary canine impaction being much more frequent than mandibular canine impaction, in a 10:1 ratio[10]; moreover, prevalence is five times higher in Caucasians compared to Asians.

As to the breakdown between palatal and buccal impactions, several studies agree that palatal impaction prevails. According to a recent review by Bedoya and Park,[9] the ratio is 2:1 in favor of palatal impaction; older studies report more extreme data, with 85% palatal impactions against 15% buccal impactions.[1,4,11]

Etiopathogenesis

Though still unclear, the etiology of canine impaction is probably multifactorial in nature.[12] Cozza[10] recently tried to classify the very numerous factors and conditions that are believed to be etiologically associated with maxillary canine impaction (Table 9-2). There are other classifications in the literature, but the one shown below has been found to be the most complete. However, in 1994 Peck et al[18] stated that buccal impaction and palatal impaction of the maxillary canine should be considered as two distinct phenomena. This view being shared by other authors,[20] we will analyze the two situations separately.

Table 9-2 Causal and predisposing factors for maxillary canine impaction[10]

	Etiopathogenesis of impacted maxillary canine		
Causal factors	Hereditary causes		
	Congenital diseases	Cleft lip and palate	
		Cleidocranial dysostosis	
		Down syndrome	
Predisposing factors	General	Endocrine dysfunctions	
		Dysmetabolic diseases	
		Prenatal infectious diseases	
	Local	Skeletal	Skeletal Class III
			Maxillary hypoplasia
			Hypodivergence
		Dental	Dental germ malposition
			Mechanical obstacles (supernumerary teeth, neoplasms, cysts, odontomes)
			Loss of space in the arch (altered eruption sequence, early extraction of the primary tooth, etc)
			Prolonged retention of the primary tooth in the arch (ankylosis)
			Ankylosis of the permanent tooth (idiopathic, traumas of the primary tooth, infectious diseases of the primary tooth)
			Dental-basal disharmony

Dislocation and Buccal Impaction

Buccal dislocation is usually linked to inadequate length of the maxillary arch and resulting lack of space. This condition frequently results in ectopic eruption of the tooth, without leading to impaction proper.[18] This clinical picture was described in 1981 by Becker et al[21] as a likely complication of a crowded maxillary arch. With the exchange of maxillary teeth, incisors and first premolars emerge in the arch before canines. Considering that the maxillary canine, in its natural eruption process, follows a buccal path that is palpable in the buccal sulcus, a crowded maxillary arch predisposes the patient to an excessive vestibularization of such a path, thus favoring canine buccal dislocation.[21] In the same line of thought and in the same year, Williams[16] drew a distinction between the usual sequence of exchange of maxillary teeth (first molar, central incisor, lateral incisor, first premolar, second premolar, canine, and second molar) and an unfavorable exchange pattern, with the latter being characterized by eruption of the second molar before the canine and, possibly, the second premolar as well.

In conclusion, it can be said that the lack of space or crowding in the maxillary area is believed to be a primary etiologic factor of canine buccal impaction,[9,10,12,22] so much that an extreme form of crowding[23] is considered as an anomaly.

Dislocation and Palatal Impaction

Palatal dislocation of the canine (PDC), instead, is an anomalous position that generally occurs in spite of there being sufficient space in the arch and typically leads to impaction of the tooth, unless it is adequately detected.[18,24]

In an attempt to understand the etiopathogenesis of this clinical picture, two main theories have been put forward:

1. *The guide theory:* This is a mechanistic theory that attributes a primary role to the function performed by the root of the lateral incisor in guiding the sliding of the canine along its distal surface; in this way, the canine deviates its eruption path from mesial to occlusal. To be an adequate guide, lateral incisors must have normal root shape and length, correct developmental timing, as well as suitable position and inclination.[10] To support this theory, Becker et al[21] investigated the association between canine palatal impaction and anomalies of the adjacent lateral incisors and found this correlation in approximately half of the cases studied. In the same paper, the authors made an interesting observation, suggesting that canine palatal dislocation can occur at two distinct times in its development: early, ie, during the formation of the roots of the lateral incisors, or late,

ie, at the end of its development, due to an obstacle represented by adjacent primary or permanent teeth.[21]

2. *Genetic theory:* This theory identifies the genetic factors underlying canine palatal impaction and the other dental anomalies commonly associated to it. This would be an inheritance of an autosomal dominant nature or linked to sexual chromosomes, with polygenic transmission and variable expressiveness.[10] The first to support this hypothesis were Peck et al,[18] who reported five categories of evidence in its favor:

- Concurrence of PDC and other dental anomalies: agenesis or malformation of other teeth, in particular lateral incisors[21,25–27]; microdontia, supernumerary teeth, and ectopic teeth[27]; late dental development[28–29]; transposition of the canine and of the first premolar.
- Bilateral PDC, with a prevalence ranging between 17% and 45%.
- Differential distribution of PDC based upon sex: Data indicate a female-to-male ratio between 3:1 and 2:1 and suggest an involvement of sexual chromosomes in the transmission of PDC.
- Family history of PDC, confirmed by three studies on families of different nationalities: Sottner and Racek,[30] Svinhufvud et al,[31] and Zilberman et al.[32]
- Uneven distribution of PDC in different populations: It would appear that PDC is much more common amongst persons of European origin than amongst those of African or Asian origin, with a ratio of approximately 5:1.

Many of the findings mentioned above have also been confirmed by more recent studies.[19,20,33-35] Baccetti[34] tried to provide further scientific support to the possible existence of significant correlations between different types of dental anomalies by studying a large group of growing patients. His findings bear out the genetic etiologic hypothesis, reporting significant mutual associations between PDC, anomalies of lateral incisors, agenesis of second premolars, infraocclusion of primary molars, and enamel hypoplasia; these five disorders could indicate the emergence of a syndrome with incomplete penetration and variable expressiveness.

One of the most recent papers relating to this theme is by Sacerdoti and Baccetti,[19] who confirmed three of the five categories of evidence proposed by Peck et al[18]: the concurrence of canine palatal malposition and microdontia of lateral incisors, bilateral PDC, and greater prevalence of the phenomenon in females. Furthermore, they have found a high percentage of hypodivergent cases in PDC patients.

Therefore, it would appear that currently there is growing scientific evidence identifying a set of disorders whose emergence is genetically controlled and which, as a result, often occur combined despite their not being correlated by a cause-and-effect relationship: PDC, microdontia, hypodontia, infraocclusion of primary molars, late dental development, ectopias, transpositions, and enamel hypoplasia.[20] The existence of these correlations is important from the etiologic as well as clinical point of view, in that early diagnosis of one of these conditions can indicate an increased risk of later appearance of the others.[19]

Diagnosis

Clinical examination and, where needed, early and accurate radiographic investigation, can help detect an altered canine eruption pattern before this causes an impaction proper; hence, the aim of early diagnosis is to take corrective actions at a low biologic cost in order to limit the likelihood of impaction or to facilitate the subsequent surgical disimpaction, where the latter is needed.[10,36]

Williams[16] effectively summarized the situation as follows: "Maxillary canine impaction is a serious issue that is frequent enough to warrant early diagnosis and action, as early as age 8 years." The intraosseous movements of the canine between 8 and 12 years of age require particular attention[16] (see Figs 9-2 and 9-3).

Clinical Examination

Based upon the preceding statements, it follows that case history plays a fundamental role in early clinical diagnosis; in particular, it is important to examine family history very accurately because, especially at a young age, it can be the most significant predictive element.[10,37]

The stages of clinical examination of interest to us for the purposes hereof are inspection and palpation.

In young patients (starting from age 7 to 10 years), during inspection the clinician should look for the following signs, which can indicate an intraosseous malposition of maxillary canines:

- Transversal contraction of the maxillary bone, possibly associated with crowding: This condition can easily cause canine buccal dislocation[2,24,38,39] (Fig 9-6).
- Other concurrent dental anomalies: These include microdontia, hypodontia, infraocclusion of primary molars, late dental development, ectopias, transpositions, and enamel hypoplasia.[20,34] These disorders can be associated with canine palatal dislocation and as such be an early indicator of impaction[19] (Fig 9-7).
- Lateral incisor anomalies: Microdontia and agenesis of these teeth are correlated with PDC (Fig 9-8). Equally important is an accurate assessment of their position and inclination, as the pressure brought to bear by a canine dislocated on the root of such an element can result in characteristic malpositions.

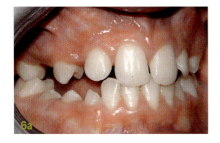 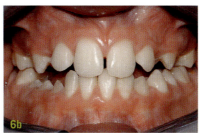 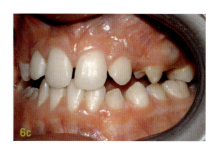

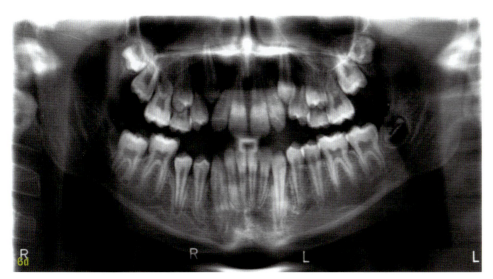

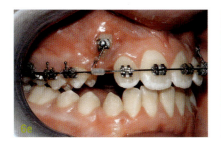 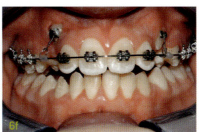 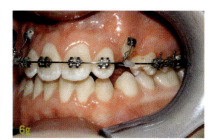

Figs 9-6a to 9-6g *(a and c)* Lateral and *(b)* frontal intraoral images of a patient with a contracted maxillary arch, especially the maxillary right arch, with loss of space for maxillary canine eruption. *(d)* The canines are palpable buccally and correspond to their position as shown on the panoramic radiograph. *(e to g)* The patient is shown after preparation of the maxillary arch and surgical exposure and bonding of the canines.

To be more precise: a lateral incisor that is too distally inclined suggests that a canine brings pressure to bear along the distoapical aspect of its root, a proclined incisor indicates a vestibularized canine that pushes its root apex palatally,[37,39] and a rotated and distally inclined incisor expresses canine palatal dislocation.[7,37]

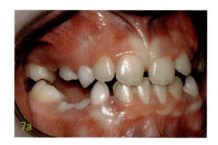
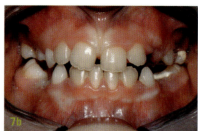
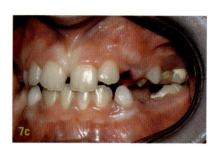

Figs 9-7a to 9-7d Intraoral situation and panoramic radiograph of an 11-year-old female patient with multiple combined dental anomalies: infraocclusion of the primary second molars in the first, third, and fourth quadrants; enamel hypoplasia; *(b and c)* especially in the permanent maxillary and mandibular left first molars; *(d)* intraosseous malposition of the permanent second premolars; and palatal dislocation of the right maxillary canine.

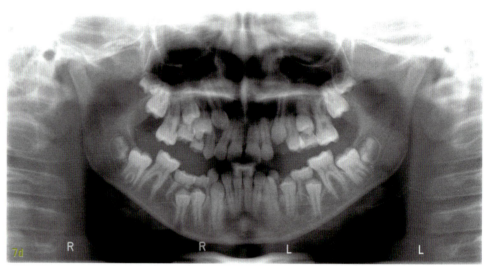

Likewise, it is very important to verify the stability of lateral incisors: excessive mobility could result from root resorption caused by a dislocated canine.[39]

- Prolonged retention or early loss of the primary canine: The former could be a mechanical obstacle to eruption of the canine while the latter could favor mesialization of the posterior sectors, resulting in space loss.[40]
- Exchange asymmetry: A significant delay in the eruption of a canine while the contralateral tooth has already erupted can indicate impaction of the former[37] (Fig 9-9).

Palpation has a twofold purpose:

- Assess the mobility of primary canines: Usually, such a finding indicates root resorption in these teeth, presumably due to a naturally erupting canine; however, mobility of the primary canine does not ensure correct eruption of the corresponding permanent tooth.[37]

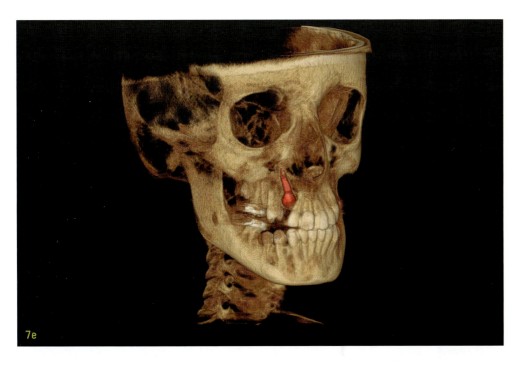

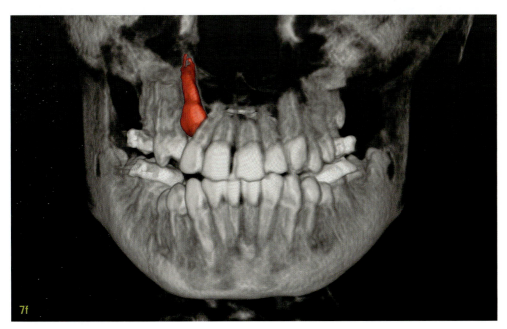

Figs 9-7e and 9-7f Follow-up at 1 year with cranial CBCT after preventive extraction of primary maxillary right canine. The position of the impacted canine appears to have improved compared to the earlier panoramic image (see Fig 9-7d), although it is still impacted and inclined palatally.

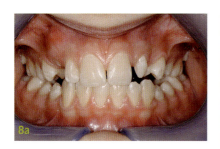

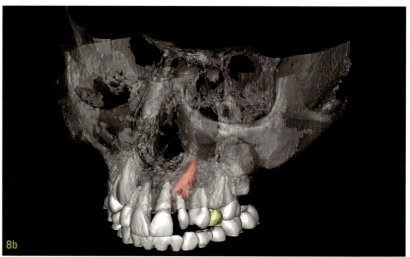

Figs 9-8a and 9-8b Microdontia of maxillary lateral incisors, particularly the left lateral incisor, concurrent with palatal dislocation of the left maxillary canine, (b) as confirmed by the 3D reconstruction.

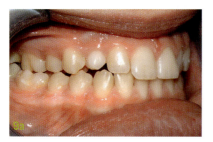
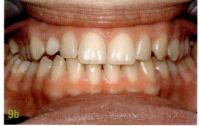
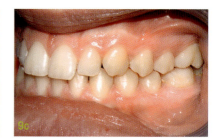

Figs 9-9a to 9-9d 13-year-old female who has completed her tooth exchange, with the primary maxillary right canine still present in the arch while the permanent contralateral canine has completely erupted. (d) In the panoramic radiograph, it appears to be impacted in a buccal position, and its bulge is palpable.

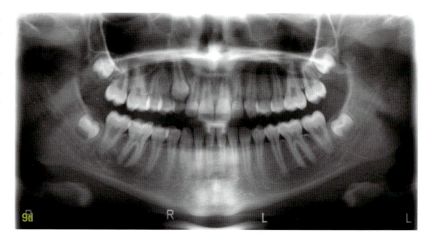

- Locate the permanent canine: The natural eruption path of a permanent maxillary canine should be buccal and palpable in the buccal sulcus in the form of a canine bulge apical to the corresponding primary tooth.[16,41] Absence of a canine bulge, particularly if asymmetric, or palpation of a canine in an anomalous position are indicative of its malposition.[37,41,42] This is particularly true of children aged 10 years and over, as in younger patients palpation is an uncertain diagnostic criterion in that the tooth still has time to correct its eruption path.[10,41]

Radiographic Investigation

Radiographic investigation is necessary in the event that, during clinical examination, one or more indicative signs of dislocation or impaction of maxillary canines are found. Ericson and Kurol[36] have identified the most appropriate time for radiographic investigation, stating that, in the absence of other indications, periodic checks and objective examination are sufficient until the age of 10 years, as radiographs before that age have been found to be scarcely predictive. Therefore, to investigate a suspected malposition of maxillary canines, the authors suggest beginning radiographic examination at the age of 10 years.

When the clinician finds a suspected case, he/she should have the patient undergo clinical checks—and, where needed, also radiographs—every 6 months; the purpose is to monitor the eruption path of the canine and, where needed, to take the most suitable corrective actions at the right time.[16]

Irrespective of the technique used, radiographic investigation has several objectives[43]:

- Assessing the anatomic relationship of the malpositioned or impacted tooth with the surrounding structures
- Highlighting any associated dental anomalies
- Measuring the size of the tooth investigated
- Locating the canine on the three planes of space
- Investigating the presence, if any, of obstacles to its normal eruption

The following instrumental examinations are useful to diagnose dislocation and/or impaction of maxillary canines[43]:

- Periapical intraoral radiograph
- Occlusal intraoral radiograph
- Panoramic radiograph
- Lateral cephalometric radiograph
- Posteroanterior (PA) cephalometric radiograph
- Traditional spiral CT or CBCT

Intraoral Radiographs

The radiographic technique classically used to locate impacted teeth is periapical intraoral radiography[16]; this being a two-dimensional (2D) image, it enables the clinician to assess the morphologic characteristics of the impacted tooth, but it requires at least two projections to give an idea of its three-dimensional (3D) position in space.[10]

To do this, the parallax radiologic principle is used, ie, the apparent shift of the object to be located, relative to another reference object, caused by the change in the angle of the x-ray beam; the image of the object that is furthest away from the source of x-rays moves in the same direction as the x-ray tube, whereas the closest object shifts in the opposite direction. This principle can be applied to a shift of the x-ray tube both horizontally (introduced by Clark[44] and known as the "Clark rule") and vertically (as proposed by Richards[45] and called the "buccal object rule"[16]).

According to Ericson and Kurol,[46] with periapical radiographs it is possible to correctly locate the impacted tooth in 92% of the cases. The same concepts can be adopted when taking intraoral occlusal radiographs, as proposed by Keur,[47] as this type of radiograph covers a broader area and allows for a greater tube shift, thus making it simpler to locate the impacted tooth, which is almost always shown in its entirety.[37] For this reason, the author has introduced the use of two new radiographic combinations:

- Two occlusal radiographs, taken with a horizontal shift of the x-ray source
- One occlusal radiograph combined with a panoramic radiograph, exploiting the principle of the vertical parallax

The advantage of the second combination is the frequent availability of panoramic imaging prior to the beginning of treatment, thus exposing the patient to just one additional radiograph (the occlusal one); moreover, the panoramic image provides a lot of information, not only on the tooth under examination, but also on the surrounding structures.[48] Despite these benefits, it should be pointed out that it is not always easy to interpret the images taken with a vertical shift of the x-ray tube.[37]

According to Jacobs,[48] the first-choice technique for locating impacted anterior teeth is a panoramic radiograph combined with a superior occlusal radiograph taken between 60 to 65 degrees and 70 to 75 degrees, using the vertical parallax principle.

Still, Mason et al,[3] in a 2001 paper, investigated the validity of this radiographic technique and reported that it correctly locates the impacted canine in only 76% of patients; therefore, the predictive capability of this method is moderate.

The second radiographic principle that can be applied to radiographic techniques is image magnification: given a defined distance between the source of x-rays and the receiver (film or sensor), the objects that are farther away from the receiver are more magnified than the closer ones.[3]

However, magnification is difficult to detect on intraoral radiographs and is more indicated in panoramic radiographs.[3,37]

In summary, the intraoral radiographs that can be used for diagnosing maxillary canine impaction are as follows[12,48]:

- Two or more periapical radiographs with horizontal shift of the x-ray tube
- Two or more periapical radiographs with vertical shift of the x-ray tube

- Two superior occlusal radiographs with horizontal shift of the x-ray tube
- One superior occlusal radiograph combined with a panoramic radiograph

The main benefits of the radiographic techniques above are low radiation dose and simplicity in taking the image, as a result of which they can be repeated over time, whereas the main disadvantages are the typical limitations of 2D radiographs, which lower their diagnostic capability, ie, overlapping of different structures and possible distortion and magnification of the image.[10]

Panoramic Radiographs

The panoramic radiograph is a routine radiologic exam, frequently already available at the beginning of treatment, that provides an overall view of the dental arches at the cost of a relatively low dose of radiation; for this reason, it has been investigated by several authors who have tried to extract from it as much diagnostic information as possible, despite the well-known limitations of this examination (image overlapping, magnification, and distortion).[10,49]

First, panoramic radiographs can highlight the concomitant occurrence of other dental anomalies possibly associated with canine palatal dislocation.[10] Furthermore, efforts to analyze the information provided by a panoramic radiograph have made available today a large number of "predictive radiographic indices" of permanent maxillary canine impaction, which can be found in any type of radiograph. Those listed below are the ones most commonly used:

- *Angle α*[50] (Fig 9-10): the angle between the long axis of the canine and the interincisal midline; an increase in this angle could indicate a worse prognosis for the tooth. In particular, Ericson and Kurol[50] highlighted that a 30-degree angle could be the threshold beyond which the likelihood of impaction increases. However, measurements show a broad diversity of this parameter that makes its predictability questionable in statistical terms. Later, Power and Short[51] also identified an angle in excess of 31 degrees as being a major negative predictive factor for canine impaction.

In 2000, Stivaros and Mandall[52] further confirmed the importance of this measurement, stating that the clinician's therapeutic choice is essentially based upon this parameter (alongside the buccopalatal position of the canine), and proposed three classes of increasing severity:

1. 0- to 15-degree angle
2. 16- to 30-degree angle
3. >30-degree angle

It should be noted that these authors considered 30 degrees as a significant threshold for predicting the severity of canine impaction.

- *Distance d*[50] (Fig 9-11): distance between canine cusp and the occlusal plane spanning from the cusp of the mandibular first molar to the incisal

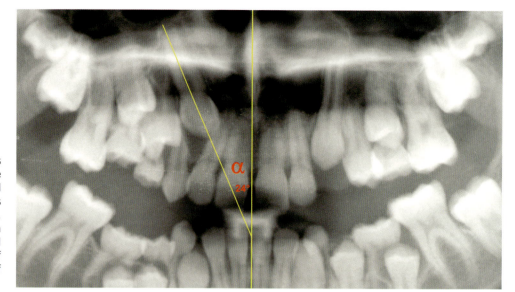

Fig 9-10 The α angle is measured by tracing the interincisal midline and extending the long axis of the impacted canine. In this patient, this is a 24-degree angle, and therefore the prognosis of the tooth appears to be of intermediate severity.

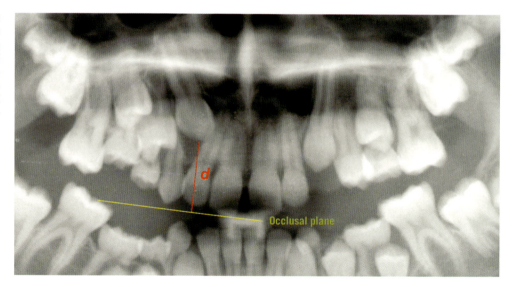

Fig 9-11 Distance (d) between the cusp of the impacted canine and the occlusal plane, obtained by tracing a line between the cusp of the mandibular molar and the incisal edge of the maxillary central incisor.

edge of the maxillary central incisor; it seems possible to assume a correlation between an increase in such distance and a worsening of canine prognosis, although measured values are broadly diverse, and they impact its predictive power.

- *Overlapping sector s*[50] (Fig 9-12): mesiodistal location of the canine cusp, as classified by drawing five sectors:
  - Between the line tangent to the distal surface of the primary canine and a line tangent to its mesial surface

- Between the line tangent to the distal surface of the lateral incisor and its long axis
- Between the long axis of the lateral incisor and the line tangent to its mesial surface
- Between the line tangent to the distal surface of the central incisor and its long axis
- Between the long axis of the central incisor and a line tangent to its mesial surface

A sector increase indicates a worse prognosis for the canine. Lindauer et al[5] reviewed these conclusions and proposed a different classification of the mesiodistal position of the canine tip relative to the root of the erupted lateral incisor. They identified four sectors:

- The area distal to the line tangent to the distal surface of the lateral incisor
- The area between the line tangent to the distal surface of the lateral incisor and its long axis
- The area between the long axis of the lateral incisor and the line tangent to its mesial surface
- The area mesial to the line tangent to the mesial surface of the lateral incisor

Also based upon this classification method, a correlation has been found between a sector increase and the likelihood of canine impaction; these findings were later confirmed in a paper by Warford et al.[53] According to these authors, the position of the canine cusp in mesiodistal sectors is the most significant parameter for predicting impaction; to be more precise, canines in sectors three and four have the highest likelihood of impaction.

A further confirmation of the importance of this parameter comes from the paper by Stivaros and Mandall,[52] who graded canine overlay relative to lateral incisors in four classes of growing severity corresponding to the sectors described by Lindauer et al.[5]

Finally, Baccetti et al[54] recently proposed a simplification of the sector breakdown so as to speed up panoramic radiograph reading using three sectors (Fig 9-13):

- Canine cusp mesial to the long axis of the central incisor
- Canine cusp between the long axis of the central incisor and that of the lateral incisor
- Canine cusp between the long axis of the lateral incisor and that of the first premolar

In this case, a predictive correlation is created between a sector decrease and a higher likelihood of impaction.

- *Vertical height of canine*[52]: vertical position of the canine crown relative to the erupted lateral incisor. There are four degrees of increasing severity (Fig 9-14): *(1)* crown occlusal to the cementoenamel junction of the lateral incisor; *(2)* crown in the occlusal half of the root of the lateral incisor; *(3)* crown in the apical half of the root of the lateral incisor; *(4)* crown apical to the root of the lateral incisor.

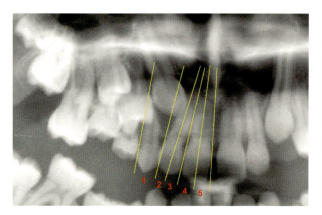

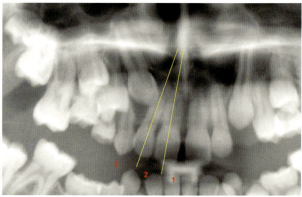

Fig 9-12 Breakdown into sectors for the mesiodistal location of the cusp of the impacted canine. In this patient, the cusp of the canine is in sector 2, bordering on sector 3.

Fig 9-13 Simplification of the mesiodistal position of the canine according to Baccetti et al.[54] In this patient, the sector decrease points to a worse prognosis for the impacted canine.

- *Horizontal position of the canine root apex*[52]: this is broken down into three degrees of increasing severity: *(1)* apex above the area of the canine; *(2)* apex above the area of first premolar; *(3)* apex above the area of the second premolar. This parameter is scarcely considered in the literature.
- *Canine axis/bicondylar line angle*[53] (Fig 9-15): angle between the canine axis and the horizontal line that passes through the most superior points of the condyles.

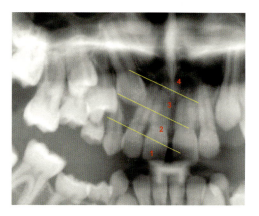

Fig 9-14 Apicocoronal location of the cusp of the impacted canine. The sector increase points to a worse prognosis for the tooth.

This type of measurement was introduced to separate the measurement of canine angle from anterior tooth relationships. Previously, this was done by taking as a reference the interincisal midline (see angle α). However, the same authors concluded that a mesial angle of the canine does not add any predictive significance to the location of the canine in the mesiodistal sectors according to the method of Lindauer et al.[5,53]

Cephalometric Radiographs

A lateral cephalometric radiograph provides a view of the skull profile. Under normal circumstances, at age 8 years, the canine crown should be viewed close to the root apex of the corresponding primary tooth, with the long axis running parallel to that of the central incisors[16] (Fig 9-16). Using this radiographic projection, the clinician can assess the location of the malpositioned or impacted canine relative to the occlusal plane and the roots of the maxillary incisors, as well as its eruption direction.[10,55]

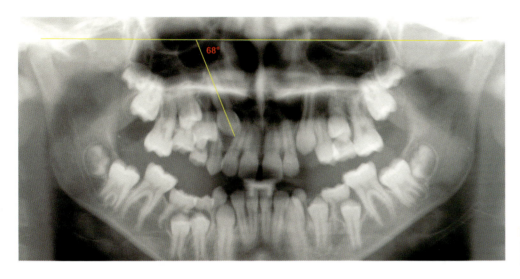

Fig 9-15 Angle between the canine long axis and bicondylar line.

Orton et al[55] studied these parameters and made several conclusions:

- The greater the distance between the canine and occlusal plane, the higher the likelihood of damage to the maxillary incisors and the worse the prognosis for the tooth.
- The more anterior a palatal canine is, the greater the risk of damage to incisors.
- The correct eruption direction of maxillary canines observed by means of a lateral cephalometric radiograph creates an angle of approximately 10 degrees with a straight line running perpendicular to the Frankfurt plane; an increase in this angle worsens the prognosis for the tooth.

However, this value becomes significant when combined with an assessment of the position of the tooth on the mesiodistal plane using a panoramic or PA cephalometric radiograph.

As suggested in Orton et al's paper, the information provided by lateral cephalometry becomes much more significant when

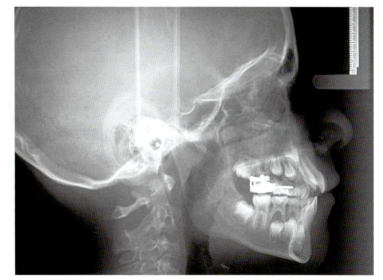

Fig 9-16 Lateral cephalometric radiograph of an 8-year-old female showing the correct position of the germs of the permanent canines, positioned apically to the primary canines and having the same inclination as the lateral incisors.

combined with a PA projection or, where appropriate, a panoramic radiograph, based on the "right angle rule," according to which two radiographs taken with an angle of 90 degrees between them allows reconstruction of the image in the three dimensions.[3]

PA cephalometry shows the midlateral position of canines, their angle, and their eruption path on a frontal plane, besides allowing for an assessment of the transverse dimension of the maxilla.[10] Normally, at age 8 years, the canine crown should be occlusal to the root apex of lateral incisors and to the floor of the nasal cavity, slightly medially inclined, and its root should lie distal to the lateral wall of the nasal cavity.[16,49]

An excessively mesial inclination of the canine, possibly associated with nonresorption of the corresponding primary tooth, should suggest its malposition.[49]

In 2004, Sambataro et al[56] investigated the dental and skeletal characteristics that can be viewed by means of PA cephalometry in patients with early mixed dentition to identify significant predictive variables for maxillary canine impaction, thus reviewing the cephalometric analysis of Ricketts et al (1972). The authors reported two predictive measures: the distance between the canine crown and the midsagittal plane, and the transversal width of the hemimaxilla of the side under investigation.

The closer the canine crown is to the midsagittal plane and the larger the hemimaxilla, the higher the likelihood of canine impaction.

As already explained in relation to the other 2D radiographic investigations, the greatest limitations of cephalometry are overlapping of structures, especially in the presence of bilateral impaction, and image distortion and magnification.[10]

Computed Tomography

CT, being the most interesting radiographic technique with respect to the purpose of this chapter, will be dealt with at length here.

Verifying the precise position of an impacted canine is crucial to determine the feasibility and the appropriate surgical technique to be adopted to salvage it and allows better planning of the direction of the orthodontic forces needed for guided eruption in the arch. Furthermore, it is strongly recommended to analyze the roots of contiguous teeth carefully, given the high percentage of root resorption caused by ectopic canines, especially in permanent lateral incisors.[9]

CT represents the actual 3D morphology of the skull and, compared to traditional radiographs, provides a more accurate representation of the bony structures when it comes to locating impacted teeth and diagnosing any associated lesions such as root resorption of the adjacent teeth[4,9,57,58] or cystic degeneration[57] of the dental follicle (Fig 9-17).

The cost-to-benefit ratio of requesting this type of radiographic investigation is a matter of controversy, especially as a result of the new stance taken vis-à-vis exposing growing patients to relatively high radiation doses. Several authors agree in justifying the request for a CT scan (irrespective of the specific radiographic technique) for patients with one or more impacted teeth.

Ericson and Kurol[59] consider it a useful tool for the 3D diagnosis of malpositioned or impacted canines, especially in cases where there is a suspicion of root resorption in adjacent teeth. According to the same authors, CT overcomes the limitations of traditional radiographic techniques (overlapping, distortion, and magnification) and is therefore useful for diagnosing and preventing complications of ectopic canines.[60]

The clinical usefulness of CT scans was investigated in 2006 by Bjerklin and Ericson,[57] who reported having made changes to the treatment plans of patients with impacted maxillary canines in 43.7% of cases subsequent to the collection of additional diagnostic information provided by a CT scan. This information relates mainly to the presence of root resorption of permanent lateral incisors adjacent to ectopic canines. Therefore, they concluded that CT is an important tool for planning an adequate treatment in cases of maxillary canine impaction.[57]

However, the high radiation exposure does not currently warrant its use in clinical practice.[4,9,58] CBCT, introduced in 1998, was specifically conceived for representing the structures of the craniofacial district.

In regard to protection from radiation, reference should always to be made to the ALARA (as low as reasonably achievable) principle and, more specifically, to the latest guidelines (currently provided by the SEDENTEXCT project[61]):

- For assessing an impacted tooth, where the reference diagnostic method is traditional CT, CBCT could be preferable because of its lower radiation dose.
- For assessing an impacted tooth, where the reference diagnostic method is traditional 2D radiography, CBCT could be requested if the information the clinician needs cannot be adequately obtained with traditional, lower-radiation-dose radiography.

The diagnosis and, possibly, orthodontic and surgical management of an impacted canine require that such a tooth be precisely located on the three planes of space and an accurate analysis be made of its relationship with the surrounding structures.[62,63]

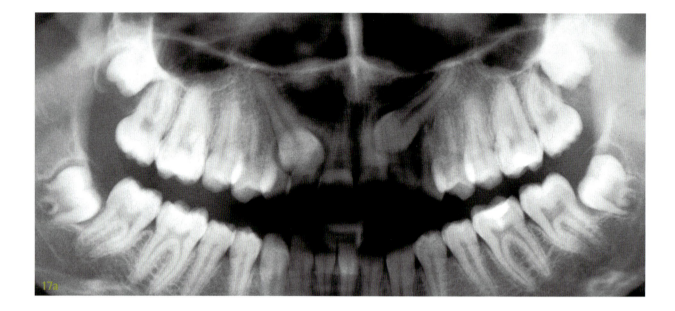

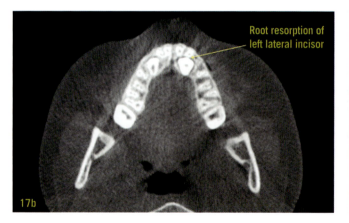

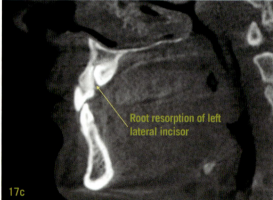

Figs 9-17a to 9-17f *(a)* The panoramic radiograph shows that both maxillary canines are impacted. Due to overlapping, it is not possible to clearly diagnose resorption in the lateral incisors, which, at a first examination, do not appear to be damaged. *(b and c)* CT provides a view on the three planes of space of the area analyzed and makes it possible to highlight root resorption of the apical third of the root of the left lateral incisor, while the right lateral incisor does not appear to be involved, *(d to f)* as confirmed by the 3D reconstruction. 3D reconstructions have been performed to highlight the relationships between lateral canines and incisors, with the remaining tissues displayed in transparence. This facilitates visual understanding of the complex three-dimensional relationships of the structures concerned; however, it is deemed more appropriate to make a diagnosis on the planar sections of the tomography itself.

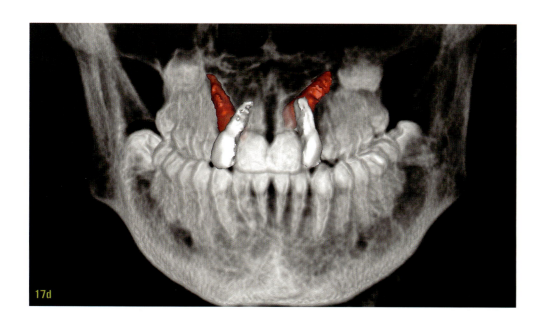

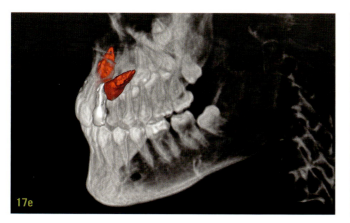
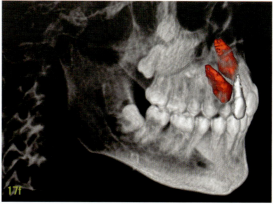

3D Diagnosis

Spatial Location of Impacted Teeth

Few papers are currently available in the literature that investigate and quantify the actual 3D position of impacted canines. Amongst these, mention should be made of the papers by Walker et al[62] and Liu et al[63] that are based on CT investigations. Both take the occlusal plane and the midsagittal plane as reference planes for their measurements; Walker et al also consider the frontal plane. The main measurements taken are:

1. *Angles:*
   - Canine axis–occlusal plane (Fig 9-18a)
   - Canine axis–midsagittal plane (Fig 9-18b)
2. *Distances:*
   - Canine cusp–occlusal plane (Fig 9-18c)
   - Canine cusp–midsagittal plane (Fig 9-18d)

Both papers report a broad variety of values, especially in regard to the angles measured; as a result, they conclude that maxillary canine impaction is broadly diverse, and no common pattern of impaction has been found.[62,63]

These considerations relate to highly diverse clinical cases of impaction and hence further support the use of radiographic investigations that allow analysis of the position of the impacted tooth on the three planes of space, like CBCT, which would be impossible with traditional 2D radiographs.[63]

Root Resorption

Root resorption of permanent maxillary incisors, in particular lateral incisors, is typically associated with ectopic canine eruption[62] (Fig 9-19).

The percentage of resorption found through CT scans in respect to lateral incisors reaches 66.7%; for central incisors, this percentage is approximately 11.1% to 23.4%.[63] This problem is extremely underestimated when using traditional 2D radiography due to the difficulty in identifying such anomalies on that type of radiograph.

Furthermore, a correlation has been found between proximity of the cusp of the impacted canine to the root of a permanent incisor and resorption of the incisor, such that it can be stated that root resorption of a tooth adjacent to an ectopic canine is caused by the pressure brought to bear by the canine cusp onto the root, without a significant mediation of the dental follicle.[62]

KPG Index

Kau et al[8] published an article in 2009 that illustrates an index called KPG (which is the acronym of the authors' surnames), the purpose of which is to provide clinicians with a method to quickly estimate the difficulty and potential effectiveness of treatment of an impacted canine. The study was made on CBCT scans as reprocessed by means of dedicated software, which made it possible to view the sagittal,

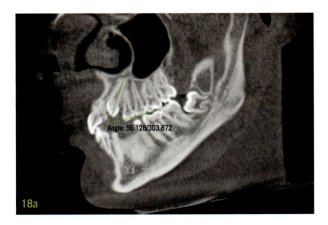
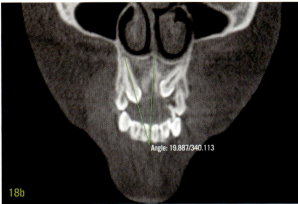
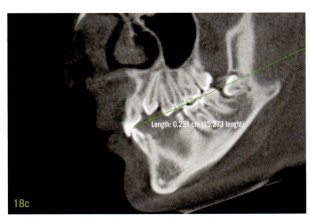
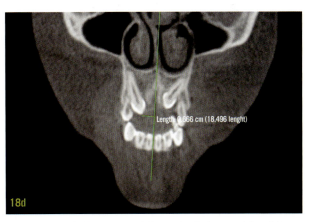

Figs 9-18a to 9-18d *(a and c)* Sagittal slice showing the angle between the long axis of the canine and the occlusal plane and the distance between the occlusal plane and the canine cusp. *(b and d)* Coronal slice showing the angle between the long axis of canine and the midsagittal plane and the distance between the canine cusp and the midsagittal plane.

coronal, and axial planes and to obtain traditional radiographic projections.

In the KPG index a value is assigned from 0 to 5 to both cusp and root apex of the impacted canine under investigation, based on their respective anatomical locations, on each of the three planes of space. Such values are then put on a grid, and their sum falls into one of the following classes of difficulty:

- 0 to 9: simple
- 10 to 14: moderate
- 15 to 19: difficult
- > 20: extremely difficult

The authors then broke down, as set out below, the three dimensions of space to analyze the position of the impacted tooth:

- *X-axis:* mesiodistal position of cusp and root apex relative to the adjacent teeth, as assessed by means of traditional panoramic radiograph (Fig 9-20a).

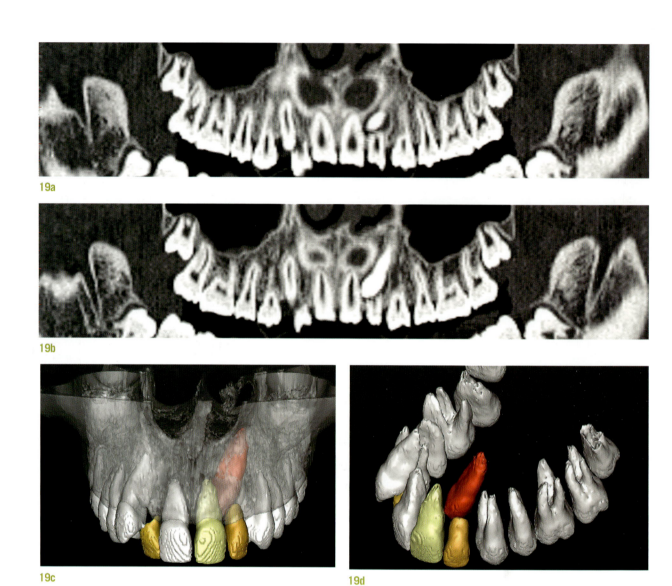

Figs 9-19a to 9-19d Severe resorption of both lateral incisors and initial involvement of the left central incisor. *(a and b)* Two pseudopanoramic images are shown in buccopalatal sequence along with *(c and d)* the 3D reconstruction.

The score assigned increases in proportion to the distance of the structure examined from its normal position. Such classification draws inspiration from the previous studies by Ericson and Kurol[50] and Lindauer et al,[5] which found that more mesialized canines have a higher likelihood of impaction.

- *y-axis:* apicocoronal position of cusp and root apex relative to the adjacent teeth, as assessed by means of conventional panoramic radiograph. In this case, because cusp and root apex are at the opposite ends of the tooth, values are assigned to the two structures in a different

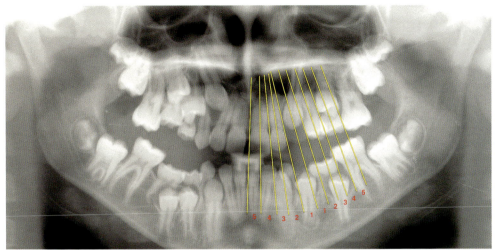

Fig 9-20a Difficulty value of the impacted canine on the x-axis according to the KPG index. The cusp of the maxillary left canine falls into sector 1. The same analysis could be done for the contralateral canine, whose cusp would fall into sector 2; therefore, the difficulty of the cusp of the right canine relative to the x-axis is greater than that of the left canine. For the apices, the score is 5 for the right canine and 3 for the left canine.

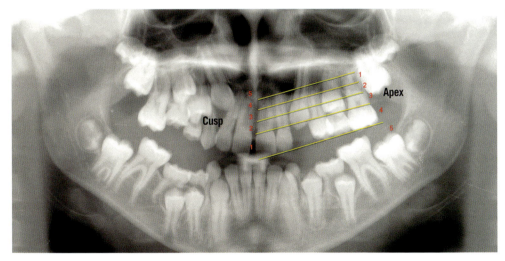

Fig 9-20b Difficulty of the impacted canine on the y-axis according to the KPG index. The left canine cusp falls into sector 1, just like its apex. The contralateral canine has its cusp at the level of the middle root third of the lateral incisor and hence falls into sector 3. The apex of the right canine is also in sector 1. Therefore, based upon the values on the y-axis, the patient's right canine is more difficult than the left canine. It should be noted that the values assigned to the cusp and the apex of the impacted tooth are opposite to those of the vertical sectors and that the root apex can hardly fall into high-difficulty sectors from the vertical point of view.

manner, as shown in Fig 9-20b. Such classification refers to the one used in 2008 by Liu et al.[63]

- *z-axis:* buccopalatal position of cusp and root apex relative to a curved line following the maxillary occlusal arch, as assessed on CBCT axial sections (Fig 9-20c). Each buccal or palatal curve is 2 mm away from the ideal occlusal arch and highlights sectors of growing difficulty ranging from 1 to 5. Hence, for every 2 mm of distance of the cusp or apex of the impacted canine from the 0 curve, the difficulty of the canine relative

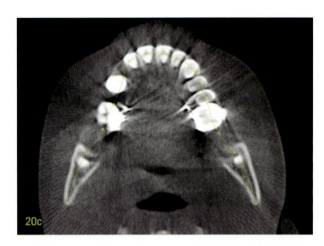

Figs 9-20c to 9-20g *(c)* Difficulty of the impacted canine on the z-axis according to the KPG index. *(d)* The cusp of the left canine is approximately 1 mm away from the ideal occlusal angle and therefore falls into the first buccal sector relative to the ideal occlusal arch. The level of difficulty is 1. *(e)* The cusp of the right canine, instead, is 3.5 mm away from the ideal occlusal angle and therefore falls into the second palatal sector relative to the ideal occlusal arch of the maxillary dental arch. The level of difficulty is 2. *(f)* The apex of the left canine is 6.3 mm away from the ideal arch and therefore falls in the fourth palatal sector (score 4). *(g)* Finally, the apex of the right canine is slightly more than 2 mm palatal to the ideal arch, and therefore the score is 2.

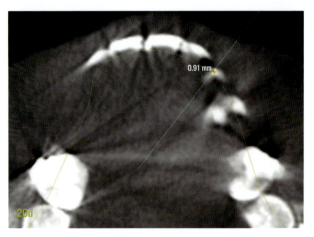
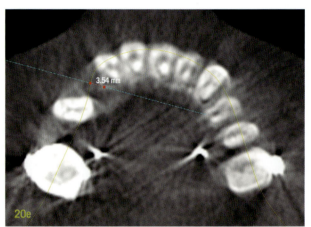
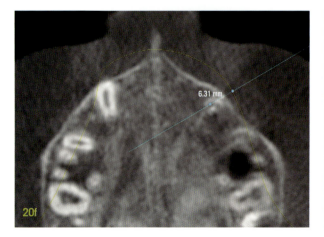
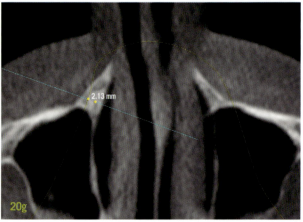

to the Z-axis increases by 1 point (Figs 9-20d to 9-20g).

Hence, upon the observation of a traditional panoramic radiograph and the axial views of a CBCT, the authors assign scores to the cusp of the canine and to its root apex, based upon their respective position in space. The difficulty of salvaging the tooth is classified based on the sum of such values (Table 9-3). According to the authors, the more difficult an impacted tooth is, the longer the time of treatment, possibly requiring the use of more advanced orthodontic techniques.

Despite its being still a work in progress, this is the first study to consider using 3D coordinates for assigning a level of difficulty to canine impaction. However, being based upon the location of points in a 3D space, this index does not consider other factors that can realistically alter the actual difficulty of treatment, such as root dilaceration of the impacted tooth or the closeness of the impacted tooth to other teeth, possibly associated with resorption of the same.

"Impacted Canines" Cephalometric Tracing

The precise location in space of impacted canines can be quantified by means of a simple 3D cephalometric tracing called "Impacted Canines."[64]

The landmarks were selected (Table 9-4), the construction planes of the tracing were determined (Table 9-5), and the measurements deemed to be most significant were taken (Table 9-6), all in light of the current literature.[62,63]

Table 9-3 Summary classification of impacted maxillary right and left canines as shown in Fig 9-20*				
	Maxillary Right Canine (13)		Maxillary Left Canine (23)	
	Cusp	Apex	Cusp	Apex
x axis	2	5	1	3
y axis	3	1	1	1
z axis	2	2	1	4
Result	15 – DIFFICULT		11 – MODERATE	

*The clinical case is the same as shown in Fig 9-7. The KPG index confirms what was already intuitively observed by means of radiographs, ie, that the maxillary right canine is more difficult than the contralateral one. Moreover, the table gives an idea of the factors underlying such difficulty, ie, mainly the distal position of the root apex and the long distance between the cusp and the occlusal plane.

Table 9-4 Impacted canine landmarks for cephalometric tracing*	
	Landmarks
Canine cusp tip (CT)	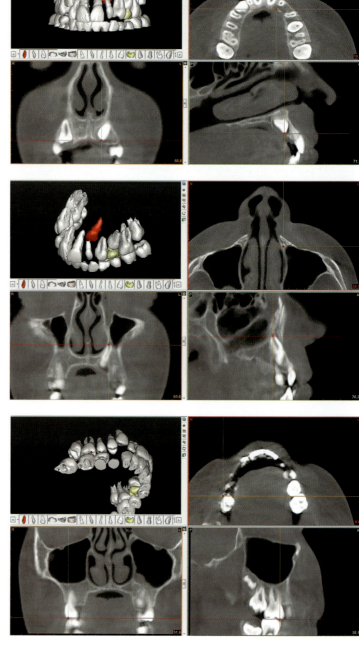
Canine cusp apex (CA)	
Mesiobuccal cusp of the maxillary right first molar (MBR)	

*As recommended in the scientific literature, the position of each landmark should be checked on each plane of space for it to be considered precise and repeatable. Mere positioning of the landmarks on the 3D reconstruction is not sufficiently reliable.

Table 9-4 (continued)

	Landmarks
Mesiobuccal cusp of the maxillary left first molar (MBL)	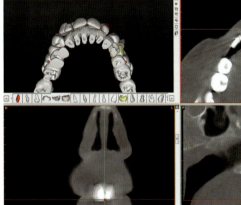
Midincisal (MI) point	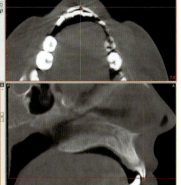
Anterior nasal spine (ANS)	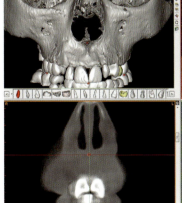

Table 9-4 (continued)

	Landmarks
Posterior nasal spine (PNS)	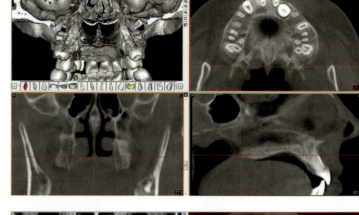
Nasopalatine foramen (NP)	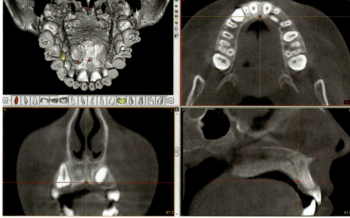

Table 9-5 Impacted canine construction planes for cephalometric tracing*

Construction planes

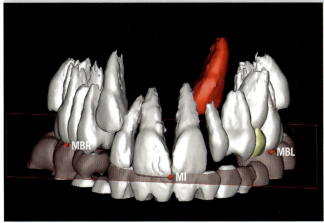

O (Occlusal plane): plane passing through MBR, MBL, and MI

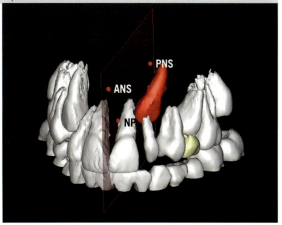

MS (Midsagittal plane): plane passing through ANS, PNS, and NP

*It should be noted that plane O is determined by dental landmarks, whereas the MS plane is determined by skeletal landmarks.

Table 9-6 Impacted canine measurements for cephalometric tracing

Construction planes

CT-O: distance (in mm) between the impacted canine cusp (CT) and the occlusal plane (O)

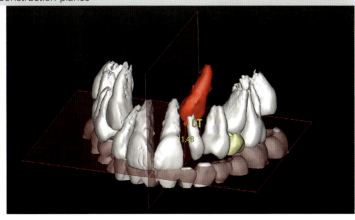

Table 9-6 (continued)

	Measurements
CT-MS: distance (in mm) between the impacted canine cusp (CT) and the midsagittal plane (MS)	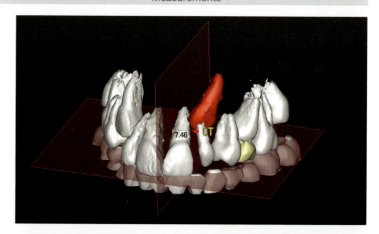
CAx^O: angle between the impacted canine axis (CAx) and the occlusal plane (O)	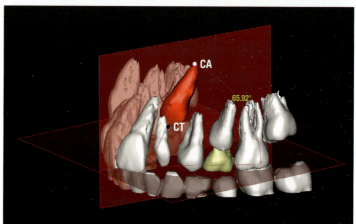
CAx^MS: angle between the impacted canine axis (CAx) and the midsagittal plane (MS)	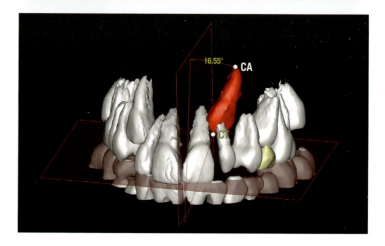

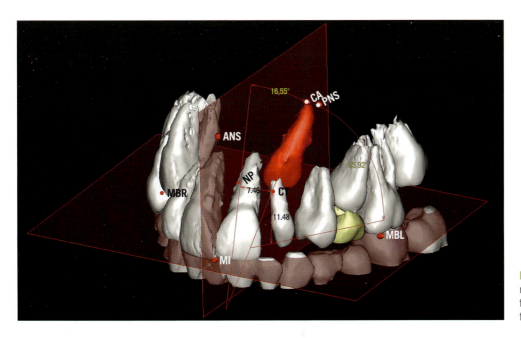

Fig 9-21 Impacted canine 3D cephalometric tracing of the same patient shown in Fig 9-8.

The resulting 3D cephalometric tracing enables the clinician to precisely determine the position in space of the impacted canine (Fig 9-21). This information is very useful in the subsequent stage of therapeutic planning, with a view to choosing the least invasive surgical technique and planning the correct orthodontic forces to be applied during guided eruption of the impacted tooth.

Simulation of Impacted Canine Orthodontic Salvage

A further possibility offered by the new 3D technologies is the simulation of the orthodontic salvage of an impacted canine by progressively shifting it from its actual position to the desired one in the arch, through transverse and rotational movements on the three planes of space. The same procedure can apply to all other teeth, with a 3D virtual setup (Fig 9-22).

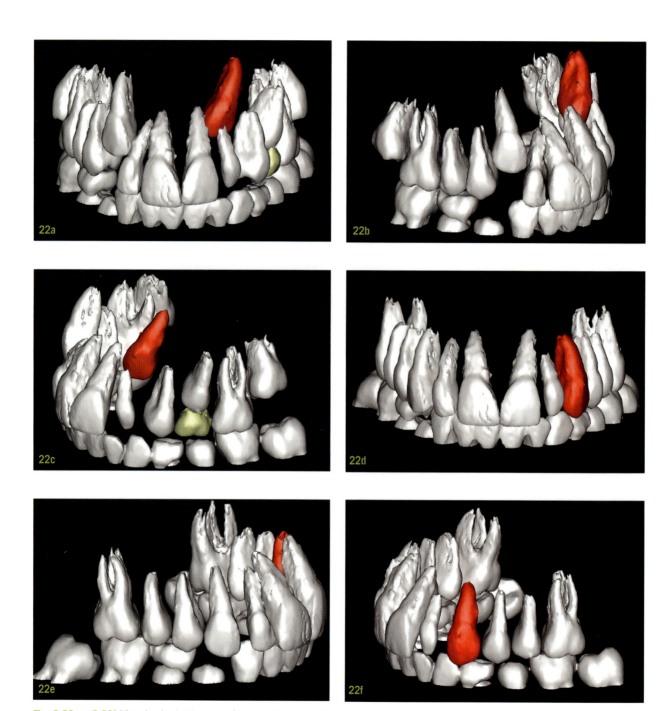

Figs 9-22a to 9-22f Virtual orthodontic setup of the maxillary arch of the patient to whom the impacted canine cephalometric tracing has been applied: *(a to c)* baseline tooth positions; *(d to f)* the final desired setup after repositioning all of the maxillary teeth.

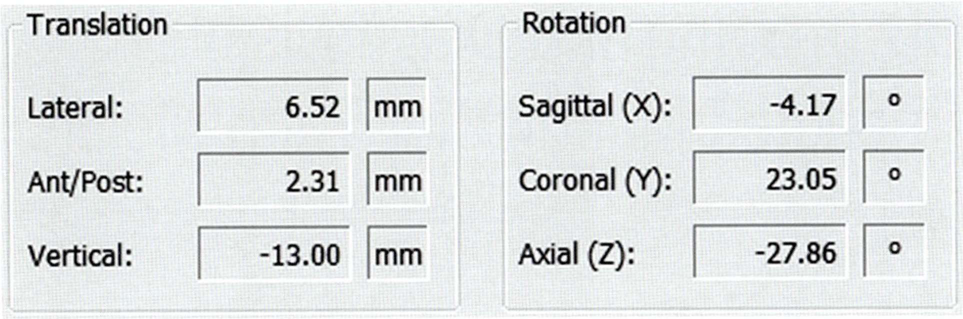

Translation			Rotation		
Lateral:	6.52	mm	Sagittal (X):	-4.17	°
Ant/Post:	2.31	mm	Coronal (Y):	23.05	°
Vertical:	-13.00	mm	Axial (Z):	-27.86	°

Fig 9-23 Summary of the simulated shift of impacted maxillary left canine, as shown in Fig 9-22.

The overall shift from the initial to the final position of each tooth is recorded and summarized by the software in terms of both translation and 3D rotation (Fig 9-23).

3D Imaging and Diagnosis of Impacted Mandibular Third Molars

Surgical extraction of mandibular third molars remains one of the most frequent oral surgeries and one that can involve major hidden dangers due to the relationship with the surrounding structures.

Normally, the follicle of mandibular third molars becomes visible at age 8 to 9 years. If, by age 14 to 16 years, the follicle is not clearly visible on radiographs, one can consider agenesis of the tooth, bearing in mind that formation of the crypt of the mandibular third molar can appear at the latest by the age of 15 years[65,66] (Figs 9-24 and 9-25).

At the time that the mandibular second molar mineralizes, it is possible to observe a posterior extension of the dental lamina and concomitant resorption of the bone exactly where the germ of the third molar will develop.

In principle, the mandibular third molar is positioned inside the ramus of the mandible with an angle of the occlusal plane of the newly formed crown that is similar to that of the mandibular plane. In order to be in the spatial position, it will have to undergo an uprighting movement during eruption (Figs 9-26 to 9-29).

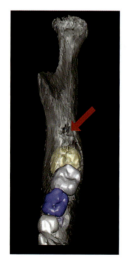

Fig 9-24a 3D rendering with view superior to the crypt of the third molar, distal to the germ of the second molar *(arrow)*; the mandible is shown in transparence, and the germ of the permanent second molar is segmented *(yellow)*.

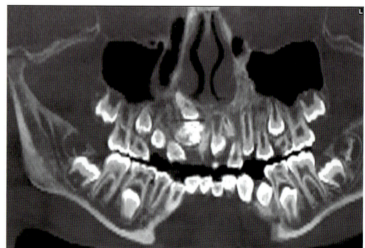

Fig 9-24b CBCT panoramic image obtained from a Digital Imaging and Communications in Medicine (DICOM) file, highlighting appearance of the follicle of the right third molar at the level of the right hemimandible.

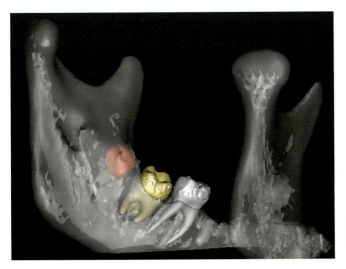

Fig 9-25 3D rendering of the mandible of a 13-year-old patient with late appearance of the follicle of the third molar *(segmented in red)*: the second molar *(segmented in yellow)* is already present in the arch.

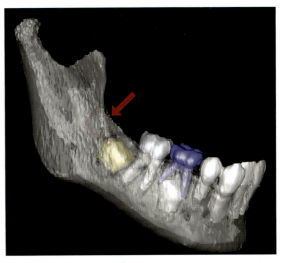

Fig 9-26 3D rendering with lateral view of the first stage of formation of the impacted third molar *(arrow)* and its follicle *(broken line)*.

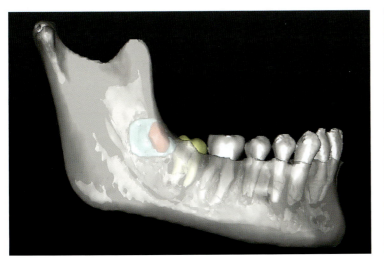

Fig 9-27a 3D rendering with lateral view of the second stage of formation of the impacted third molar: the crown has been reconstructed *(red)*, and the remaining portion of the follicle has been highlighted *(light blue)*.

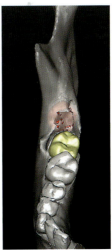

Fig 9-27b 3D rendering with occlusal view of the second stage of formation of the impacted third molar: the crown of the third molar *(red)* is highlighted by the transparency of the mandibular bone.

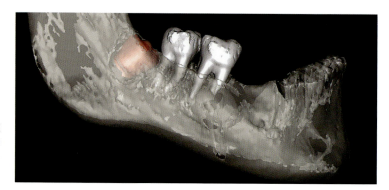

Fig 9-28 3D rendering with lateral view of the third stage of maturation of the impacted third molar.

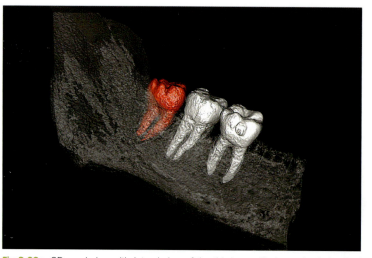

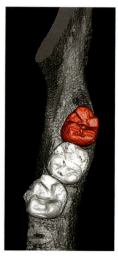

Fig 9-29b 3D rendering with occlusal view of the third molar after its emergence from the mandibular bone.

Fig 9-29a 3D rendering with lateral view of the third mandibular molar in its final stage of growth.

The germ of the third molar remains in position until the crown is in its formation stage, and then it begins to erupt, detaching from the mandibular canal when the coronal portion of the root is formed.

If the tooth finds resistance during eruption, its maturation will continue close to the mandibular canal, with formation of indentations and/or notches, apex deflections, and, in rare instances, circumferential growth of the roots around the mandibular canal, to the effect that the inferior alveolar neurovascular bundle passes through a sort of tunnel (Figs 9-30 and 9-31).

Changes in the eruption direction usually lead to root deflection, thus resulting in a curved eruption of the mandibular third molar, taking into account that growth of this tooth within the mandible causes the root apices to diverge (Fig 9-32).

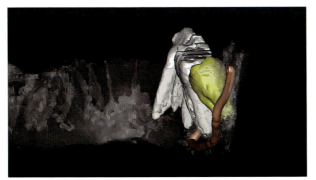

Fig 9-30 3D rendering with posterior view of a semi-impacted third molar, with lingual course of the mandibular canal in close contact.

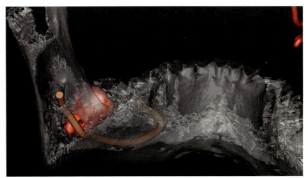

Fig 9-31 3D rendering with posterior view of a mandibular third molar with the root being indented by the course of the mandibular canal.

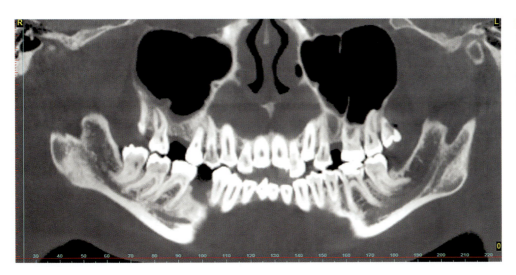

Fig 9-32a CBCT panoramic image of a patient presenting a third molar with strongly deflected roots and close contact with the mandibular canal.

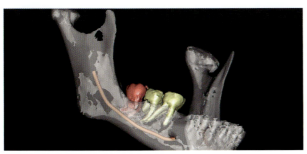

Fig 9-32b 3D rendering of the mandible with the third molar segmented in red.

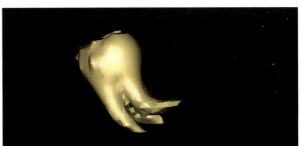

Fig 9-32c Detail of third molar showing the degree of root deflection.

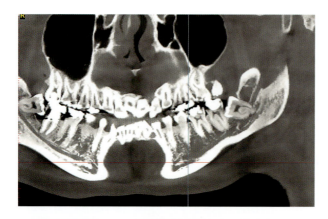

Fig 9-33 CBCT panoramic image of a patient showing the mandibular third molar with fused roots in contact with the mandibular canal.

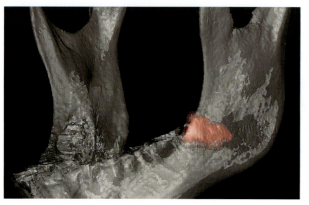

Fig 9-34a 3D rendering of partially impacted third molar with fused roots.

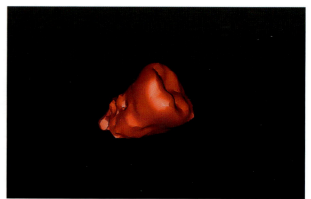

Fig 9-34b Detail of impacted tooth clearly showing fused roots.

Another phenomenon that can change root morphology and anatomy is the formation of excess cementum in semi-impacted or fully impacted molars, an occurrence that leads to fusion of the roots that were originally separate or to swelling of the middle portion of the roots (Figs 9-33 and 9-34).

Etiology of Impaction

The etiologic cause of third molar impaction comprises multiple factors:

- *Lack of space in the region of the third molar*[67,68]: The growth of the ramus of the mandible is associated with resorption of the anterior surface of the ramus and deposition of newly formed bone on the posterior surface. Without this balance, mandibular third molars will not have enough space to erupt[69,70] (Fig 9-35).

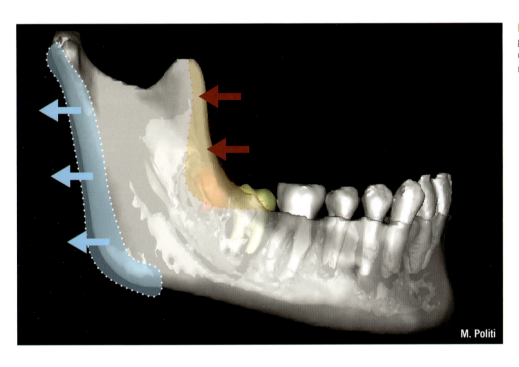

Fig 9-35 Mandibular growth favoring an increase in space in the retromandibular region.

- Obstruction of the eruption path: The presence of odontomas, cysts, supernumerary teeth, or particularly dense bone can hamper the eruption into the arch of the mandibular third molar.

  - *Angle of third molar:* If the tooth is angulated medially during the initial stages of calcification and root development, the direction of eruption will not be a favorable one[71] (Fig 9-36).

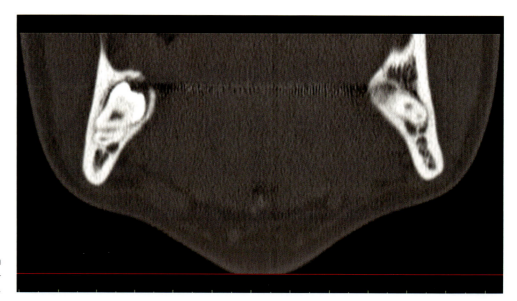

Fig 9-36 Coronal section showing the medial angle of the left third molar.

- *Vertical growth pattern*[72–75]: Dolichocephalic patients, with posteriorly rotated mandibular growth associated with reduced growth of the ramus, would appear to be more at risk for third molar impaction. Similarly, brachycephalic patients, with horizontal mandibular growth and good vertical growth of the ramus, would appear to be less exposed to this risk.[74] The studies carried out by Nanda[76] show that brachycephalic patients present prolonged growth compared to dolichocephalic patients; thus, possible residual growth of the mandible in brachycephalic patients would also appear to favor formation of the correct space for eruption of the mandibular third molar[72] (Fig 9-37).
- *Ectopic position of the follicle*
- *Poor eruptive force of third molars* and the phylogenetic theory of the reduction in the size of the mandible[73,74]
- *Late mineralization of third molar/ early physical maturity*

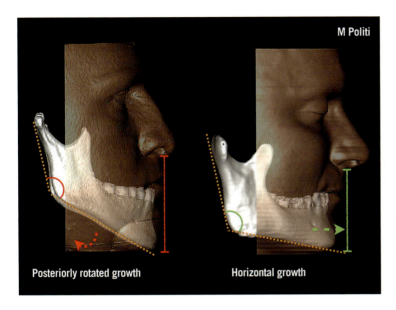

Fig 9-37 Comparison of two different growth patterns: brachycephalic patient *(right)* with horizontal growth of the mandible and dolichocephalic patient *(left)* with posteriorly rotated growth of the mandible and an increase in vertical dimension of the lower third of the face *(red line)*.

Anatomical Structures of Interest in the Region of the Third Molar

The critical structures to be considered when extracting the mandibular third molar are as follows: alveolar bone surrounding the tooth, periodontal ligament on the distal surface of the second molar, inferior alveolar neurovascular bundle, and lingual nerve.

A deep knowledge of the anatomy and position of these structures and of their interrelationships allows the clinician to choose amongst different surgical approaches (Fig 9-38).

Alveolar Bone

The third molar is positioned in a portion of alveolar bone that is medial and anterior to the ramus of the mandible. This implies that the mandibular third molar is often covered by more bone buccally than lingually (Fig 9-39). In most cases, the lingual bone is comprised of a very thin cortical layer, and when attempting to extract a fractured apex, it may happen that the latter is inadvertently dislocated to the submandibular space.[77]

The bony septum between the second and third molars can be very thin or even absent. In these cases, it is absolutely necessary to use caution while using the elevator so as to avoid damaging the integrity of the periodontal ligament of the second molar, which might lead to a loss of bony support[78] (Figs 9-40 and 9-41).

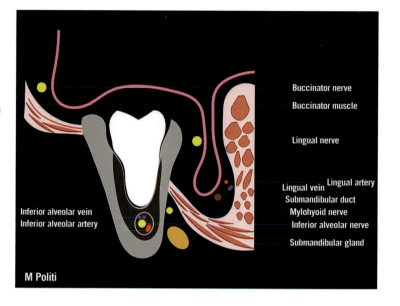

Fig 9-38 Frontal view of the anatomy of the region of the third molar.

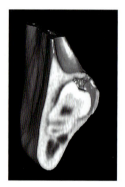

Fig 9-39 3D rendering of mandibular coronal section showing the amount of buccal alveolar bone compared to the lingual alveolar bone.

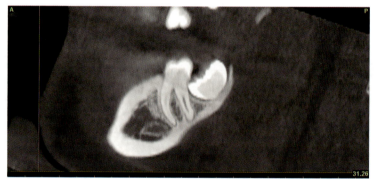

Fig 9-40 Sagittal section in a patient showing the bone septum between the second and third molars.

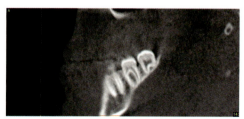

Fig 9-41a Sagittal section in a patient without an infraosseous septum between the second and third molars.

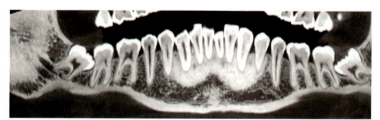

Fig 9-41b CBCT panoramic image of patient without an infraosseous septum between the second and third molars.

Mandibular Canal

The mandible is traversed by a principal canal, the mandibular canal, which, beginning at the ramus, crosses the mandibular body and exits through the mental foramen. The canal can be buccal or lingual to the mandibular third molar or between its roots. Inside the canal is the inferior alveolar neurovascular bundle, composed of the inferior alveolar artery, the inferior alveolar nerve, and three or more inferior alveolar veins (Fig 9-42).

In view of correct surgical management, it is useful to know the spatial relationships between the various structures of the inferior alveolar neurovascular bundle. The inferior alveolar artery is always inferior to the nerve and in a more lingual position, while superior to the nerve, in a more buccal position, is the alveolar vein, which is composed of three to five vessels.[79]

This implies that, in the event of the tooth and the mandibular canal being contiguous, injury of the alveolar artery during extraction of the third molar, with the resulting bleeding, is associated with nerve damage, with the nerve being necessarily traumatized before a tool can reach the underlying artery. Only with a lingual approach to the mandibular canal is it possible to damage the artery and spare the nerve.

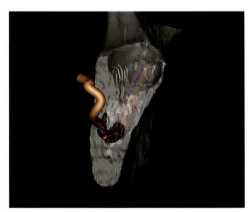

Fig 9-42 3D reconstruction of dissected mandible highlighting the components of the inferior alveolar neurovascular bundle: the inferior alveolar nerve, the inferior alveolar artery, and two to three veins.

Nervous Component

The inferior alveolar nerve stems from the mandibular nerve (third branch of the trigeminal nerve), while the lingual nerve originates near the foramen ovale (approximately 5 to 10 mm from the skull base) and runs close to the main branch; both nerves pass toward the medial surface of the ramus of the mandible. Close to the lingula of the mandible (also referred to as spine of Spix), a new branch, the mylohyoid nerve, departs from the inferior alveolar nerve, which instead enters into the mandibular canal (Fig 9-43). Near the third molar, the lingual nerve

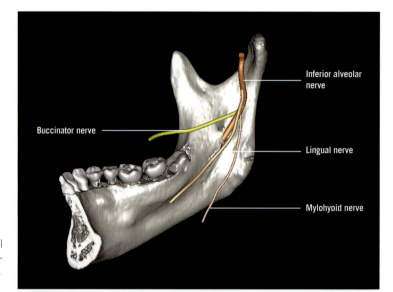

Fig 9-43 3D rendering of the nervous structures: all the terminal branches of the mandibular nerve depart from its main trunk, beyond the foramen ovale.

Fig 9-44 Reconstruction of the course of the lingual nerve, with measurement of its distance from the alveolar crest and from the lingual surface.

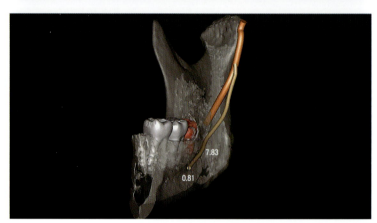

usually comes into close contact with the lingual surface of the mandible. This nerve is frequently located about 0.8 mm medial to the mandible and 7.8 mm below the alveolar crest (with some degree of variation, depending on the degree of atrophy of the mandible as well)[80] (Fig 9-44).

The inferior alveolar nerve enters the ramus of the mandible and runs in the mandibular body until it splits into the incisive branch, which continues to the incisors, and the mental branch, which exits at the mental foramen (Fig 9-45).

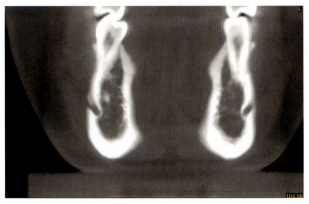

Fig 9-45a Coronal slice of the mental foramen, from which the mental branch of the inferior alveolar nerve exits.

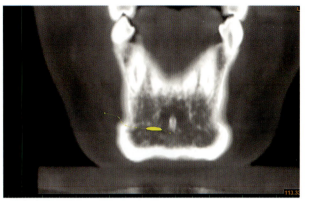

Fig 9-45b Coronal slice highlighting the course *(yellow)* of the incisive-branch portion of the inferior alveolar nerve.

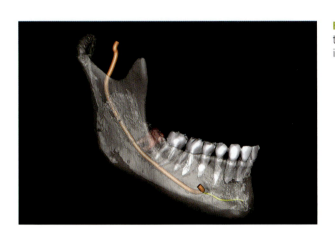

Fig 9-45c 3D rendering of mandibular innervation: reconstruction of the courses of the inferior alveolar nerve, the mental branch, and the incisive branch.

Bony Trabeculae

The visibility of the mandibular canal can vary from patient to patient as well as from one area of the mandible to the other. The canal is more easily identified in the posterior area, and its visibility tends to decrease gradually as it reaches the mental foramen due to the reduction in trabecular bone[81] (Fig 9-46).

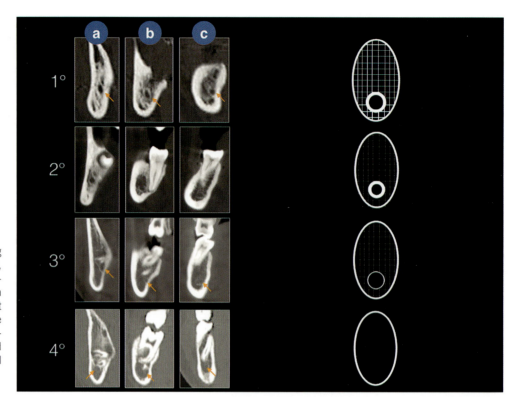

Fig 9-46 Image showing four different mandibles, with decreasing trabeculae, as captured through three cross sections at the same points: *(a)* close to the third molar, *(b)* mesial to the first molar, and *(c)* close to the mental foramen.

Accessory Canals

Though typically described as a single canal, in some cases the mandibular canal can be bifid or even trifid, and the presence of such variations requires careful clinical assessment. Such branches can originate when the inferior alveolar nerve is already within the canal or may originate in the infratemporal fossa and then enter the mandible as separate branches. Inadequate anesthesia can be explained by the presence of an additional mandibular canal or an accessory foramen. During surgery, the presence of two or three neurovascular bundles can lead to damage of one of them, causing paresthesia, development of a neuroma, or bleeding. Naioth et al[82] suggested that mandibular canals be classified into four types:

1. *Retromolar (type 1):* Also called Robinson's canal, this type is defined as the branch in which the foramen is in the bone surface of the retromolar region; then it extends distally to the second molar or up to the third molar, depending on the dental formula (agenesis of the third molar) and the severity of impaction of the third molar. The incidence of this canal is 7.7% to 25%,[83,84] and it can be associated with an accessory mandibular foramen. Histopathologic studies have enabled identification of the contents of the retromolar canal, which comprises myelinated nerve fibers, one arterial vessel, and several venous vessels[84,85] (Fig 9-47).
2. *Anterior (type 2):* This type is present when the canal ends in the apices of the second or third molar (Fig 9-48).

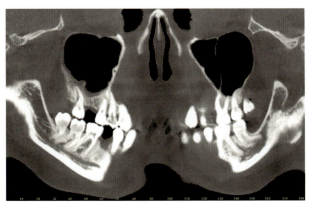

Fig 9-47a CBCT panoramic image obtained from a DICOM file showing the presence on the right hemimandible of a retromolar accessory canal (type 1).

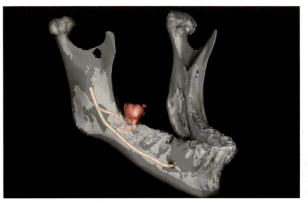

Fig 9-47b 3D rendering showing the course of the alveolar canal and the retromolar canal *(orange)* and the mandibular third molar *(red)*.

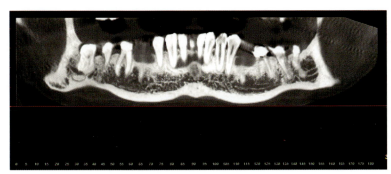

Fig 9-48a CBCT panoramic image: the arrow indicates the start of the bifurcation of the anterior accessory canal (type 2).

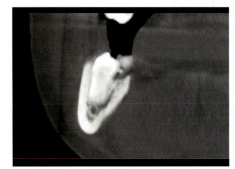

Fig 9-48b Coronal slice highlighting the superolingual course of the accessory canal.

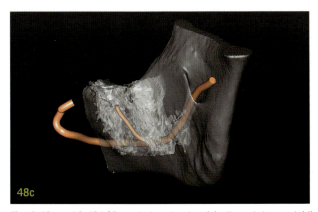

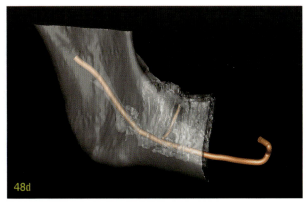

Figs 9-48c and 9-48d 3D rendering showing *(c)* a lingual view and *(d)* a buccal view of the course of the anterior accessory canal.

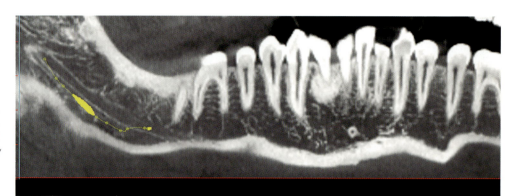

Fig 9-49a CBCT panoramic image of a mandible with a buccolingual accessory canal *(yellow line)* (type 3).

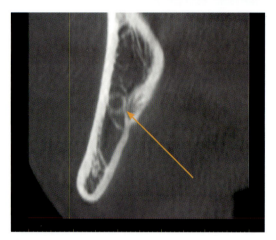

Fig 9-49b Coronal slice highlighting the presence of two canals *(orange arrow)*.

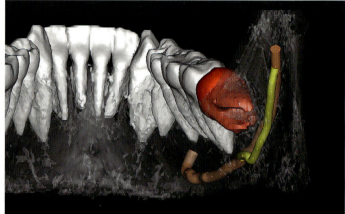

Fig 9-49c 3D rendering showing, from a posterolingual view, the course of the buccolingual accessory canal.

3. *Buccolingual (type 3):* This accessory canal detaches from the superior wall of the main canal with or without confluence of the latter (Fig 9-49).
4. *Dental (type 4):* The accessory canal detaches lingually or buccally from the main canal (Fig 9-50).

Serres' canal is a temporary canal that is only present at a young age and allows passage of a vascular bundle only; it tends to disappear with the loss of the last primary teeth (age 8 to 9 years).[19]

Preoperative Assessment

An accurate preoperative assessment is fundamental when considering the surgical extraction of the third molar impacted in the mandibular jaw. In particular:

- Plan adequate surgical time.
- Inform the patient before surgery of the possible risk of complications.
- Assess the degree of difficulty, especially in relation to the experience of the surgeon.

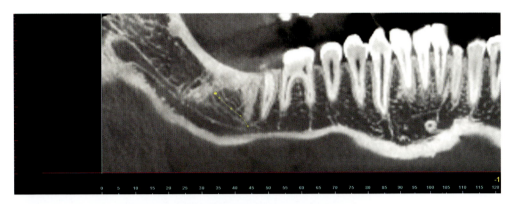

Fig 9-50a CBCT panoramic image of mandible with dental accessory canal (yellow line) (type 4).

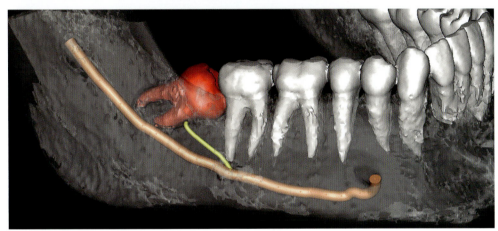

Fig 9-50b 3D rendering, from a buccal view, of the course of the dental accessory canal.

It is fundamental for the clinician to assess the difficulty of the surgery; in particular, less experienced surgeons should refrain from performing surgeries that may be too demanding. Various attempts have been made to build a reliable model to assess surgical difficulty, but, although several have been defined, none of them has yet been universally adopted.

The most well-known classification systems, both based on radiologic findings, are that of Winter[86] and that of Pell and Gregory[87] (Figs 9-51 to 9-53).

These classifications were only based on radiographic variables, while recent research has shown an association with other clinical and demographic variables as well.[88–90]

In a recent literature review, Akadiri et al[91] state that demographic, radiographic, and clinical variants are strongly associated with the difficulty of the surgery. Therefore, several pieces of information need be gathered to predict with reasonable accuracy the difficulty of the surgical extraction of an impacted third molar.

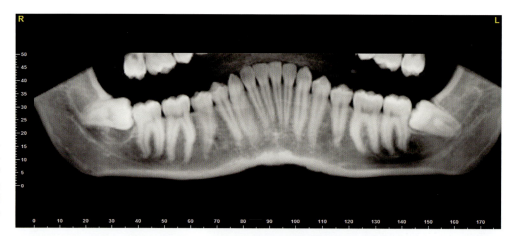

Fig 9-51a CBCT panoramic image of a mesially inclined mandibular right third molar with increased pericoronal space due to pericoronitis.

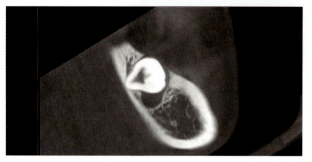

Fig 9-51b Sagittal slice showing a broadening of the pericoronal space due to tooth angle.

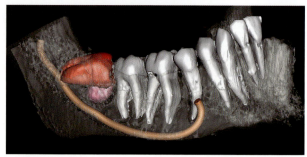

Fig 9-51c 3D rendering of mandible with a mesially inclined third molar leading to inflammation *(pink)* inferior to the crown.

Some data are patient-related factors:

- Overall health status
- Age
- Body mass index
- Accessibility of the surgical site and degree of opening of the mouth
- Degree of collaboration of the patient

Five points must be evaluated in detail to correctly predict the difficulty of the surgery in anatomical/radiologic terms:

- Pericoronal space
- Periodontal space
- Impaction
- Root morphology
- Relationship with the mandibular canal

The pericoronal space can be thin, as is the case with healthy young adults, and then broaden during development or after episodes of pericoronitis, or absent, as is often the case with the edentulous elderly (see Fig 9-51).

The periodontal ligament[92] can be radiotransparent or radiopaque, as well as with normal width, broadened, or absent.

Several variables describe impaction:

- *Type of impaction*[93]: erupted/partial mucosa, mucosa/partial bony, or full bony; this variable indicates to the clinician not just the type of surgical procedure to be used,[94] but also the duration of surgery.

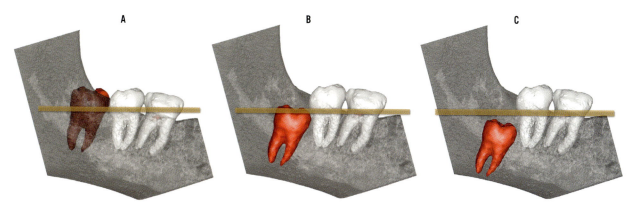

Fig 9-52 Classification of surgical difficulty according to Pell and Gregory based on the position of the third molar relative to the cementoenamel junction of the second molar.

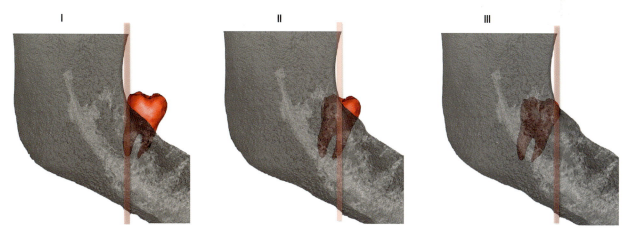

Fig 9-53 Classification of surgical difficulty according to Pell and Gregory based on the position of the third molar relative to the anterior edge of the mandibular ramus.

- *Depth:* distance between the occlusal plane passing through the crown of the second molar and the crown of the third molar (Pell and Gregory[87]) (see Fig 9-52).
- *Image of the crown of the impacted tooth overlapping that of the ramus of the mandible:* no overlapping, partial overlapping, ramus overlapping the entire crown (Pell and Gregory[87]) (see Fig 9-53).
- *Angle:* measured by calculating the angle between the axis of the second molar and that of the third molar; the angle may be mesial, vertical, distal, horizontal, or inverted (Winter[86]) (Fig 9-54).
- *Rotation:* buccal, axial, or lingual (Fig 9-55).
- *Proximity to second molar*[95]: presence or absence of a bone septum or of a radiotransparent space between the second and the third molar.

Root morphology is fundamental to evaluate the difficulty of surgery.

Several factors comprise the evaluation of root morphology:

- Degree of formation (Fig 9-56)[94,95]
- Number of roots[94–96]
- Angle between roots: parallel, convergent, divergent[95]
- Length of the root trunk[94,95]
- Curvature of the lower third of the root[94,97,98] (Fig 9-57)

A 3D examination enables a more complete assessment of root morphology, given that over 10% of third molars have three to four roots that are difficult to define with traditional radiography.[99]

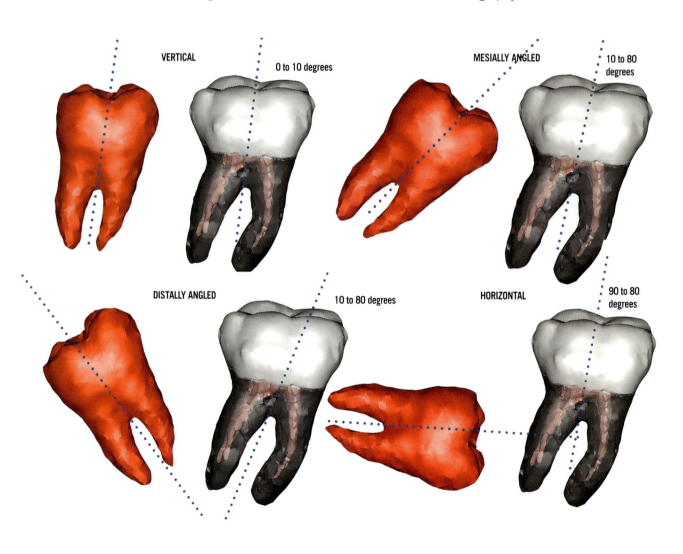

Fig 9-54 Classification of difficulty of the surgery according to Winter,[86] based on the inclination of the third molar *(red)* relative to the second molar.

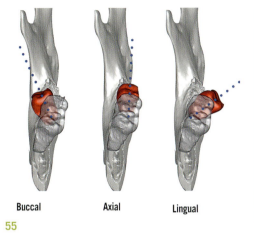

Buccal Axial Lingual

55

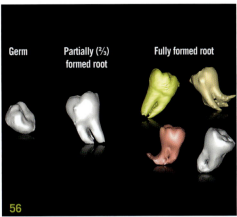

56

Fig 9-55 Representation of the three possible rotations of the third molar.
Fig 9-56 Illustration of third molars in different stages of maturation: root maturation, as shown, can be varied.

Relationship Between the Mandibular Canal and the Mandibular Third Molar

A panoramic radiograph cannot provide information on buccolingual spatial relationships between the mandibular canal and the third molar when their images are overlapped. Panoramic radiography only enables the clinician to exclude with certainty any contact when the images of the mandibular canal and the impacted tooth are neither in contact nor overlapped.[100] Closeness of the mandibular canal is a factor of difficulty, as it reduces the operating range of the surgical instruments, especially rotating ones, which must not damage the inferior alveolar neurovascular bundle.

Direct contact between tooth and the mandibular canal can be excluded with certainty when the distance between the two is ≥ 0.5 mm as shown by panoramic radiography.[100]

SEPARATE	**> 0.5 mm** between apex and mandibular canal
IN CONTACT	**−0.5 mm to 0.5 mm** between apex and mandibular canal
OVERLAPPING	**< −0.5 mm**

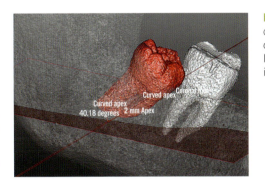

Fig 9-57 Analysis of the curvature of the root apex of a mandibular third molar, performed using dedicated imaging software.

Nakagawa et al[101] and Szalma et al[94] state that women with an absence of the cortical surface of the mandibular canal, as shown by panoramic radiographs, are strongly associated with an increased risk of paresthesia of the inferior alveolar nerve. One of the possible reasons is that the mandible in the area of the third molar is thinner (buccolingually) in women, and this determines a shorter distance between tooth and canal, thus increasing the risk of lesion.[71]

In 1990 Rood and Sheehab[102] defined the indicators of risk of complications for the inferior alveolar nerve that can be seen with panoramic radiography. Of course, when panoramic radiography does not show these specific signs, one should not necessarily rule out contact between the molar and the canal,[100] but this fact does not diminish the capability of the indicators to predict damage. However, in the absence of conclusive evidence, it can be maintained that surgeons find in 3D images valuable information for preventing damage, which allows for a more rational planning of surgery in the cases at risk. The European Commission recently launched a project (SEDENTEXCT) to codify the indications for requesting 3D images and, in particular, for the use of CBCT. The team of experts in charge of preparing the guidelines based on scientific evidence has established that routine radiographic study of impacted mandibular third molars is based on 2D images. Only after the decision has been made to extract the impacted tooth, and in the presence of risk factors found in panoramic radiographs, is the use of CBCT warranted. Then, the surgeon can deem 3D images to be necessary every time the surgical plan provides that instruments will come very close to—or even go beyond—the alveolar canal, given that the buccolingual position of the canal cannot be established with 2D images.

The indicators of risk of contact between the third molar and the mandibular canal identified by Rood and Shehab[102] are the following:

- Increased root radiolucency
- Interruption of the opaque line that marks the boundary of the canal
- Sharp deflection of the root
- Decoupled apex (bifid root)
- Sharp deviation of the direction of the canal
- Narrowing of the canal

The data provided by Rood and Shehab has been essentially confirmed by subsequent literature[103–105] and also validated by 3D imaging data, with the latter having confirmed the association between these signs and a spatial relationship of close proximity.[100,106–108]

For example, curved roots were associated with a higher frequency of paresthesia (24.4% vs 10%) with an odds ratio of 2.65.[94] Also, Tay and Go[97] stated that teeth with curved roots represent a high risk for paresthesia (odds ratio, 2.54). However, panoramic radiographs do not enable the anatomy of the impacted tooth to be defined in detail, and root curvatures can be over- or underestimated.[98]

Palma-Carrió et al[109] compared the sensitivity and specificity of CT versus panoramic radiography, which were measured to be, respectively, 93% and 77% (CT) against 70% and 63% (panoramic). This indicates that 3D examination is significantly better than panoramic radiography in predicting nerve exposure during the extraction of the mandibular third molar, even though a nerve lesion is rare despite exposure of the neurovascular bundle.[79] In other words, the predictive value of radiographic indicators is very low, in both 2D and 3D images. Luckily, however, the negative predictive value is high: neurologic damage is quite rare in the absence of specific signs of risk.

Patients have been split into high-risk and low-risk groups, based on the sum of the radiologic signs that have been validated in different studies[97,98,100,109,110] (Fig 9-58).

NERVE COMPLICATIONS
RELATIONSHIP WITH THE MANDIBULAR CANAL

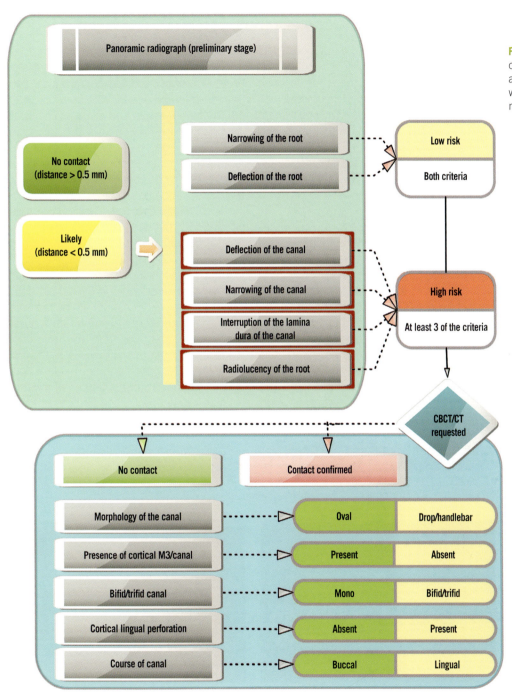

Fig 9-58 Decision flowchart for the extraction of a mandibular third molar when it is close to the mandibular canal.

Conclusion

A 3D examination enables a more complete assessment of root morphology, given that more than 10% of third molars have three to four roots that are difficult to define with conventional radiography.[99] Only 3D imaging can provide surgeons with information on the spatial relationships between the impacted tooth and the mandibular canal. Low-dose tomography (CBCT) with an adequate field of view (for the molar region, a 5 × 5–cm field of view is adequate) so as to further reduce exposure to radiation provides clinicians with much more information compared to a 2D image. It is very important to determine the thickness of the slice to be requested from the radiology center, which cannot exceed 0.2 mm to avoid poor sharpness of the image and to prevent missing anatomical details that can be important.[111]

In some cases, the following considerations can be useful for a more complete preoperative assessment, because they enable the clinician to make various judgements when planning surgery:

- *Relationship between root apex and mandibular canal:* The possibility to accurately identify the relationship between these two structures can lead to a different surgical approach (Fig 9-59).
- *Presence or absence of bone between impacted tooth and canal:* (The radiopaque line that marks the boundary of the mandibular canal is not cortical, but just a layer of parallel trabeculae crossed by the beam)
- *Buccolingual relationship between the third molar and the mandibular canal:* Knowing the position of the canal relative to the tooth, it is possible to identify the patients that are at high risk for inferior alveolar nerve lesions in the event that instrumentation is needed in deep structures, eg, to extract a root fragment after fracture. For example, the course of the buccal canal relative to the third molar or presence of grooves on the root of the third molar (and hence close contact with the mandibular canal) are crucial knowledge.[112] It is critical to know whether the canal runs close to the bifurcation of the roots of the impacted tooth where there is an indication to separate the roots (Figs 9-60 to 9-62).

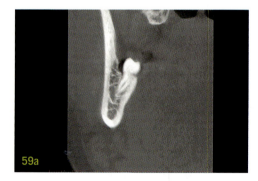
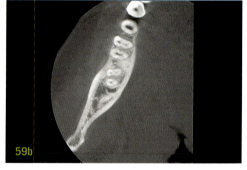

Figs 9-59a and 9-59b *(a)* Coronal and *(b)* axial slices of the root apex of a mandibular third molar in close contact with the mandibular canal.

- *Perforation of the lingual cortical plate*: This piece of information can be helpful to predict a potential risk of damaging the lingual nerve[99] and of dislocating the root apex into the sublingual space.[113]
- *Accessory canals*: Variations of the mandibular canal, as in bifid cases, in previous studies carried out by means of panoramic radiography show an incidence < 1%,[114,115] whereas the studies based on CBCT-derived images show an increase in incidence from 15.6% to 65%.[82,116] Identifying aberrant courses of the inferior alveolar nerve and hence recognizing possible surgical traps becomes easier with CBCT. The causes that can lead to incorrect interpretation of a "false double canal" using conventional panoramic radiography can include the imprint of the mylohyoid nerve on the inner surface of the mandible or an increase in density due to the insertion of the mylohyoid muscle running parallel to the mandibular canal[100] (Fig 9-63).

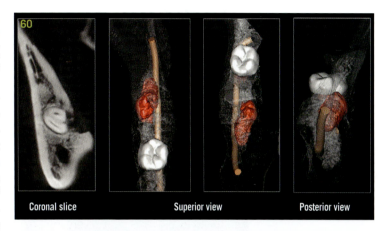

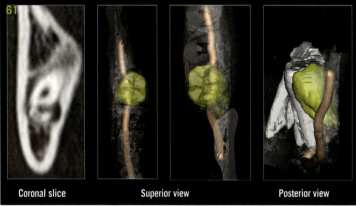

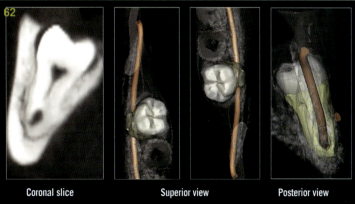

Fig 9-60 A third molar showing no contact with the mandibular canal.

Fig 9-61 Record of a third molar showing close contact with the mandibular canal.

Fig 9-62 A third molar with the mandibular canal crossing the roots of the tooth.

Fig 9-63a CBCT panoramic image: Reconstruction based on a DICOM file showing no accessory canal of the mandibular canal.

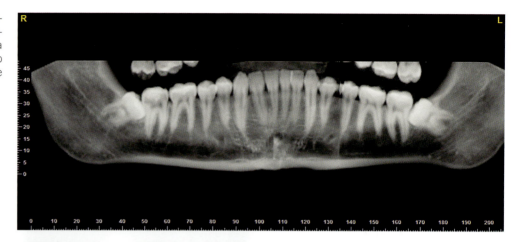

Fig 9-63b Coronal slice highlighting the presence of a bifid mandibular canal.

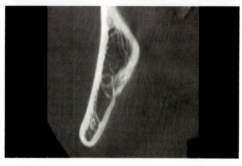

Fig 9-64 Coronal slices showing various canal shapes.

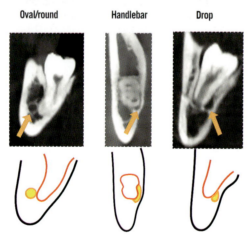

- *Assessment of the shape of the canal*: Knowing the morphology of the canal enables better planning of the surgery and, by surfing through the coronal tomography sections, it is possible to see how the shape varies from the foramen onwards. The "drop" and "handlebar" canal shapes are the ones showing most frequently a close correlation with the third molar and which, as a result, are associated with a higher risk of damage[117] (Fig 9-64).

References

1. Abron A, Mendro RL, Kaplan S. Impacted permanent maxillary canines: Diagnosis and treatment. N Y State Dent J 2004;70(9):24–28.
2. Thilander B, Jakobsson SO. Local factors in impaction of maxillary canines. Acta Odontol Scand 1968;26:145–168.
3. Mason C, Papadakou P, Roberts GJ. The radiographic localization of impacted maxillary canines: A comparison of methods. Eur J Orthod 2001;23:25–34.
4. Richardson G, Russell KA. A review of impacted permanent maxillary cuspids—Diagnosis and prevention. J Can Dent Assoc 2000;66:497–501.
5. Lindauer SJ, Rubenstein LK, Hang WM, Andersen WC, Isaacson RJ. Canine impaction identified early with panoramic radiographs. J Am Dent Assoc 1992;123:91–92, 95–97.
6. Suri L, Gagari E, Vastardis H. Delayed tooth eruption: Pathogenesis, diagnosis, and treatment. A literature review. Am J Orthod Dentofacial Orthop 2004;126:432–445.
7. Kuftinec MM, Shapira Y. The impacted maxillary canine: I. Review of concepts. ASDC J Dent Child 1995;62:317–324.
8. Kau CH, Pan P, Gallerano RL, English JD. A novel 3D classification system for canine impactions—The KPG index. Int J Med Robot 2009;5:291–296.
9. Bedoya MM, Park JH. A review of the diagnosis and management of impacted maxillary canines. J Am Dent Assoc 2009;140:1485–1493.
10. Cozza P. Il Canino Superiore Incluso. Diagnosi e Terapia Basate Sull'evidenza Scientifica. Testo Atlante. Bologna: Martina, 2010.
11. Coulter J, Richardson A. Normal eruption of the maxillary canine quantified in three dimensions. Eur J Orthod 1997;19:171–183.
12. McSherry PF. The ectopic maxillary canine: A review. Br J Orthod 1998;25:209–216.
13. Hurme VO. Ranges of normalcy in the eruption of permanent teeth. J Dent Child 1949;16(2):11–15.
14. Becker A, Chaushu S. Dental age in maxillary canine ectopia. Am J Orthod Dentofacial Orthop 2000;117:657–662.
15. Baccetti T, Franchi L, De Lisa S, Giuntini V. Eruption of the maxillary canines in relation to skeletal maturity. Am J Orthod Dentofacial Orthop 2008;133:748–751.
16. Williams BH. Diagnosis and prevention of maxillary cuspid impaction. Angle Orthod 1981;51:30–40.
17. McSherry P, Richardson A. Ectopic eruption of the maxillary canine quantified in three dimensions on cephalometric radiographs between the ages of 5 and 15 years. Eur J Orthod 1999;21:41–48.
18. Peck S, Peck L, Kataja M. The palatally displaced canine as a dental anomaly of genetic origin. Angle Orthod 1994;64:249–256.
19. Sacerdoti R, Baccetti T. Dentoskeletal features associated with unilateral or bilateral palatal displacement of maxillary canines. Angle Orthod 2004;74:725–732.
20. Langberg BJ, Peck S. Tooth-size reduction associated with occurrence of palatal displacement of canines. Angle Orthod 2000;70:126–128.
21. Becker A, Smith P, Behar R. The incidence of anomalous lateral incisors in relation to palatally-displaced cuspids. Angle Orthod 1981;51:24–29.
22. Cozza P, Chimenti C, Gatto R. Eziopatogenesi e terapia delle inclusioni dentarie. Dent Cadmos 1999;7:11–28.
23. Al-Nimri K, Gharaibeh T. Space conditions and dental and occlusal features in patients with palatally impacted maxillary canines: An aetiological study. Eur J Orthod 2005;27:461–465.
24. Jacoby H. The etiology of maxillary canine impactions. A clinical and radiologic study. Am J Orthod 1983;84:125–132.
25. Becker A. Etiology of maxillary canine impactions. Am J Orthod 1984;86:437–438.
26. Bass TB. Observations on the misplaced upper canine tooth. Dental Practitioner 1967;18:25–33.

27. Racek J, Sottner L. Heredity of canine teeth retention [in Czech]. Cesk Stomat 1977;77:209–213.
28. Newcomb MR. The recognition and interception of aberrant canine eruption. Angle Orthod 1959;29:161–168.
29. Garn SM, Lewis AB, Vicinus JH. Third molar polymorphism and its significance to dental genetics. J Dent Res 1963;42:1344–1363.
30. Sottner L, Racek J. Determination of heritability of the character; Model: Retention of canines [in Czech]. Cas Lek Cesk 1978;117:1060–1062.
31. Svinhufvud E, Myllarniemi S, Norio R. Dominant inheritance of tooth malpositions and their association to hypodontia. Clin Genet 1988;34:373–381.
32. Zilberman Y, Cohen B, Becker A. Familial trends in palatal canines, anomalous lateral incisors, and related phenomena. Eur J Orthod 1990;12:135–139.
33. Peck S, Peck L, Kataja M. Prevalence of tooth agenesis and peg-shaped maxillary lateral incisor associated with palatally displaced canine (PDC) anomaly. Am J Orthod Dentofacial Orthop 1996;110:441–443.
34. Baccetti T. A controlled study of associated dental anomalies. Angle Orthod 1998;68:267–274.
35. Peck S, Peck L, Kataja M. Concomitant occurrence of canine malposition and tooth agenesis: Evidence of orofacial genetic fields. Am J Orthod Dentofacial Orthop 2002;122:657–660.
36. Ericson S, Kurol J. Radiographic assessment of maxillary canine eruption in children with clinical signs of eruption disturbance. Eur J Orthod 1986;8:133–140.
37. Jacobs SG. Localization of the unerupted maxillary canine: How to and when to. Am J Orthod Dentofacial Orthop 1999;115:314–322.
38. McConnell TL, Hoffmann DL, Forbes DP, Janzen EK, Weintraub NH. Maxillary canine impaction in patients with transverse maxillary deficiency. ASDC J Dent Child 1996;63:190–195.
39. Schindel RH, Duffy SL. Maxillary transverse discrepancies and potentially impacted maxillary canines in mixed-dentition patients. Angle Orthod 2007;77:430–435.
40. Bishara SE. Impacted maxillary canines: A review. Am J Orthod Dentofacial Orthop 1992;101:159–171.
41. Ericson S, Kurol J. Longitudinal study and analysis of clinical supervision of maxillary canine eruption. Community Dent Oral Epidemiol 1986;14:172–176.
42. Becker A. Trattamento ortodontico dei denti inclusi. Torino: UTET, 1998.
43. Chaushu S, Chaushu G, Becker A. The role of digital volume tomography in the imaging of impacted teeth. World J Orthod 2004;5:120–132.
44. Clark CA. A method of ascertaining the relative position of unerupted teeth by means of film radiographs. Proc R Soc Med 1910;3:87–90.
45. Richards AG. Roentgenographic localization of the mandibular canal. J Oral Surg 1952;10:325–329.
46. Ericson S, Kurol J. Incisor resorption caused by maxillary cuspids: A radiographic study. Angle Orthod 1987;57:332–346.
47. Keur JJ. Radiographic localization techniques. Aust Dent J 1986;31:86–90.
48. Jacobs SG. Radiographic localization of unerupted teeth: Further findings about the vertical tube shift method and other localization techniques. Am J Orthod Dentofacial Orthop 2000;118:439–447.
49. Shapira Y, Kuftinec MM. Early diagnosis and interception of potential maxillary canine impaction. J Am Dent Assoc 1998;129:1450–1454.
50. Ericson S, Kurol J. Early treatment of palatally erupting maxillary canines by extraction of the primary canines. Eur J Orthod 1988;10:283–295.
51. Power SM, Short MB. An investigation into the response of palatally displaced canines to the removal of deciduous canines and an assessment of factors contributing to favorable eruption. Br J Orthod 1993;20:217–223.

52. Stivaros N, Mandall NA. Radiographic factors affecting the management of impacted upper permanent canines. J Orthod 2000;27:169–173.
53. Warford JH Jr, Grandhi RK, Tira DE. Prediction of maxillary canine impaction using sectors and angular measurement. Am J Orthod Dentofacial Orthop 2003;124:651–655.
54. Baccetti T, Crescini A, Nieri M, Rotundo R, Pini Prato GP. Orthodontic treatment of impacted maxillary canines: An appraisal of prognostic factors. Prog Orthod 2007;8:6–15.
55. Orton HS, Garvey MT, Pearson MH. Extrusion of the ectopic maxillary canine using a lower removable appliance. Am J Orthod Dentofacial Orthop 1995;107:349–359.
56. Sambataro S, Baccetti T, Franchi L, Antonini F. Early predictive variables for upper canine impaction as derived from posteroanterior cephalograms. Angle Orthod 2004;75:28–34.
57. Bjerklin K, Ericson S. How a computerized tomography examination changed the treatment plans of 80 children with retained and ectopically positioned maxillary canines. Angle Orthod 2006;76:43–51.
58. Cattaneo PM, Melsen B. The use of cone-beam computed tomography in an orthodontic department in between research and daily clinic. World J Orthod 2008;9:269–282.
59. Ericson S, Kurol J. CT diagnosis of ectopically erupting maxillary canines—A case report. Eur J Orthod 1988;10:115–120.
60. Ericson S, Kurol J. Resorption of incisors after ectopic eruption of maxillary canines. A CT study. Angle Orthod 2000;70:415–423.
61. SEDENTEXCT Project. Radiation Protection: Cone Beam CT for Dental And Maxillofacial Radiology. Evidence-Based Guidelines (2011). http://www.sedentexct.eu/system/files/.
62. Walker L, Enciso R, Mah J. Three-dimensional localization of maxillary canines with cone-beam computed tomography. Am J Orthod Dentofacial Orthop 2005;128:418–23.
63. Liu DG, Zhang WL, Zhang ZY, Wu YT, Ma XC. Localization of impacted maxillary canines and observation of adjacent incisor resorption with cone-beam computed tomography. Oral Surg Oral Med Oral Pathol Oral Radiol Endod 2008;105:91–98.
64. Ferrario S, Perrotti G, Weinstein RL. "Impacted canines": Proposta di analisi cefalometrica 3D. Rivista CAD-CAM Italy 2013;1:26–29.
65. Garn SM, Lewis AB, Bonne B. Third molar formation and its development course. Angle Orthod 1962;32:270–279.
66. Barnett DP. Late development of a lower third molar. A case report. Br J Orthod 1976;3:111–112.
67. Bishara SE, Andreasen G. Third molars: A review. Am J Orthod 1983;83:131–137.
68. Hattab FN, Abu Alhaija ES, Jordan I. Radiographic evaluation of mandibular third molar eruption space. Oral Surg Oral Med Oral Pathol Oral Radiol Endod 1999;88:285–291.
69. Grover PS, Lorton L. The incidence of unerupted permanent teeth and related clinical cases. Oral Surg Oral Med Oral Pathol 1985;59:420–425.
70. Björk A. Prediction of mandibular growth rotation. Am J Orthod 1969;55:585–599.
71. Richardson M. Changes in lower third molar position in the young adult. Am J Orthod Dentofacial Orthop 1992;102:320–327.
72. Richardson M. The development of third molar impaction. Br J Orthod 1975;2:231–234.
73. Bermúdez de Castro JM. Third molar agenesis in human prehistoric populations of the Canary Islands. Am J Phys Anthropol 1989;79:207–215.
74. Breik O, Grubor D. The incidence of mandibular third molar impactions in different skeletal facial types. Aust Dent J 2008;53:320–324.
75. Lytle JJ. Etiology and indications for the management of impacted teeth. Northwest Dent 1995;74(6):23–32.
76. Nanda SK. Patterns of vertical growth in the face. Am J Orthod Dentofac Orthop 1988;93:103–116.
77. Tulloch JF, Antczak AA, Wilkes JW. The application of decision analysis to evaluate the need for extraction of asymptomatic third molars. J Oral Maxillofac Surg 1987;45:855–865.

78. Schroeder C, Cecil JC 3rd, Cohen ME. Retention and extraction of third molars in naval personnel. Milit Med 1983;148:50–53.
79. Poegrel MA, Dorfman D, Fallah H. The anatomic structure of the inferior alveolar neurovascular bundle in the third molar region. J Oral Maxillofac Surg 2009;67:2452–2454.
80. Hölzle FW, Wolff KD. Anatomic position of the lingual nerve in the mandibular third molar region with special consideration of an atrophied mandibular crest: An anatomical study. Int J Oral Maxillofac Surg 2001;30:333–338.
81. Oliveira-Santos C, Rubira-Bullen IR, Dezzoti MSG, Capelozza ALA, Fischer CM, Poleti ML. Visibility of the mandibular canal on CBCT cross-sectional images. J Appl Oral Sci 2011;19:130–133.
82. Naitoh M, Hiraiwa Y, Aimiya H, Ariji E. Observation of bifid mandibular canal using cone-beam computerized tomography. Int J Oral Maxillofac Implants 2009;24:155–159.
83. Sawyer DR, Kiely ML. Retromolar foramen: A mandibular variant important to dentistry. Ann Dent 1991;50:16–18.
84. Bilecenoglu B, Tuncer N. Clinical and anatomical study of retromolar foramen and canal. J Oral Maxillofac Surg 2006;64:1493–1497.
85. Schejtman R, Devoto FC, Arias NH. The origin and distribution of the elements of the human mandibular retromolar canal. Arch Oral Biol 1967;12:1261–1268.
86. Winter GB. Principles of exodontia as applied to the impacted third molar. St Louis: American Medical Books, 1926.
87. Pell GJ, Gregory GT. Impacted third molars: Classification and modified technique for removal. Dent Digest 1933;39:330–338.
88. Susarla SM, Dodson TB. Risk factors for third molar extraction difficulty. J Oral Maxillofac Surg 2004;62:1363–1371.
89. Renton T, Smeeton N, McGurk M. Factors predictive of difficulty of mandibular third molar surgery. Br Dent J 2001;190:607–610.
90. Pogrel M, Dodson T, Swift J, et al. White paper on third molar data. American Association of Oral and Maxillofacial Surgeons. March 2007. http://www.aaoms.org/docs/third_molar_white_paper.pdf.
91. Akadiri OA, Obiechina AE. Assessment of difficulty in third molar surgery—A systematic review. J Oral Maxillofac Surg 2009;67:771–774.
92. Santamaria J, Arteagoitia I. Radiologic variables of clinical significance in the extraction of impacted mandibular third molars. Oral Surg Oral Med Oral Pathol Oral Radiol Endod 1997;84:469–473.
93. Baqain ZH, Karaky AA, Sawair F, Khaisat A, Duaibis R, Rajab LD. Frequency estimates and risk factors for postoperative morbidity after third molar removal: A prospective cohort study. J Oral Maxillofac Surg 2008;66:2276–2283.
94. Szalma J, Lempel E, Jeges S, Szabó G, Olasz L. The prognostic value of panoramic radiography of inferior alveolar nerve damage after mandibular third molar removal: Retrospective study of 400 cases. Oral Surg Oral Med Oral Pathol Oral Radiol Endod 2010;109:294–302.
95. Carvalho RW, Vasconcelos BC. Assessment of factors associated with surgical difficulty during removal of impacted lower third molars. J Oral Maxillofac Surg 2011;69:2714–2721.
96. Kugelberg CF. Impacted lower third molars and periodontal health. An epidemiological, methodological, retrospective and prospective clinical study. Swed Dent J Suppl 1990;68:1–52.
97. Tay AB, Go WS. Effect of exposed inferior alveolar neurovascular bundle during surgical removal of impacted lower third molars. J Oral Maxillofac Surg 2004;62:592–600.
98. Bell GW, Rodgers JM, Grime RJ, et al. The accuracy of dental panoramic tomographs in determining the root morphology of mandibular third molar teeth before surgery. Oral Surg Oral Med Oral Pathol Oral Radiol Endod 2003;95:119–125.
99. Lubbers HT, Matthews F, Damerau G, et al. Anatomy of impacted lower third molars evaluated by computerized tomography: Is there an indication for 3-dimensional imaging? Oral Surg Oral Med Oral Pathol Oral Radiol Endod 2011;111:547–550.

100. Nakamori K, Fujiwara K, Miyazaki A, et al. Clinical assessment of the relationship between the third molar and the inferior alveolar canal using panoramic images and tomography. J Oral Maxillofac Surg 2008;66:2308–2313.
101. Nakagawa Y, Nomura Y, Watambe NY, Hoshiba D, Kobayashi K, Ishibashi K. Third molar position: Reliability of panoramic radiography. J Oral Maxillofac Surg 2007;65:1303–1308.
102. Rood JP, Shehab BA. The radiological prediction of inferior alveolar nerve injury during third molar surgery. Br J Oral Maxillofac Surg 1990;28:20–25.
103. Queral-Godoy E, Figueiredo R, Valsameda-Castellón E, Berini-Aytés, Gay-Escoda C. Frequency and evolution of lingual nerve lesions following third molar extraction. J Oral Maxillofac Surg 2006;64:402–407.
104. Leung YY, Cheung LK. Correlation of radiographic signs, inferior dental nerve exposure, and deficit in third molar surgery. J Oral Maxillofac Surg 2011;69:1873–1879.
105. Blaeser BF, August MA, Donoff RB, Kaban LB, Dodson TB. Panoramic radiographic risk factors for inferior alveolar nerve injury after third molar extraction. J Oral Maxillofac Surg 2003;61:417–421.
106. Mahasantipiya PM, Savage NW, Monsour PA, Wilson RJ. Narrowing of the inferior dental canal in relation to the lower third molars. Dentomaxillofac Radiol 2005;34:154–163.
107. De Melo Albert DG, Gomes AC, do Egito Vasconcelos BC, de Oliveira e Silva ED, Holanda GZ. Comparison of orthopantomographs and conventional tomography images for assessing the relationship between impacted lower third molars and the mandibular canal. J Oral Maxillofac Surg 2006;64:1030–1037.
108. Nakagawa Y, Ishii H, Nomura Y, et al. Third molar position: Reliability of panoramic radiography. J Oral Maxillofac Surg 2007;65:1303–1308.
109. Palma-Carrió C, García-Mira B, Larrazabal-Morón C, Peñarrocha-Diago M. Radiographic signs associated with inferior alveolar nerve damage following lower third molar extraction. Med Oral Patol Oral Cir Bucal 2010;15:e886–e890.
110. Tantanapornkul W, Okouchi K, Fujiwara Y, et al. Comparative study of cone beam computed tomography and conventional panoramic radiography in assessing the topographic relationship between the mandibular canal and impacted third molars. Oral Surg Oral Med Oral Pathol Oral Radiol Endod 2007;103:253–259.
111. De Olivera-Santos C, Souza PH, De Azambuja Berti-Couto S, et al. Assessment of variations of the mandibular canal through cone beam computed tomography. Clin Oral Invest 2012;16:387–393.
112. Ghaeminia H, Meijer GJ, Soehardi A, Borstlap WA, Mulder J, Berg SJ. Position of the impacted third molar in relation to the mandibular canal. Diagnostic accuracy of cone beam computed tomography compared with panoramic radiography. Int J Oral Maxillofac Surg 2009;38:964–971.
113. Aznar-Arasa L, Figuereido R, Gay-Escoda C. Iatrogenic displacement of lower third molar roots into the sublingual space: Report of 6 cases. J Oral Maxillofac Surg 2012;70:e107–e115.
114. Nortj CJ, Farman AG, Grotepass FW. Variations in the anatomy normal of the inferior dental (mandibular) canal: A retrospective study of panoramic radiographs from 3612 routine dental patients. Br J Oral Surg 1977;15:55–63.
115. Sanchis JM, Peñarrocha M, Soler F. Bifid mandibular canal. J Oral Maxillofac Surg 2003;61:422–424.
116. Kuribayashi A, Watanabe H, Imaizumi A, Tantanapornkul W, Katakami K, Kurabayashi T. Bifid mandibular canals: Cone beam computed tomography evaluation. Dentomaxillofac Radiol 2010;39:235–239.
117. Ueda M, Nakamori K, Shiratori K, et al. Clinical significance of computed tomographic assessment and anatomic features of the inferior alveolar canal as risk factors for injury of the inferior alveolar nerve at third molar surgery. J Oral Maxillofac Surg 2012;70:514–520.

F Bianchi

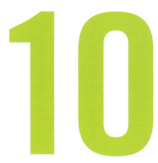

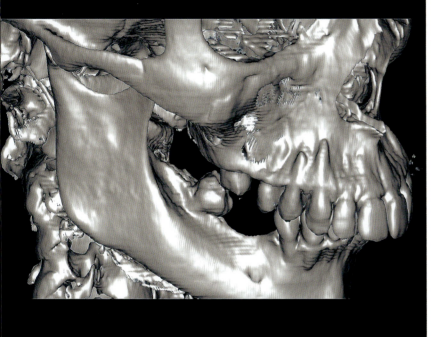

Conventional radiographic techniques present limitations in the periodontal field in regard to imaging of three-dimensional structures such as furcation defects, intraosseous defects, root anatomy, and determination of buccal and lingual bone loss.
For this reason, the diagnostic potential of dental cone beam computed tomography (CBCT) has been analyzed as an alternative to traditional methods of investigation

CBCT
in Periodontology

The diagnosis of periodontal defects has traditionally relied upon two-dimensional (2D) imaging complemented by probing to reconstruct the architecture of periodontal tissues indirectly.

Radiographs help identify the amount of bone destruction and the type of defect (horizontal or vertical) and provide information on the lamina dura and the periodontal space.

However, 2D radiographic investigation is at times limited in terms of correctly identifying the buccal and lingual architecture and vertical defects, in particular shallow defects or the defects of reduced buccolingual width. The diagnosis of teeth with furcation involvement can present further problems (and sometimes discrepancies between the clinical and radiographic findings), in particular because of difficulty in accessing interproximal furcations using the periodontal probe and overlapping anatomical structures, such as, for example, the palatal root overlapping the residual bone structure in a maxillary molar (Fig 10-1a).[1]

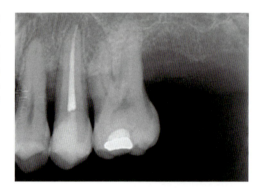

Fig 10-1a Periapical 2D radiograph taken digitally. The overlapping of structures in the buccopalatal direction masks the bony defect at the level of the furcation of the maxillary left first molar.

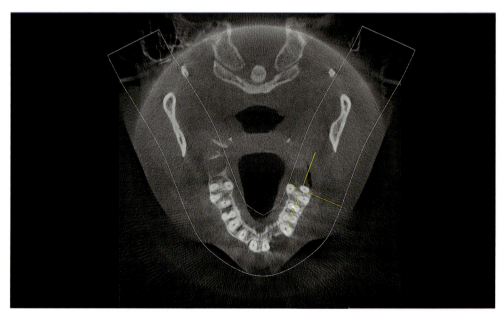

Fig 10-1b Axial image acquired with CBCT. The axial sections at different levels complete the visualization of the defect morphology.

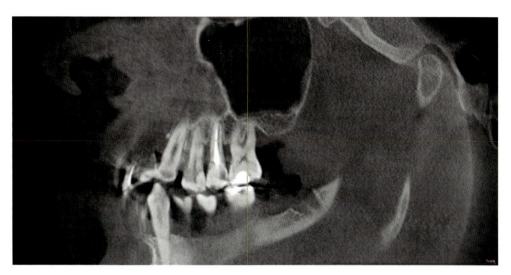

Fig 10-1c Tangential CBCT image. The defect affecting the furcation of the maxillary left first molar is evident. The presence of highly radiopaque endodontic filling and restoration materials causes a certain level of image disturbance.

Given the limitations of conventional radiographic techniques, it has been necessary to consider new and more accurate techniques, with an emphasis on the imaging of three-dimensional (3D) structures such as furcation defects, intraosseous defects, root anatomy, and the determination of the buccal and lingual bone loss (Figs 10-1b to 10-1d).

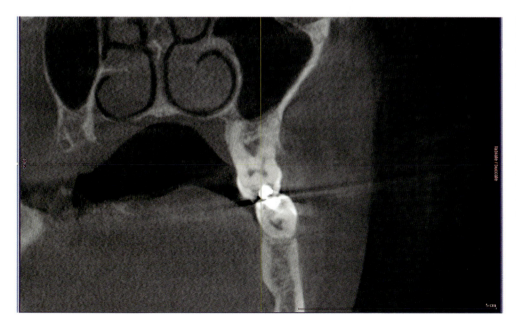

Fig 10-1d Transversal CBCT image. In the cross section the morphology and extension of intraroot loss are well displayed. The latter affects about half the length of the palatal and distal root, influencing tooth prognosis. Unlike the 2D image, in this image it is also possible to view the degree of bone resorption on the buccal and palatal aspects.

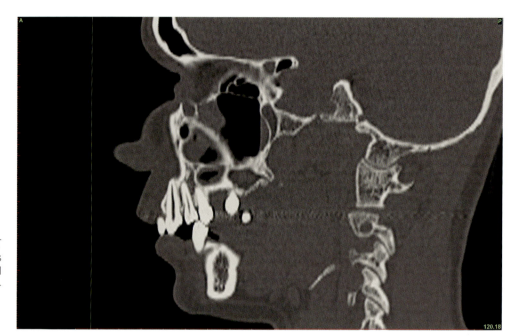

Fig 10-2a Sagittal CBCT image. The section allows visualization of the buccal fenestration of the maxillary left canine.

Use of conventional CT for determining destruction of periodontal tissues has been evaluated in vitro and been found to be very effective in representing periodontal defects. In a study[2] of intraosseous defects artificially created buccally and lingually after removal of soft tissues and metallic restorations, a comparison was made of the results of detection, classification, and vertical depth of intraosseous defects. The study has concluded that if there are no significant differences between CT and intraoral radiography as to the accuracy of the imaging for horizontal bone loss, only 60% of intraosseous defects have been detected with intraoral radiography as opposed to 100% in the case of high-resolution CT, the latter being a method that enables identification of bone morphology without overlapping of structures.

Moreover, in further in vitro studies, conventional CT has been found to be by far superior to 2D radiography in detecting furcation defects (21% using 2D radiography versus 100% using CT)[3] and interproximal bone defects (60% using 2D radiography using 100% using CT).[4]

Despite the significant accuracy and precision of traditional CT, the use of this method of investigation for periodontal diagnosis is not indicated for reasons of cost, accessibility, and radiation dose.

With the advent of the CBCT technology in the dental field, the diagnostic potential of this imaging method has been investigated as an alternative to conventional methods of investigation (Fig 10-2). The undoubted advantage of this method lies in the possibility of obtaining a 3D view of periodontal defects, including intraosseous defects and

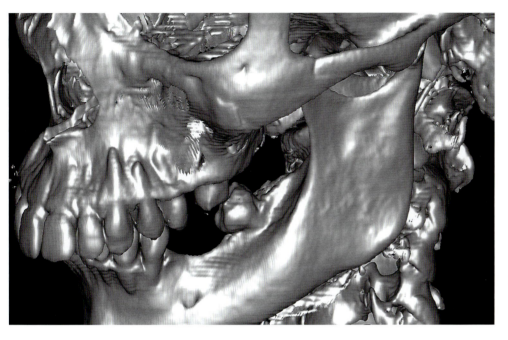

Fig 10-2b Surface rendering showing dehiscence of the maxillary left canine.

furcation involvement, where the morphology of the defect has a significant impact on the treatment plan and on the prognosis of the tooth involved.[5]

One of the first investigations of the use of CBCT in periodontal diagnosis[6] compared intraoral radiographs, panoramic radiographs, traditional CT images, and CBCT images to stereomicroscopy histologic findings in swine and human mandibles. This study examined dehiscences; fenestrations; defects on two and three walls; and Class I, II, and III furcations as created artificially in a standardized manner in swine and human mandibles. Both CT and CBCT proved to be very accurate in imaging the intraosseous defects, showing their superiority in accuracy as compared to intraoral radiography and panoramic radiographs.

In another investigation done in vitro,[7] CBCT was compared to analog intraoral radiographs and clinical probing; the level of accuracy of CBCT was similar to that of bone probing, even though the measurement of defects was more precise, in a statistically significant manner, with CBCT. Differences were found between the two methods in detection of interproximal defects; intraoral radiographs have been found to be absolutely inadequate for the purpose of detecting buccal and lingual defects. The use of CBCT has enabled detection of 100% of the intraosseous defects, whereas intraoral radiographs detected only 67%. This study concluded that CBCT is superior to the other periodontal diagnostic techniques in that it allows detection of defects in the three dimensions. Further investigations compared the CBCT method to intraoral radiographs taken using charge-coupled

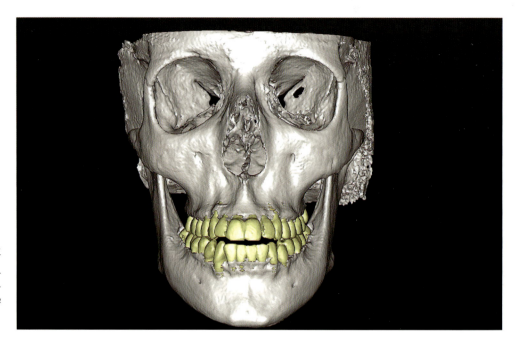

Fig 10-3a 3D rendering, frontal view. The CBCT taken for orthodontic purposes shows the buccalization of the teeth in the maxilla and mandible.

device (CCD) digital sensors.[8,9] Here again, CBCT was proven to be superior in the imaging of defect morphology and the involvement of furcations, even though digital intraoral radiographs were superior for their level of detail relating to bone quality and representation of the lamina dura.

These findings were confirmed by a cadaver study[10] in which CBCT was found to be more accurate for imaging of periodontal defects compared to a complete series of intraoral radiographs, although, interestingly, the diagnostic accuracy of CBCT progressively decreases in the anterior regions. While it was reported that CBCT imaging compared to intraoperative measurements at reentry has an accuracy of 84% in determining defects such as furcations in maxillary molars, CBCT underestimated the extent of the defect in about 15% of the cases and overestimated it in 1% of the cases.[11]

Another investigation[12] was conducted to quantify the levels of circumferential bone using the CBCT method. This study used dedicated software to take measurements between the cementoenamel junction and the bone crest medially, centrally, and distally for different teeth, with single or multiple roots, in a human skull. The measurements were then compared to the clinical measurements taken by probing. The study confirmed the hypothesis that the CBCT method allows accurate determination of bone levels and intraosseous defects, thus confirming the findings of other studies[7,9] that had concluded that, unlike intraoral radiographs, CBCT allows detection of 100% of craterlike defects and furcation involvements. It is necessary to highlight that in the model used in this study there were no soft tissues or equivalent substitutes or highly opaque metallic restorations that

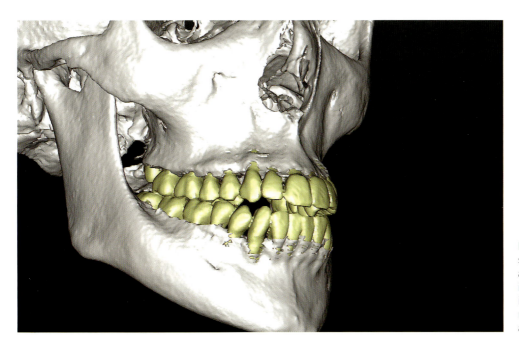

Fig 10-3b 3D rendering, side view. Dehiscences and fenestration affecting the teeth of the maxillary right arch and the mandibular right canine are evident.

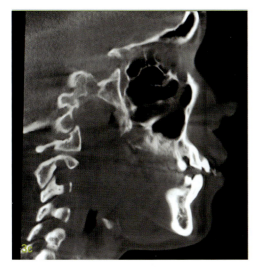

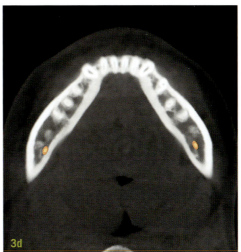

Fig 10-3c Sagittal CBCT image.

Fig 10-3d Axial CBCT image. The buccal cortical bone of the mandibular left canine is missing.

could cause significant problems in image quality and accuracy of diagnosis.

A further periodontal application of CBCT concerns the postoperative assessment of bone regeneration procedures. A study[13] compared the accuracy of CBCT to that of intraoral radiographs with respect to periodontal defects treated with bone grafting, showing that the values of CBCT are close to the clinical measurements taken at surgical reentry.

The potential of dentoalveolar CBCT scans has been studied for its ability to provide important periodontal information in orthodontics, based on the presence and the extent of pretreatment buccal dehiscences. Dehiscences and fenestrations cannot be detected with conventional intraoral radiography due to the superimposition of the lingual cortical bone or the dental root. With the advent of CBCT, multiplanar 2D images of the sagittal, axial, and coronal sections have been used for studying these periodontal defects (Fig 10-3). More recently, 3D surface rendering has become a popular imaging method for dehiscences. A study[14] conducted on 2D multiplanar reconstructions and on 3D surface rendering derived from CBCT scans with a voxel size of 0.2 mm has proven the accuracy of both imaging methods in the diagnosis of dehiscences. Another study,[15] however, questioned the accuracy of CBCT in measuring the dehiscences of mandibular incisors based on voxel resolution. This parameter, as well as the presence of soft tissues, is said to influence the accuracy of data in that a 0.125-mm voxel appears unable to precisely describe the presence of particularly thin buccal bone, exposing the risk of overestimating fenestrations and dehiscences. A further study on the accuracy and reliability of CBCT in detecting fenestrations and dehiscences[16] reported a discrepancy between the measurements taken directly on the dry skulls examined and those taken using CBCT, stating that the cause is the limited spatial resolution of CBCT images. According to other authors[17] the less-accurate estimates of bone dimensions for thin bone (eg, buccal bone at the coronal level) is ascribable to the fact that thin bone is particularly susceptible to partial volume averaging, as already documented for CT, which occurs when the voxel size exceeds that of the object to be represented. To reduce the influence of partial volume averaging, it is necessary to reduce the voxel size, which, in turn, requires a higher radiation dose and increases the risk of image disturbance. With CBCT, the level of disturbance increases as the field of view (FOV) increases; for this reason, large FOVs, such as those used in scans for orthodontic purposes, are contraindicated for an accurate diagnosis of the thickness of thin buccal bone. Moreover, in general, it can be stated that spatial resolution and the factors that determine it must be accurately studied to determine clinical protocols for CBCT when assessing alveolar bone alterations.[18]

In conclusion, the use of CBCT appears to have significant potential in periodontology, taking into account the variables that can have an impact on the quality of the investigation (image acquisition parameters in terms of kV, mA, size of voxels, and FOV; software parameters in terms of threshold and reconstruction algorithms). Further research is required to establish the ideal exposure parameters to optimize the quality of the image without loss of definition, as well as consideration of a number of variables that occur in vivo such as the presence of soft tissues, metallic restorations, and the patient's movement during scanning.

As should be the rule in the medical field, the appropriateness of a diagnostic method should be determined on the basis of the cost- and risk-to-benefit ratios. With this in mind, and in light of the criteria described above, the appropriateness of CBCT imaging as a diagnosis and follow-up tool in periodontology is at present debatable, save in selected cases in which CBCT is required to obtain information other than of a strictly periodontal nature, for example, in view of a preoperative diagnosis in surgery, orthodontics, or implant placement, as already documented in other sections of this book.

References

1. Lindhe J, Lang NP, Karring T. Parodontologia Clinica ed Implantologia Orale, ed 5. Milan: Ermes, 2009.
2. Fuhrmann RA, Bucker A, Diedrich PR. Assessment of alveolar bone loss with high resolution computed tomography. J Periodontal Res 1995;30:258–263.
3. Fuhrmann RA, Bucker A, Diedrich PR. Furcation involvement: Comparison of dental radiographs and HR-CT-slices in human specimens. J Periodontal Res 1997;32:409–418.
4. Fuhrmann RA, Wehrbein H, Langen HJ, Diedrich PR. Assessment of the dentate alveolar process with high resolution computed tomography. Dentomaxillofac Radiol 1995;24:50–54.
5. du Bois AH, Kardachi B, Bartold PM. Is there a role for the use of volumetric cone beam computed tomography in periodontics? Aust Dent J 2012;57(suppl 1):103–108.
6. Mengel R, Candir M, Shiratori K, Flores-de-Jacoby L. Digital volume tomography in the diagnosis of periodontal defects: An in vitro study on native pig and human mandibles. J Periodontol 2005;76:665–673.
7. Misch KA, Yi ES, Sarment DP. Accuracy of cone beam computed tomography for periodontal defect measurements. J Periodontol 2006;77:1261–1266.
8. Vandenberghe B, Jacobs R, Yang J. Diagnostic validity (or acuity) of 2D CCD versus 3D: CBCT images for assessing periodontal breakdown. Oral Surg Oral Med Oral Pathol Oral Radiol Endod 2007;104:395–401.
9. Vandenberghe B, Jacobs R, Yang J. Detection of periodontal bone loss using digital intraoral and cone beam computed tomography images: An in vitro assessment of bony and/or infrabony defects. Dentomaxillofac Radiol 2008;37:252–260.
10. Mol A, Balasundaram A. In vitro cone beam computed tomography imaging of periodontal bone. Dentomaxillofacial Radiol 2008;37:319–324.
11. Walter C, Weiger R, Zitzmann NU. Accuracy of three-dimensional imaging in assessing molar furcation involvement. J Clin Periodontol 2010;37:436-441.
12. Fleiner J, Hannig C, Schulze D, Stricker A, Jacobs R. Digital method for quantification of circumferential periodontal bone levels using cone beam CT. Clin Oral Invest 2013;17:389–396.
13. Ising N, Kim KB, Araujo VE, Buschang P. Evaluation of dehiscences using cone beam computed tomography. Angle Orthod 2012;82:122–130.
14. Hassan B, Couto Souza P, Jacobs R, de Azambuja Berti S, van der Stelt P. Influence of scanning and reconstruction parameters on quality of three-dimensional surface models of the dental arches from cone beam computed tomography. Clin Oral Investig 2010;14:303–310.
15. Patcas R, Müller L, Ullrich O, Peltomäki T. Accuracy of cone-beam computed tomography at different resolutions assessed on the bony covering of the mandibular anterior teeth. Am J Orthod Dentofacial Orthop 2012;141:41–50.
16. Leung C, Palomo L, Griffith R, Hans MG. Accuracy and reliability of cone-beam computed tomography for measuring alveolar bone height and detecting bony dehiscences and fenestrations. Am J Orthod Dentofacial Orthop 2010;137:S109–S119.
17. Molen AD. Considerations in the use of cone beam computed tomography for buccal bone measurements. Am J Orthod Dentofacial Orthop 2010;137:S130–S135.
18. Braut V, Bornstein MM, Belser U, Buser D. Thickness of the anterior maxillary facial bone wall–A retrospective radiographic study using cone beam computed tomography. Int J Periodontics Restorative Dent. 2011;31:125–131.

G Ferrara
M Del Fabbro
S Taschieri

11

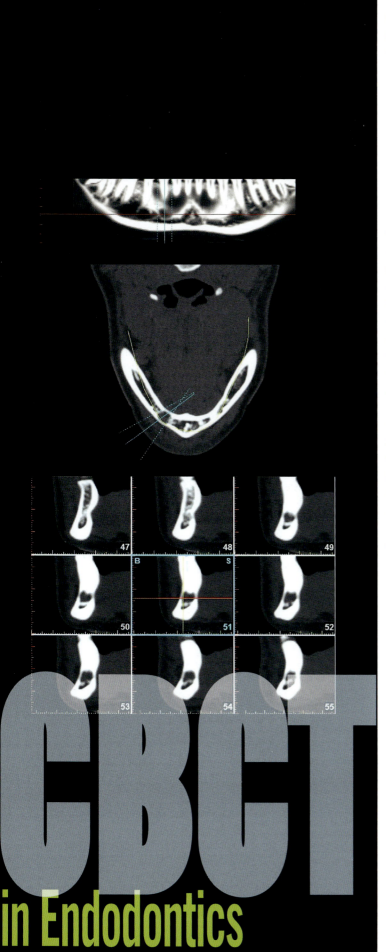

Use of cone beam computed tomography (CBCT) in endodontics can overcome the limitations of two-dimensional (2D) radiography and can obtain accurate three-dimensional (3D) images, while the patient is exposed to much less radiation as compared to traditional volumetric tomography.

CBCT is a second-level diagnostic test that should only be used in complex cases. It is indicated for in-depth diagnoses of complex morphologies, root resorptions, iatrogenic perforations, periapical lesions, traumas, fractures, and in endodontic surgery. To optimize the image quality, it is important to know the technical features of the CBCT equipment. Indeed, high spatial resolution is required in endodontics, which can be achieved by setting a narrow field of view (FOV) and by reducing the voxel size.

This chapter shall investigate the clinical indications and benefits of using CBCT in endodontics.

CBCT in Endodontics

The growing interest in using CBCT in endodontics stems from classic studies carried out by Bender and Seltzer[1,2] on the limitations of 2D radiology for diagnosing periapical lesions. These papers showed that, for an endoosseous lesion to be visible on intraoral radiographs, at least some cortical bone should be involved. This finding, which highlighted some diagnostic issues in managing periapical lesions, has been verified and confirmed in a large number of studies.[3–11]

Imaging in Endodontics

Radiographs are fundamental in all stages of endodontic therapy, from diagnosis, to treatment planning, to intraoperative controls and postoperative assessment.[12–14]

1. *Preoperative evaluation:* In the diagnostic phase, the dentoalveolar morphology is examined, and potential pathologic alterations are identified—location and number of root canals, width of the pulp chamber and degree of calcification, structure and bending radius of the roots, fractures, iatrogenic errors, and size of the caries lesion.
2. *Intraoperative control:* Radiographs are taken to confirm the working length and to test the gutta percha cones.
3. *Postoperative assessment:* Radiographs are used to confirm canal obturation and as a baseline for evaluating mid- and long-term periapical healing.

Limitations of 2D Radiology

The image obtained with an intraoral radiograph is a 2D representation of a 3D structure. This kind of imaging technique provides limited information.
Following are the main factors that contribute to deforming the image.
Compression of the third dimension: The anatomy of a tooth and of surrounding tissues is only viewed on the mesiodistal plane, while the characteristics of the buccolingual plane (ie, the third dimension) may not be fully appreciated.[15–17] The same applies to the spatial relationship of the root with anatomical structures or with any periapical lesion.[18,19] Similarly, the location, nature, and form of structures or abnormalities inside the root, such as root resorptions or iatrogenic perforations, might be hard to assess.[17,20–22]

In endodontic surgery, relying only on a 2D image will not allow proper assessment of the thickness of the cortical bone, the angle of the root, and the relationship with crucial anatomical structures, such as the inferior alveolar nerve, the mental foramen, and the maxillary sinus.

In an attempt to overcome such limitations, multiple images can be taken by moving the horizontal angle of the x-ray tube by 10 to 15 degrees.[21,23,24] This technique is also used for diagnosing fractures and dislocations in trauma patients, as well as for viewing roots that are located on the same plane as the x-ray beam so as to identify any anatomical peculiarities such as a second mesiobuccal canal in maxillary molars[23,25] (Fig 11-1). However, such radiographic images cannot guarantee that all anatomical or pathologic components are identified and might not give much more information than a single image.[26,27]

Geometrical distortion: Intraoral radiographs should be taken by using a Rinn film holder and the parallel-ray technique so as to obtain images that are geometrically more accurate than those obtained with the bisecting angle technique.[28] To achieve an accurate anatomical image, the detector (film or digital sensor) should be placed parallel to the vertical axis of the tooth, while the beam emitted by the x-ray tube should be perpendicular to the detector and to the investigated tooth.

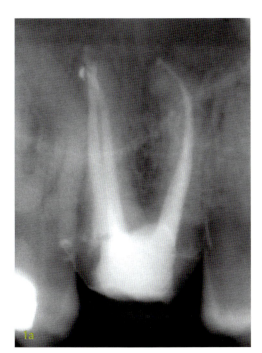
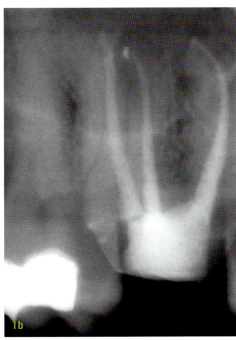

Figs 11-1a and 11-1b *(a)* In many cases, the distobuccal root of maxillary molars appears to overlap the palatal root on the buccolingual plane. *(b)* Shifting the horizontal angle of the x-ray tube by 10 to 15 degrees allows one to view both anatomical structures correctly.

This is normally feasible in the posterior mandibular region.[29] In the maxilla, however, a shallow palatal dome may hinder an ideal positioning of the film or sensor, thus generating geometric distortion. Overangled or underangled radiographs may respectively reduce or increase the root length,[21] increase or reduce the width of a periapical lesion, or even conceal it.[30]

Anatomical distortion: Some anatomical structures may overlap and hide the area of interest, which sometimes makes it difficult to interpret radiographic images.[31] Among the factors that affect this phenomenon are anatomical overlaps of the zygomatic process, mental foramen, and maxillary sinus, which may mask the root morphology (Fig 11-2). In the evaluation and diagnosis of periapical lesions, an overlap of the cortical bone may partly or totally conceal conditions that are confined to the medullary bone.[32,33]

One of the criteria for endodontic success is the lack of radiolucent lesions on radiographs. A study carried out by Goldman et al[34] with the goal of evaluating the healing of periradicular lesions on 2D radiographs only achieved 47% consensus among six selected examiners. Moreover, a review of the images by the same examiners at a later time showed that the two evaluations only matched in 19% to 80% of cases.

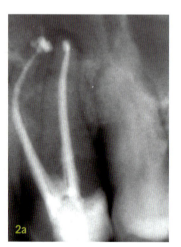 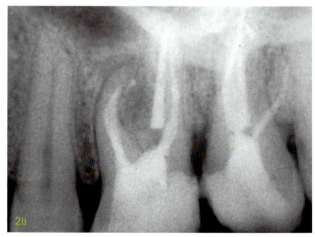

Figs 11-2a and 11-2b The overlapping of some anatomical structures such as the maxillary sinus and the zygomatic process may conceal the area of interest. *(a)* A radiograph was taken at an angle on the mesiodistal plane to get a clearer view of the anatomy of the maxillary left second premolar, which requires endodontic treatment. However, the overlapping maxillary sinus makes it difficult to perform a preoperative morphologic examination of the tooth. *(b)* Evaluating the maxillary left first and second molars is difficult because of the overlapping base of the zygomatic process, which masks the apical region of some roots and hampers the interpretation of potential periapical lesions.

Cone Beam Computed Tomography in Endodontics

The need to have accurate images on the three spatial planes for preimplant planning and at the same time the desire to work with a lower amount of radiation as compared to traditional computed tomography are some of the reasons that led to the development of a new imaging system: CBCT. The technology and functioning of CBCT have already been described in this book and shall not be repeated in this chapter. CBCT can be performed with a wide, medium, or narrow image-acquisition field, depending on the size of the FOV of the device. The FOV is the extension of the irradiated volume and depends on the size and shape of the detector, on the field of projection of the beam, and on the collimation of the beam. An appropriate collimation of the beam allows reduction of radiation exposure to the area of interest. The following is a description of some of the CBCT systems available on the market.[35]

Units with a wide FOV—between 15 and 23 cm—are mainly used in maxillofacial surgery, in orthodontic diagnosis and treatment planning, in the evaluation of temporomandibular joints, in craniofacial trauma, and maxillary diseases. NewTom 3G and 5G (Quantitative Radiology), i-CAT Next Generation (Imaging Sciences), and the CS 9300 (Carestream Dental) are only some examples. These devices can also be used with a narrower FOV.

Units with a medium FOV—between 10 and 15 cm—provide images of the maxillary and mandibular regions and are mainly used for implant preplanning. This category includes Galileos (Sirona), GX CB-500 (Gendex), NewTom VGi, 3D Accuitomo 170 (Morita), and Skyview (My-Ray).

Units with a narrow FOV—less than 10 cm and in some cases as narrow as 4 × 4 cm—are becoming increasingly popular. These devices are suitable for providing dentoalveolar images and are also indicated for endodontic purposes. Some examples include CS 9000 3D (Carestream Dental), Orthophos XG 3D (Sirona), Veraviewepocs 3D (Morita), and 3D Accuitomo 80 (Morita). The size of the FOV affects the image quality: the smaller the scanned volume, the higher the spatial resolution that can be obtained. Because the first sign of a periapical disease is discontinuity in the lamina dura and a widening of the space of the periodontal ligament, the optimal resolution for using CBCT in endodontics is 200 μm, ie, the average width of the periodontal ligament space. The advantages offered by a narrow FOV are mainly the ability to obtain images with a very high voxel spatial resolution of 0.076 mm, while exposing the patient to a limited dose of ionizing radiation, as opposed to systems based on a wide FOV. Moreover, a narrow FOV reduces the examined volume that the operator should then interpret in the report.[36]

Liedke et al[37] recommend a minimum voxel resolution of 0.3 mm to diagnose external root resorption. An ex vivo study[38] highlighted the effect of the voxel size on the ability of the observer to identify the presence or absence of secondary canals in the mesiobuccal root of the maxillary first molar on

CBCT. The observer's diagnostic accuracy increased as resolution increased. Indeed, it exceeded 93% when observing images taken with a voxel resolution of 0.12 mm. Conversely, the ability to diagnose any secondary canal on the images of the same teeth with a voxel resolution of 0.4 mm dropped to 60%. Several papers have demonstrated the accuracy of CBCT. Kobayashi et al[39] compared narrow-FOV CBCT and spiral CT in measuring the width of endosseous lesions that were artificially produced in cadaver mandibles and obtained accurate measurements. These results overlap those obtained by Lascala et al,[40] who analyzed the accuracy of linear measurements obtained with CBCT. Pinsky et al[41] documented an average linear accuracy of 0.1 mm in resin blocks and of less than 0.3 mm in the mandible.

Case Selection Criteria

The American Association of Endodontics and the American Academy of Oral and Maxillofacial Radiology have recently published a paper on the use of CBCT in endodontics.[42] Their recommendations for obtaining high-resolution images while minimizing the quantity of radiation delivered to the patient are: select a narrow FOV and minimum voxel size (0.076 mm); select the lowest settings both for electricity intensity supplied to the machine (milliamperes) and for exposure time; and use a pulsed exposure mode.

CBCT is a second-level diagnostic test and therefore should not be administered as a screening test to all patients. Eligible cases should be selected based on the patient's history, the clinical examination, and already available radiographs so as to make sure that the diagnostic benefits outweigh the radiation risk. CBCT should only be performed in complex endodontic cases if 2D radiographs do not provide sufficient diagnostic information:

- Identification of accessory canals in teeth with complex morphology or abnormalities in the canal system
- Diagnosis of periapical diseases in patients presenting contradictory or nonspecific signs and symptoms, or who report poorly localized symptoms involving previously treated or intact teeth, when no pathologic signs can be identified on 2D images, or some anatomical structures overlap
- Diagnosis of diseases of nonendodontic origin so as to establish the extension of the lesion and the effects generated on surrounding structures
- Assessment of intraoperative or postoperative complications—apical extrusion of filling material, broken endodontic instruments, identification of calcified canals, location of perforations
- Diagnosis and management of dentoalveolar lesions (especially root fractures, dislocations, alveolar fractures)

- Location and differential diagnosis of internal, external, and cervical root resorption
- Preoperative planning in surgical endodontics: location of root apexes with reference to cortical bone, identification and extension of periapical lesions, and proximity of anatomical structures

Applications of CBCT in Endodontics

One of the key benefits of CBCT in endodontics is the ability for the operator to interactively manipulate the images on the three spatial planes on a computer screen. Using dedicated software allows viewing of the relevant structures on the axial, sagittal, and coronal planes, moving through different sections within the reconstructed volume. Depending on the diagnostic requirements, the operator may select and modulate the sectional planes on the image, which can also be placed on different planes other than standard orthogonal planes. Several software products provide nonaxial images obtained from multiplanar reconstructions of the data volume. Through computerized processing of Digital Imaging and Communications in Medicine (DICOM) data, it is possible to obtain images similar to a panoramic radiograph and transverse sections. The latter can also be used to make distortion-free measurements and magnifications and to accurately view the relationships between specific teeth and any related disease or crucial anatomical structures such as the maxillary sinus, the inferior alveolar nerve canal, and the mental foramen.

Some studies[43–47] advocate that the quality of CBCT images is higher than the quality of spiral and multislice CT images for assessing hard tissues and high-contrast structures such as the mandibular canal and the mental foramen. However, one limitation of CBCT is that it offers poor contrast in the representation of structures with lower radiopacity. This can be seen on images produced with a low definition of soft tissues and is confirmed by the limited ability to represent subtle grey hues attributable to the broad range of radiopacity values of different tissues. This has a clinical impact when it comes to determining the nature of the content in periapical lesions or in the maxillary sinus.

A significant problem, which may affect the quality and the diagnostic accuracy of CBCT images, is the presence of highly radiopaque structures such as posts and metal-based restorations.[48,49] The resulting artifacts appear as a distorted representation of metallic components and the presence of bands on surrounding structures, which may undermine the diagnostic value of the examination.[4–6,50] The main areas of application of CBCT shall be discussed in depth in this chapter.

Preoperative Morphologic Assessment

An endodontic therapy can only be successful if it leads to identification of all root canals in order to shape, clean, and seal the entire endodontic system[51] (Fig 11-3). The prevalence of a second mesiobuccal canal (MB2) in the first maxillary molar ranges from 69% to 93% depending on the studies taken into account and on the investigation method employed. This variability in the diagnosis of the accessory canals may be related to the overlapping of anatomical structures on the buccolingual plane, which makes it difficult to appreciate some morphologic details, especially on 2D images.[16,52] Indeed, an examination of intraoral radiographs can identify the presence of MB2 in approximately 50% of the patients.[53] Matherne et al[27] conducted an ex vivo study comparing the ability of three experienced endodontists to identify the number of root canals in 72 extracted teeth, using digital intraoral radiographs or, alternatively, CBCT. On an average, by observing the intraoral radiographs the observers failed to identify a canal in 40% of the analyzed teeth. Conversely, when using CBCT, a larger number of canals were identified, with the observers indicating an average of 3.58 canals in maxillary molars, 1.21 in mandibular premolars, and 1.5 in mandibular incisors. The accuracy of CBCT in the identification of canal morphology was compared to the staining and clearing techinques.[54] Out of 95 teeth examined with CBCT, the root canals were correctly identified in 99.71% of cases, while an observation of the intraoral radiographs led to missing two or more canals in 23.8% of cases. Another study[55] compared CBCT images with histologic sections of the same teeth as observed under an optical microscope. Closely correlated data were obtained from the two methods, which confirms that CBCT is an accurate, minimally invasive method for investigating canal anatomy.

The accuracy in identifying accessory canals increases if high voxel resolution is used. Indeed, the diagnostic ability of the operator may even increase from 60% to 93.3% when comparing images with an increasingly higher resolution.[38] This suggests the use of images with a voxel size of 0.12 mm or less for investigating root morphology.

CBCT images are helpful when evaluating teeth with a complex morphology such as dens in dente (dens invaginatus) or dens evaginatus or teeth with an unusual number of roots,[56,57] studying marked root curvatures, and managing calcified canals[58] (Figs 11-4 to 11-6). Another field of application of CBCT is the management of iatrogenic conditions such as fractures and root perforations (Fig 11-7). Viewing the exact position of an instrument fragment in a root, its relationship with the canal walls, and especially the residual root thickness allows the clinician to plan safer extraction, thus minimizing the risk of stripping or excessive thinning of root walls. In managing iatrogenic perforations of the pulp chamber or of the roots, examining the size, location, and periradicular pathology that may be associated with the perforation allows a more accurate prognosis to be made. In doubtful cases, a CBCT analysis may provide additional details to gear treatment towards maintenance or extraction of the tooth.

A study[59] reported using CBCT for presurgical planning of the removal of a fractured instrument whose location on the buccolingual plane could not be seen on the intraoral radiograph. CBCT allowed exact location of the fragment and the use of a more conservative surgical approach. Conversely, another ex vivo study[60] does not show any statistically significant difference between using intraoral radiographs or CBCT for managing broken instruments and root perforations. CBCT is a useful diagnostic system, but the clinical and prognostic help that it might offer has to be assessed on a case-by-case basis and should be limited to cases where 2D imaging does not provide sufficient information for optimal therapeutic management.

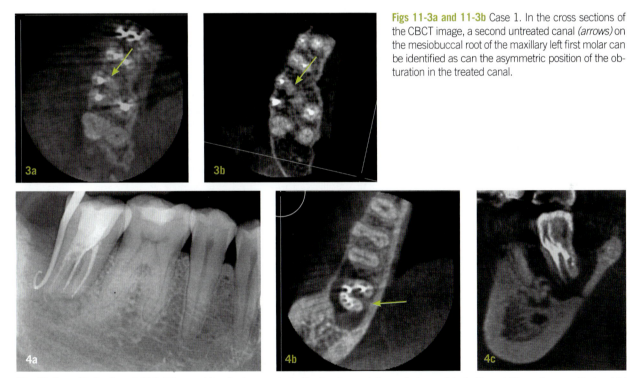

Figs 11-3a and 11-3b Case 1. In the cross sections of the CBCT image, a second untreated canal *(arrows)* on the mesiobuccal root of the maxillary left first molar can be identified as can the asymmetric position of the obturation in the treated canal.

Figs 11-4a to 11-4c Case 2. This 56-year-old patient presented with chewing and discomfort associated with mobility on the mandibular right second molar, which had been endodontically treated by another dentist a few years before. *(a)* The fistulous tract was traced, which identified a large periapical lesion. Because the anatomy of this tooth was not clearly represented on the periapical radiograph, a CBCT scan was performed to better investigate the morphologic nature of this tooth and the extension and location of the lesion. *(b)* The CBCT images clearly show the C-shaped anatomy of the tooth, which increases the difficulty in cleaning and sealing the canal space during initial treatment. The lesion extended apically and longitudinally to the tooth and had partly eroded the buccal cortical bone. *(c)* The longitudinal section shows that the apical margins of the lesion are very close to the inferior alveolar neurovascular bundle.

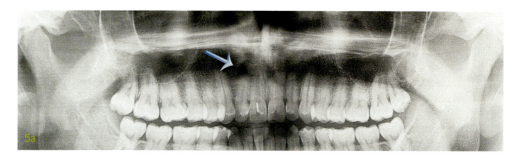

Figs 11-5a to 11-5g
Case 3. This 42-year-old patient reported undefined symptoms in the area of the maxillary right central and lateral incisors, discomfort under vestibular palpation, and signs of a prior fistula apical to the lateral incisor, which was more sensitive to percussion as compared to the other teeth. *(a)* The panoramic radiograph shows a periapical lesion between the roots of the right incisors, which seems to mostly affect the lateral incisor. *(b to d)* Conversely, CBCT images show that the lesion affects the central incisor, which was necrotic. *(e to g)* The root canal therapy done on this tooth, which had two canals, led to complete resolution of symptoms and healing of the periapical tissues.

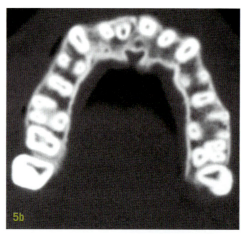
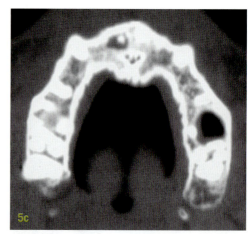
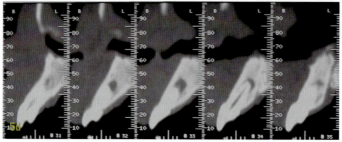
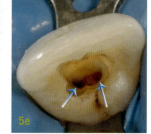
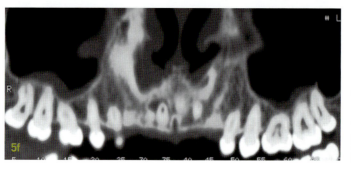
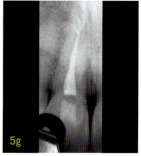

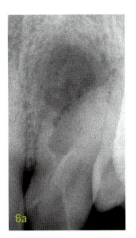 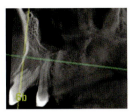 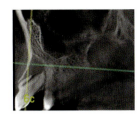 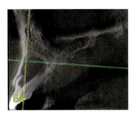 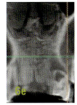

Figs 11-6a to 11-6e Case 4. *(a)* The intraoral radiograph shows that the maxillary left lateral incisor is affected by a periapical endodontic lesion, and an altered anatomy can be assumed. *(b to d)* The CBCT images allow for 3D reconstruction of the tooth, which is classified as a dens invaginatus Type III B. *(e)* The 3D examination established the relationship of the endodontium with the periodontal space and the exact extension and location of the endodontic lesion. (Courtesy of Dr Fabio Gorni, Milan, Italy.)

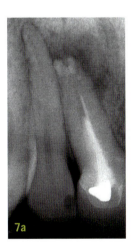 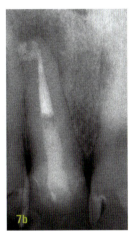 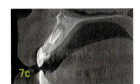

Figs 11-7a to 11-7c Case 5. *(a)* The preoperative intraoral radiograph of the maxillary right central incisor, which had been previously treated endodontically, shows a periapical endodontic lesion combined with a lateral lesion of the middle third of the root. The images showed some radiopaque material extruded from the root apex and an incomplete canal seal. The tooth was retreated nonsurgically. *(b)* The postoperative intraoral radiograph shows a complete canal seal. The therapy also allowed repair of a buccal perforation of the root, which could not be seen on the 2D radiograph. *(c)* The CBCT slice clearly shows the perforation repaired with mineral trioxide aggregate and the actual extent of the intraosseous lesion. (Courtesy of Dr Fabio Gorni, Milan, Italy.)

Periapical Pathologies

Periapical periodontitis may involve both necrotic and endodontically treated teeth. The affected teeth may be symptomatic or show no symptoms at all. Ørstavik and Pitt Ford,[61] Friedman,[62] and Trope[63] identified prevention and/or healing of apical periodontitis as the goals of any endodontic therapy. Based on this statement, endodontic treatment is targeted at shaping, cleaning, and sealing the canal space and the coronal access, so as to allow for appropriate healing of the periradicular tissues and for maintenance of physiologic healthy conditions of the tooth over time.[64]

As already discussed, 2D radiographic systems offer limited accuracy in identifying periapical lesions when there are overlapping anatomical structures or cortical bone. Using CBCT when the patient reports contradictory or nonspecific symptoms on one or more teeth allows diagnosis of periapical lesions in many instances in which no pathologic signs can be identified on 2D

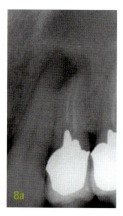 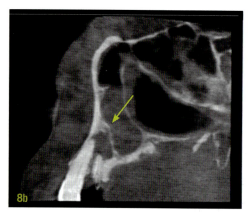 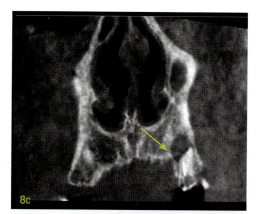 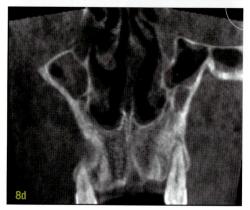

Figs 11-8a to 11-8d Case 6. The patient, a 46-year-old woman, presented as an urgent case due to pain under pressure on the maxillary left canine and first premolar, with a swelling present at the height of the vestibule. *(a)* The intraoral radiograph showed a large lesion located apical to the two teeth. The pulp sensitivity test provided an ambiguous answer on all teeth in the anterior sector, especially the canines. *(b and c)* A CBCT scan was performed, which allowed accurate location of the lesion around the roots of first premolar extending mesially towards the canine, which, however, *(d)* was not affected by the pathology.

images[65] (Figs 11-8 and 11-9). A study[4] assessed the accuracy of three observers in diagnosing periapical diseases on 46 teeth, comparing high-resolution low-FOV CBCT with intraoral radiographs. The latter allowed detection of 53 lesions on the basis of individual roots, while 86 lesions were identified on CBCT images. Other studies also confirmed the higher accuracy of CBCT as compared to intraoral radiographs in diagnosing periapical lesions.[5,6,8–10] Depending on the authors, CBCT images allowed identification of 34% to 54% more lesions than 2D radiographs. Using an ex vivo model, Patel et al[11] reported a diagnosis percentage of 24.8% and 100% for intraoral radiographs and CBCT, respectively. The accuracy of CBCT was proved to be comparable to that of traditional CT.[65] For this reason, and because of the lower dose of radiation administered to the patient, CBCT should be the first-line 3D examination in those instances in which 2D radiographs cannot solve diagnostic issues, or the patient reports poorly localized pain and symptoms with no disease being identified by conventional radiographs.[66–68]

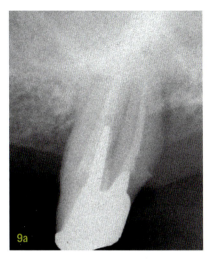
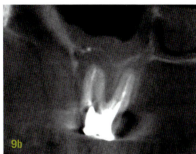
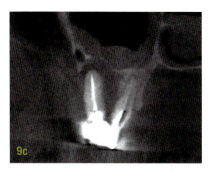

Figs 11-9a to 11-9c Case 7. *(a)* The intraoral radiograph shows a combined endodontic-periodontal lesion with diffuse margins on the maxillary left second molar. It is hard to establish the actual size of the bone defect. *(b)* The CBCT section defines the extension of the bone defect as involving the mesial root with partial disappearance of the buccal cortical bone in its distant coronal portion. *(c)* Another slice shows the morphology of the bone defect, which involves the distal root and the furcation between it and the palatal root. (Courtesy of Dr Manuela Uberti, Como, Italy.)

Assessment of Dentoalveolar Traumas and of Root Fractures

The advantages of using CBCT in trauma patients has been largely documented.[17,24,66,69] Used as a support to clinical examination, CBCT offers the opportunity to evaluate, with a single radiographic test, the exact nature, severity, and location of a trauma (Figs 11-10 and 11-11). The extraoral radiologic examination (panoramic radiograph, CBCT) is indicated in those clinical situations where the patient reports pain or limitations in functional movements. With dislocations or alveolar fractures, performing intraoral or occlusal radiographs may be painful, and it may be hard to place the film correctly. The resulting images may turn out to be misaligned or distorted. On the other hand, CBCT allows selection of multiplanar views with no geometric distortion or dispersion of anatomical structures. When diagnosing horizontal root fractures, CBCT[70] can replace the series of intraoral radiographs that are normally taken from different angles, which do not guarantee accurate viewing and may actually cause discomfort to the patient, especially in case of recent trauma. Moreover, CBCT images may show possible cortical fractures, which are very difficult to identify on conventional radiographs. Root fractures are hard to diagnose on 2D radiographs, unless the beam goes directly through the fracture line.[71]

With vertical root fractures (VRFs), the clinician is forced to rely on a number of vague symptoms and clinical signs, such as fistulas and isolated deep pockets upon probing, which may or may not be present, and would lead the clinician to suspect a fracture.[72–74] A systematic review of literature conducted by Tsesis et al[75] analyzed all the articles written on VRF from 1971 to 2010. The most frequently detected characteristic was a series of apical and/or lateral radiolucencies on one or both sides of the root and/or in the area of the furcation, which could be mistaken for endodontic and/or periodontal pathologies.

The only type of specific radiologic image is the so-called halo sign (Fig 11-12). The authors, however, concluded that there is a shortage of sound, evidence-based data in the current literature concerning the clinical and radiographic signs that might clearly lead to a diagnosis of VRF. The contribution of CBCT to the diagnostic process consists of locating the site and extension of the lesion accurately, but it presents limitations in identifying the presence or absence of a VRF with certainty. If the size of the VRF is smaller than the resolution of the machine used for the test, it will not be visible. Consequently, it might be very challenging to recommend a treatment plan without a sure and specific diagnosis and, indeed, the recommendation in doubtful cases is to reflect a so-called explorative flap.[76] Another study[77] compared the ability of the operators to identify VRFs on intraoral radiographs and on CBCT images. The latter showed much higher accuracy, albeit limited due to a suboptimal voxel resolution (0.25 mm) and to the presence of radiopaque material in the canal lumen.

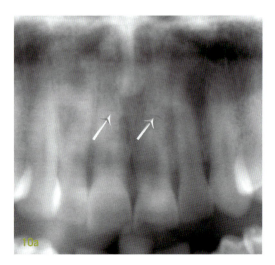
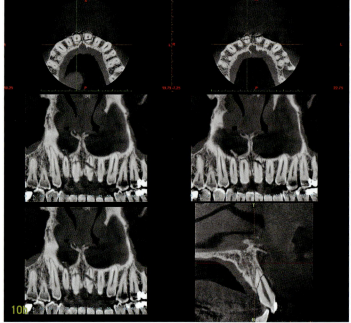

Figs 11-10a and 11-10b Case 8. This 19-year-old patient was referred to the dental practice due to trauma to the anterior teeth. (a) The panoramic radiograph shows a fracture line involving the apical segments of the two central incisors. (b) The CBCT images clearly show the location and nature of the fracture and the involvement of the buccal cortical bone. (Courtesy of Dr Sandro De Nardi, Milan, Italy.)

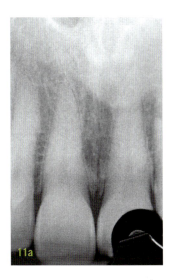 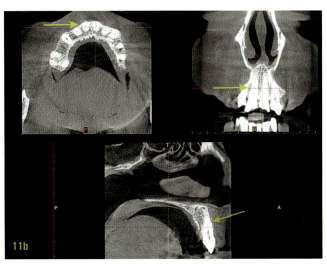

Figs 11-11a and 11-11b Case 9. This 28-year-old patient reported vague, diffuse symptoms around the maxillary central incisors and showed a marked response to the bite test on the right central incisor. *(a)* The intraoral radiograph identified no pathologic signs, *(b)* while the CBCT images show an incomplete root fracture in the middle third of the right central incisor.

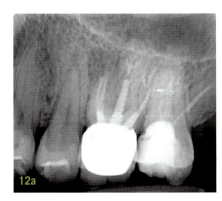 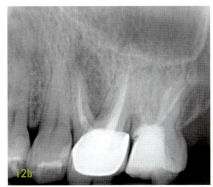 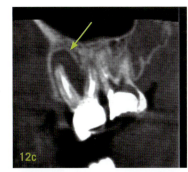 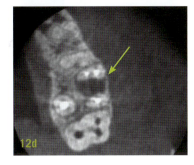

Figs 11-12a to 11-12d Case 10. This 33-year-old patient was referred for root canal re-treatments of the maxillary left first and second molars, which showed incomplete restorations and poor previous endodontic therapy. The patient did not report any symptoms on those teeth, except for some discomfort under percussion on both teeth. *(a and b)* The intraoral radiographs show a radiolucency around the palatal root of the first molar and a large radiolucent area around the mesial root. Periodontal probing, which was within the physiologic range of periodontal health around the perimeter of the tooth, revealed a narrow 12-mm pocket on the buccal side. *(c and d)* A CBCT scan was performed to investigate a suspected VRF, which was confirmed by the halo sign around the lesion extending apically to the mesial root and longitudinally and also involving the furcation area.

Root Resorptions

It may be very challenging to arrive at a correct diagnosis and management of root resorption. In these cases, CBCT offers valuable help (Fig 11-13). The data gathered from 3D images actually provide information on the size of the defect, the distance from the root canal, and the prognosis of the tooth.[17,60]

Two studies by Patel et al[78,79] evaluated the use of CBCT in the management of root resorption as compared to intraoral radiographs. Traditional radiography allows the clinician to attempt to establish the position of a resorption and whether the process has an internal or external origin by using a series of intraoral radiographs taken by changing the angle of the x-ray tube. However, this technique does not allow one to establish the depth and extension of the defect. On the radiographs, the internal root resorption appears as a sharp radiolucent area with a clearly defined margin, which may have a tapered shape and is located adjacent to the root canal. Another characteristic of internal resorption can be appreciated by comparing two intraoral radiographs taken at different angles: the position of the defect with reference to the root will actually be the same on both films. On the other hand, an external resorption does not show similarly clear margins. The unchanged profile of the root canal can be seen through the radiolucent area, and the lesion seems to change location if one looks at it on two radiographs taken from different angles.

The author concluded that CBCT, in addition to showing the actual extension of the lesion, also allows the operator to formulate a more

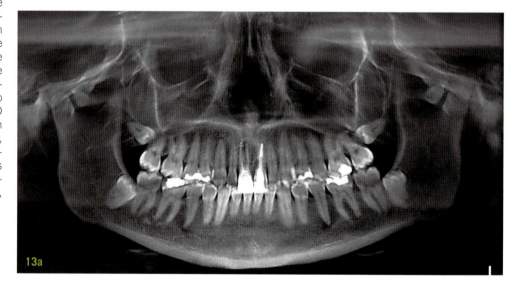

Figs 11-13a-c Case 11. *(a)* This patient reported vague signs and symptoms in the anterior sector that were exacerbated during mastication. Periodontal probing on the maxillary right central incisor showed a depth of 6 mm on the buccal side and a large dehiscence. There was also a fistula located apical to the cementoenamel junction. The periapical radiograph shows an incomplete canal seal, especially in the apical third, and an open apex. *(b)* A lesion of endodontic origin can be identified in the apical area and a horizontal root fracture in the middle third. *(c to e)* On the left central incisor, external root resorption can be observed around the root axis in the middle third. The CBCT image clearly shows the pathologic alteration of the two teeth and provides a 3D image of root resorption of the left central incisor, thus confirming the diagnosis and poor prognosis for the two teeth. (Courtesy of Dr Tiziano Testori, Como, Italy.)

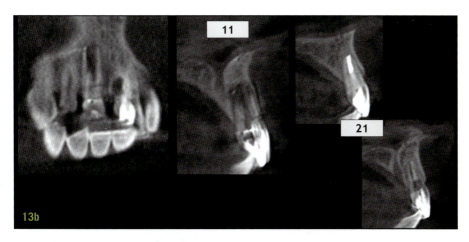
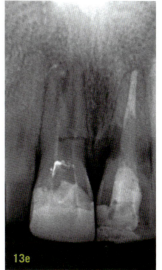
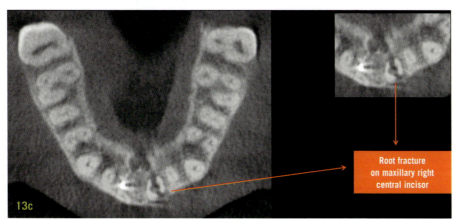

Root fracture on maxillary right central incisor

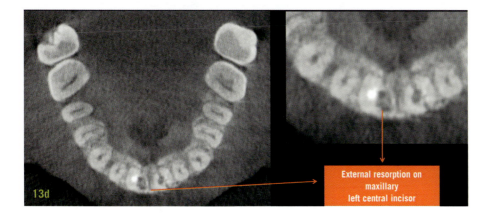

External resorption on maxillary left central incisor

reliable therapeutic approach and diagnosis for each tooth. A study published by the same author in 2009,[79] which examined the accuracy of CBCT in diagnosing both internal and external resorption, was the first to consider the impact of CBCT in designing a correct treatment plan for the patient. CBCT proved to be

Figs 11-14a to 11-14c Case 12. This 38-year-old patient reported pain upon percussion on the maxillary left second molar, which had been endodontically treated in another dental practice. The coronal restoration was intact and esthetically acceptable. Therefore, a surgical approach was recommended. *(a)* The intraoral radiograph did not clearly show whether the lesion surrounded the mesial roots or whether it affected the palatal root, and the maxillary sinus seemed to be adjacent to but separated from the lesion by a portion of cortical bone (Oberli Class II). *(b and c)* CBCT images clearly show the lesion around the two buccal roots, while the palatal root does not seem to be involved. They also confirm the separation between the lesion and the maxillary sinus.

extremely accurate in diagnosing different types of resorption. The ability of the observers to select an ideal treatment plan for each tested tooth was 60% and 80%, respectively, when using intraoral radiographs or CBCT as diagnostic tools.

Endodontic Surgery

Endodontic surgery may present some challenges, especially in the posterior quadrants near anatomical structures such as the maxillary sinus, the mandibular canal, and the mental foramen (Figs 11-14 and 11-15). In these patients, CBCT offers valuable help in the presurgical planning stage.[67] Rigolone et al[80] were among the first to describe the contribution of CBCT to planning endodontic surgery. The authors measured the average distance between the palatal root of the maxillary first molar and the buccal cortical bone on 43 CBCT images of 31 patients in order to decide whether to take a buccal surgical approach to the palatal root or to opt for a more complex palatal access. The average distance was 9.73 mm. The authors also calculated how often the lateral recess of the maxillary sinus occupied the space between the buccal roots and the palatal root, ie, in 25% of the cases. The authors concluded that CBCT plays an important role in optimizing the surgical access to the palatal root, which, in most patients, can be performed from the buccal cortical bone. Other authors came to similar conclusions on the importance of CBCT in the surgical management of teeth that are adjacent to the maxillary sinus.[59,68]

Another paper[81] evaluated the thickness of the sinus membrane on CBCT images of 100 patients referred for endodontic surgeries on maxillary molars. The sinus membrane was significantly thickened near the roots affected by periapical lesions as compared to the roots that were not involved.

Due to the 2D nature of intraoral radiographs, it is hard to foresee whether a root that appears to be overlapping the maxillary sinus floor actually protrudes into the sinus cavity or whether it is just a radiographic projection.[82,83]

Oberli et al[82] evaluated the correlation between intraoral radiographs taken in the preoperative stage and the intraoperative clinical evidence collected during endodontic surgery on maxillary premolars and mo-

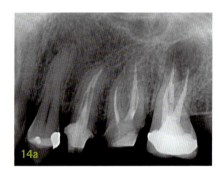
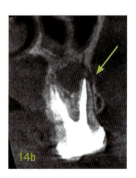
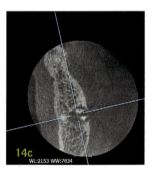

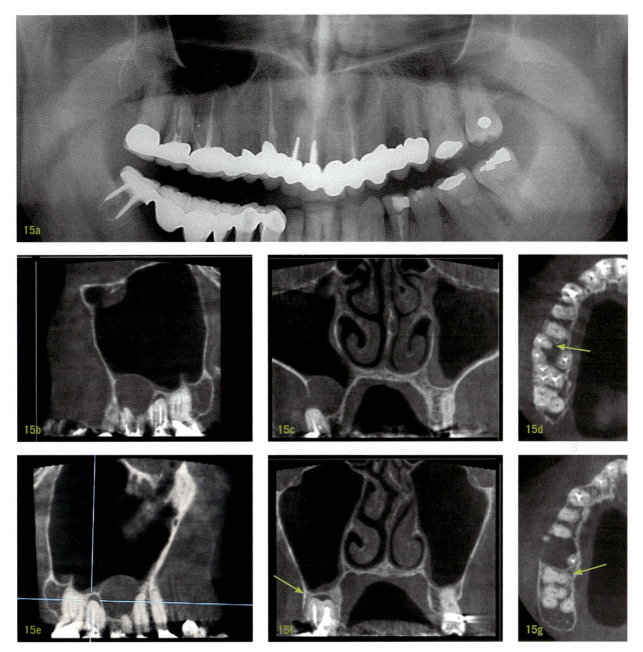

Figs 11-15a to 11-15g Case 13. This 56-year-old patient reported radiating pain in the maxillary right quadrant and sinusitis. *(a)* The panoramic radiograph shows a large lesion of endodontic origin affecting the maxillary right first molar, which seems to invade the maxillary sinus. *(b and c)* The CBCT images confirm that the lesion extends into the maxillary sinus (Oberli Class III) and that the buccal cortical bone around the first molar is completely eroded. *(d)* The cross-sectional view of the mesial root shows the asymmetric location of the root filling material, which may indicate the presence of a second, untreated, mesiobuccal canal. *(e to g)* On the second molar, an apical lesion can be identified involving the buccal and palatal roots, which is separate from the lesion on the first molar and is separated from the sinus by a thin layer of cortical bone (Oberli Class II). All slices show an absence of apical seal.

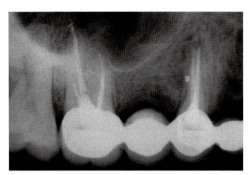

Fig 11-16 Oberli Class I: The root apex and the maxillary sinus are separated by a distinct space.

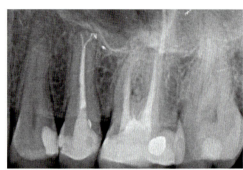

Fig 11-17 Oberli Class II: The root apex almost touches the floor of the maxillary sinus.

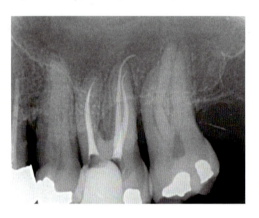

Fig 11-18 Oberli Class III: The root apex overlaps the floor of the maxillary sinus.

lars in regard to the exposure of the maxillary sinus membrane. The authors then suggested a radiologic classification based on the relationship between the roots (and the lesions associated with them) and the maxillary sinus. Oberli's classification (Figs 11-16 to 11-18) is applied on intraoral radiographs and is based on three subgroups: Class I includes teeth where a space separating the root apex and the maxillary sinus floor can be clearly observed; Class II includes teeth where the root apex seems to almost touch the sinus floor; Class III includes teeth where the root apexes overlap the maxillary sinus floor (see Figs 11-16 to 11-18). A similar classification was applied to periapical lesions, based on whether they were separate from, adjacent to, or overlapping the maxillary sinus (Class I, II, and III, respectively). From a clinical standpoint, Class I lesions are very likely to leave the maxillary sinus unaffected during endodontic surgery. In Class II and III lesions, the use of 3D technology can be helpful. In these patients, CBCT allows a more accurate diagnosis of the location of the lesion with reference to the maxillary sinus,[84] so as to reduce the risk of creating an oroantral communication and to evaluate the surgical time and techniques necessary, should the lesion reach into the antrum.[85]

Postoperative Evaluation

The parameters to be used for evaluating the success of endodontic treatment are lack of symptoms in the treated teeth and healing of the existing periapical lesions. Intraoral radiographs are commonly used to monitor

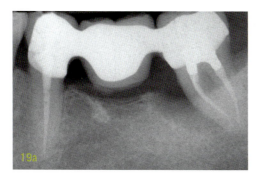 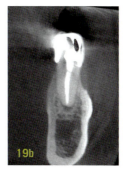 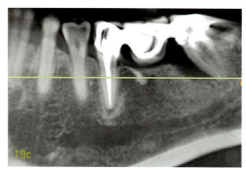

Figs 11-19a to 11-19c Case 14. *(a)* An intraoral radiograph was taken of the mandibular left quadrant of a 56-year-old patient who reported chewing discomfort around the prosthetic restoration from the second premolar to the second molar. The second molar was affected by a large periodontal defect, while no pathologic alterations were identified around the second premolar. *(b)* The CBCT images showed a periapical endodontic lesion on the premolar, which could not be seen on traditional radiographs. *(c)* The frontal section clearly shows a periapical lesion on the premolar and a periodontal lesion on the molar. (Courtesy of Dr Manuela Uberti, Como, Italy.)

the health of periradicular tissues and the absence of discontinuities in the periodontal ligament (Figs 11-19 and 11-20).

However, several studies[4,5,7,65,86] have shown that a high percentage of teeth considered to have healed based on intraoral radiographs indeed show residual periapical pathologies when examined on CBCT and/or histologically. Intraoral images used to be the gold standard to evaluate the success of root canal treatment radiologically. Nowadays, with the development of CBCT technology, better understanding of endodontic pathologies has been achieved.[87] According to Wu et al,[87] success criteria and rates for endodontic treatments should be reevaluated by long-term longitudinal trials using CBCT images. The authors believe that the success rate of endodontic therapies reported in literature based on the assessment of intraoral radiographic images overestimates the percentage of truly healed periapical lesions. However, using intraoral radiographs for medium- and long-term postoperative assessment of endodontically treated teeth is a valuable strategy for predicting the survival of a tooth.[88,89] This suggests that the success of an endodontic therapy is not necessarily linked to complete healing as diagnosed on radiographs; the recovery of the chewing function of the tooth involved and the lack of signs and symptoms should also be considered. It should therefore be clarified whether using CBCT instead of intraoral radiographs in the postoperative assessment may offer benefits to the patient, or whether it is a form of overtreatment.

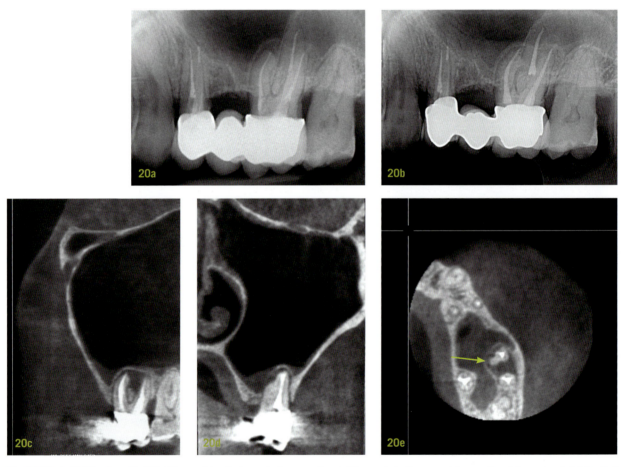

Figs 11-20a to 11-20e Case 15. This 58-year-old patient reported recurrent and diffuse pain in the area of the maxillary left quadrant. *(a)* The first molar was mildly painful under percussion and showed a periapical lesion on the mesial root. Before replacing the prosthesis, which had both esthetic and functional problems, the patient underwent nonsurgical re-treatment. After initial resolution of symptoms, radiating diffuse discomfort reappeared after a few months. *(b)* Follow-up radiograph at 10 months indicates that the apical lesion is still there, but the distortion of the anatomical structures makes it difficult to locate its boundaries. *(c to e)* The CBCT images clearly show the extent of the lesion, which appears to be much larger. The cross-sectional views show asymmetric placement of the filling material on the mesiobuccal root, which indicates the presence of an additional, untreated canal (MB2).

References

1. Bender I, Seltzer S. Roentgenographic and direct observation of experimental lesions in bone: I. J Endod 2003;29:702–706.
2. Bender I, Seltzer S. Roentgenographic and direct observation of experimental lesions in bone: II. J Endod 2003;29:707–712.
3. Huumonen S, Kvist T, Gröndahl K, Molander A. Diagnostic value of computed tomography in re-treatment of root fillings in maxillary molars. Int Endod J 2006;39:827–833.
4. Lofthag-Hansen S, Huumonen S, Gröndahl K, Gröndahl HG. Limited cone beam CT and intraoral radiography for the diagnosis of periapical pathology. Oral Surg Oral Med Oral Path Oral Radiol Endod 2007;103:114–119.
5. Estrela C, Bueno MR, Leles CR, Azevedo B, Azevedo JR. Accuracy of cone beam computed tomography and panoramic and periapical radiography for detection of apical periodontitis. J Endod 2008;34:273–279.
6. Estrela C, Bueno MR, Azevedo BC, Azevedo JR, Pécora JD. A new periapical index based on cone beam computed tomography. J Endod 2008;34:1325–1331.
7. Vandenberghe B, Jacobs R, Yang J. Detection of periapical bone loss using digital intraoral and cone beam computed tomography images: An in vitro assessment of bony and/or infrabony defects. Dentomaxillofac Radiol 2008;37:252–260.
8. Stavropoulos A, Wenzel A. Accuracy of cone beam dental CT, intraoral digital and conventional film radiography for the detection of periapical lesion. An ex vivo study in pig jaws. Clin Oral Invest 2007;11:101–106.
9. Özen T, Kamburoglu K, Cebeci AR, Yüksel SP, Paksoy CS. Interpretation of chemically created periapical lesions using 2 different dental cone-beam computerized tomography units, an intraoral digital sensor, and conventional film. Oral Surg Oral Med Oral Path Oral Radiol Endod 2009;107:426–432.
10. Low KMT, Dula K, Bürgin W, von Arx T. Comparison of periapical radiography and limited conebeam tomography in posterior maxillary teeth referred for apical surgery. J Endod 2008;34:557–562.
11. Patel S, Dawood A, Mannocci F, Wilson R, Pitt Ford T. Detection of periapical bone defects in human jaws using cone beam computed tomography and intraoral radiography. Int Endod J 2009;42:507–515.
12. Forsberg J. Radiographic reproduction of endodontic "working length" comparing the paralleling and the bisecting-angle techniques. Oral Surg Oral Med Oral Path Oral Radiol Endod 1987;64:353–360.
13. Forsberg J. A comparison of the paralleling and bisecting-angle radiographic techniques in endodontics. Int Endod J 1987;20:177–182.
14. Walton RE. Diagnostic imaging. A: Endodontic radiography. In: Ingle JI, Bakland LK, Baumgartner JC (eds). Ingle's Endodontics, ed 6. Hamilton, Ontario: BC Decker, 2008:554–572.
15. Webber RL, Messura JK. An in vivo comparison of digital information obtained from tuned-aperture computed tomography and conventional dental radiographic imaging modalities. Oral Surg Oral Med Oral Path 1999;88:239–247.
16. Nance R, Tyndall D, Levin LG, Trope M. Identification of root canals in molars by tuned-aperture computed tomography. Int Endod J 2000;33:392–396.
17. Cohenca N, Simon JH, Roges R, Morag Y, Malfaz JM. Clinical indications for digital imaging in dento-alveolar trauma. Part 1: Traumatic injuries. Dent Traumatol 2007;23:95–104.
18. Cotti E, Vargiu P, Dettori C, Mallarini G. Computerized tomography in the management and follow-up of extensive periapical lesion. Endod Dent Traumatol 1999;15:186–189.
19. Cotti E, Campisi G. Advanced radiographic techniques for the detection of lesions in bone. Endod Topics 2004;7:52–72.
20. Patel S, Dawood A. The use of cone beam computed tomography in the management of external cervical resorption lesions. Int Endod J 2007;40:730–737.

21. Whaites E. Periapical radiography. In: Essentials of Dental Radiology and Radiography, ed 4. Philadelphia: Churchill Livingston Elsevier, 2007:97–124.
22. Whaites E. Alterative and specialized imaging modalities. In: Essentials of Dental Radiology and Radiography, ed 4. Philadelphia: Churchill Livingston Elsevier, 2007:223–242.
23. Glickman GW, Pettiette MT. Preparation for treatment. In: Cohen S, Hargreaves KM (eds). Pathways of the Pulp, ed 9. St Louis: Mosby Elsevier, 2006:97–135.
24. Patel S, Pitt Ford T. Is the resorption external or internal? Dent Update 2007;34:218–229.
25. Manogue M, Patel S, Walker R. Diagnosis and treatment planning. In: Manogue M, Patel S, Walker R (eds). The Principles of Endodontics. Oxford: Oxford University Press, 2005:31–46.
26. Barton DJ, Clark SJ, Eleazer PD, Scheetz JP, Farman AG. Tuned-aperture computed tomography versus parallax analog and digital radiographic images in detecting second mesiobuccal canals in maxillary first molars. Oral Surg Oral Med Oral Pathol Oral Radiol Endod 2003;96:223–228.
27. Matherne RP, Angelopoulos C, Kulilid JC, Tira D. Use of cone-beam computed tomography to identify root canal systems in vitro. J Endod 2008;34:87–89.
28. Forsberg J, Halse A. Radiographic simulation of a periapical lesion comparing the paralleling and the bisecting-angle techniques. Int Endod J 1994;27:133–138.
29. Walker RT, Brown JE. Radiography. In: Stock C, Walker R, Gulabivala K (eds). Endodontics, ed 3. Philadelphia: Mosby, 2005:77–92.
30. Huumonen S, Ørstavik D. Radiological aspects of apical periodontitis. Endod Topics 2002;1:3–25.
31. Gröndahl H-G, Huumonen S. Radiographic manifestations of periapical inflammatory lesions. Endod Topics 2004;8:55–67.
32. Bender IB, Seltzer S. Roentgenographic and direct observation of experimental lesions in bone: I. J Am Dent Assoc 1961;62:152–160.
33. Schwartz SF, Foster JK. Roentgenographic interpretation of experimentally produced bony lesions. Part 1. Oral Surg Oral Med Oral Pathol 1971;32:606–612.
34. Goldman M, Pearson AH, Darzenta N. Endodontic success—Who's reading the radiograph? Oral Surg Oral Med Oral Pathol 1972;33:432–437.
35. Tyndall DA, Kohltfarber H. Application of cone beam volumetric tomography in endodontics. Aust Dent J 2012;57(suppl 1):72–81.
36. Farman AG, Levato C, Scarfe WC, Chenin D. Cone beam CT trends towards hybrid systems and third party software utilization. Inside Dentistry 2008;4:102–105.
37. Liedke GS, Da Silveira HED, Da Silveira HLD, Dutra V, De Figueiredo JAP. Influence of voxel size in the diagnostic ability of cone beam tomography to evaluate simulated external root resorption. J Endod 2009;35:233–235.
38. Bauman M. The effect of cone beam computed tomography voxel resolution on the detection of canals in the mesiobuccal roots of permanent maxillary first molars [thesis]. Louisville, Kentucky: University of Louisville School of Dentistry, 2009.
39. Kobayashi K, Shimoda S, Nakagawa Y, Yamamoto A. Accuracy in measurement of distances using limited cone-beam computerized tomography. Int J Oral Maxillofac Implants 2004;19:228–231.
40. Lascala C, Panella J, Marques MM. Analysis of the accuracy of linear measurements obtained by cone beam computed tomography (CBCT-NewTom). Dentomaxillofac Radiol 2004;33:291–294.
41. Pinsky HM, Dyda S, Pinsky RW, Misch KA, Sarment DP. Accuracy of three-dimensional measurements using cone-beam CT. Dentomaxillofac Radiol 2006;35:410–416.
42. American Association of Endodontists and American Academy of Oral and Maxillofacial Radiology. Use of cone-beam computed tomography in endodontics. Joint Position Statement of the American Association of Endodontists and the American Academy of Oral and Maxillofacial Radiology. Oral Surg Oral Med Oral Pathol 2011;111:234–237.
43. Bartling SH, Majdani O, Gupta R, et al. Large scan field, high spatial resolution flat-panel detector based volumetric CT of the whole human skull base and for maxillofacial imaging. Dentomaxillofac Radiol 2007;36:317–327.

44. Hirsch E, Graf H-L, Hemprich A. Comparative investigation of image quality of three different X-ray procedures. Dentomaxillofac Radiol 2003;32:201–211.
45. Hashimoto K, Yoshinori Y, Iwai K, Araki M, Kawashima S, Terakado M. A comparison of a new limited cone beam computed tomography machine for dental use with a multidetector row helical CT machine. Oral Surg Oral Med Oral Pathol Oral Radiol Endod 2003;95:371–377.
46. Hashimoto K, Kawashima S, Araki M, Sawada K, Akiyama Y. Comparison of image performance between cone-beam computed tomography for dental use and four-row multidetector helical CT. J Oral Sci 2006;48:27–34.
47. Hashimoto K, Kawashima S, Kameoka S, et al. Comparison of image validity between cone beam computed tomography for dental use and multidetector row helical computed tomography. Dentomaxillofac Radiol 2007;36:465–471.
48. Mora MA, Mol A, Tyndall DA, Rivera E. In vitro assessment of local computed tomography for the detection of longitudinal tooth fractures. Oral Surg Oral Med Oral Pathol Oral Radiol Endod 2007;103:825–829.
49. Sogur E, Baksi BG, Gröndahl H-G. Imaging of root canal fillings: A comparison of subjective image quality between limited cone-beam CT, storage phosphor and film radiography. Int Endod J 2007;40:179–185.
50. Estrela C, Leles CR, Hollanda AC, Moura MS, Pécora JD. Prevalence and risk factors of apical periodontitis in endodontically treated teeth in a selected population of Brazilian adults. Braz Dent J 2008;19:34–39.
51. Vertucci FJ. Root canal anatomy of the human permanent teeth. Oral Surg Oral Med Oral Pathol 1984;58:589–599.
52. Pineda F. Roentgenographic investigation of the mesiobuccal root of the maxillary first molar. Oral Surg Oral Med Oral Pathol 1973;36:253–260.
53. Ramamurthy R, Scheetz JP, Clark SJ, Farman AG. Effects of imaging system and exposure on accurate detection of the second mesiobuccal canal in maxillary molar teeth. Oral Surg Oral Med Oral Pathol Oral Radiol Endod 2006;102:796–802.
54. Neelakantan P, Subbarao C, Subbarao CV. Comparative evaluation of modified canal staining and clearing technique, cone beam computed tomography, peripheral quantitative computed tomography, spiral computed tomography, and plain and contrast medium enhanced digital radiography in studying root canal morphology. J Endod 2010;36:1547–1551.
55. Michetti J, Maret D, Mallet JP, Diemer F. Validation of cone beam computed tomography as a tool to explore root canal anatomy. J Endod 2010;36:1187–1190.
56. Tu MG, Huang HL, Hsue SS, et al. Detection of permanent three-rooted mandibular first molars by cone-beam computed tomography imaging in Taiwanese individuals. J Endod 2009;35:503–507.
57. Cleghorn BM, Christie WH, Dong CCS. Anomalous mandibular premolars: A mandibular first premolar with three roots and a mandibular second premolar with a C-shaped canal system. Int Endod J 2008;41:1005–1014.
58. Estrela C, Bueno MR, Sousa-Neto MD, Pécora JD. Method for determination of root curvature radius using cone-beam computed tomography images. Braz Dent J 2008;19:114–118.
59. Tsurumachi T, Honda K. A new cone beam computerized tomography system for use in endodontic surgery. Int Endod J 2007;40:224–232.
60. D'Addazio P, Campos C, Özcan M, Teixeira H, Passoni R, Carvalho A. A comparative study between cone-beam computed tomography and periapical radiographs in the diagnosis of simulated endodontic complications. Int Endod J 2011;44:218–224.
61. Ørstavik D, Pitt Ford TR. Apical periodontitis: Microbial infection and host responses. In: Ørstavik D, Pitt Ford TR (eds). Essential Endodontology. Oxford: Blackwell Science, 1998:1–8.
62. Friedman S. Considerations and concepts of case selection in the management of post-treatment endodontic disease (treatment failure). Endod Topics 2002;1:54–78.

63. Trope M. The vital tooth—Its importance in the study and practice of endodontics. Endod Topics 2003;5:1–11.
64. Wu M-K, Dummer PMH, Wesselink PR. Consequences of and strategies to deal with residual post-treatment root canal infection. Int Endod J 2006;39:343–356.
65. Jorge EG, Tanomaru-Filho M, Goncalves M, Tanomaru MG. Detection of periapical lesion development by conventional radiography or computed tomography. Oral Surg Oral Med Oral Path ol Oral Radiol Endod 2008;106:e56–e61.
66. Cotton TP, Geisler TM, Holden DT, Schwartz SA, Schindler WG. Endodontic applications of cone-beam volumetric tomography. J Endod 2007;33:1121–1132.
67. Patel S, Dawood A, Pitt Ford T, Whaites E. The potential applications of cone beam computed tomography in the management of endodontic problems. Int Endod J 2007;40:818–830.
68. Nakata K, Naitoh M, Izumi M, Inamoto K, Ariji E, Nakamura H. Effectiveness of dental computed tomography in diagnostic imaging of periradicular lesion of each root of a multirooted tooth: A case report. J Endod 2006;32:583–587.
69. Tsukiboshi M. Optimal use of photography, radiology and micro computed tomography scanning in the management of traumatized teeth. Endod Topics 2008;12:4–19.
70. Terakado M, Hashimoto K, Arai Y, Honda M, Sekiwa T, Sato H. Diagnostic imaging with newly developed ortho cubic super-high resolution computed tomography (Ortho-CT). Oral Surg Oral Med Oral Pathol Oral Radiol Endod 2000;89:509–518.
71. Özer Y. Detection of vertical root fractures of different thicknesses in endodontically enlarged teeth by cone beam computed tomography versus digital radiography. J Endod 2010;36:1245–1249.
72. Tamse A, Fuss Z, Lustig J, Kaplavi J. An evaluation of endodontically treated vertically fractured teeth. J Endod 1999;25:506–508.
73. Meister F Jr, Lommel TJ, Gerstein H. Diagnosis and possible causes of vertical root fractures. Oral Surg Oral Med Oral Path 1980;49:243–253.
74. Testori T, Badino M, Castagnola M. Vertical root fractures in endodontically treated teeth: A clinical survey of 36 cases. J Endod 1993;19:87–91.
75. Tsesis I, Rosen E, Tamse A, Taschieri S, Kfir A. Diagnosis of vertical root fractures in endodontically treated teeth based on clinical and radiographic indices: A systematic review. J Endod 2010;36:1455–1458.
76. Tamse A. Vertical root fractures in endodontically treated teeth: Diagnostic signs and clinical management. Endod Topics 2006;13:84–94.
77. Hassan B, Metska ME, Ozok AR, van der Stelt P, Wesselink PR. Detection of vertical root fractures in endodontically treated teeth by a cone beam computed tomography scan. J Endod 2009;35:719–722.
78. Patel S, Dawood A. The use of cone beam computed tomography in the management of external cervical resorption lesions. Int Endod J 2007;40:730–737.
79. Patel S, Dawood A, Wilson R, Horner K, Mannocci F. The detection and management of root resorption lesions using intraoral radiography and cone beam computed tomography—An in vivo investigation. Int Endod J 2009;42:831–838.
80. Rigolone M, Pasqualini D, Bianchi L, Berutti E, Bianchi SD. Vestibular surgical access to the palatine root of the superior first molar: "low-dose cone-beam" CT analysis of the pathway and its anatomic variations. J Endod 2003;29:773–775.
81. Bornstein M, Wasmer J, Sendi P, et al. Characteristics and dimensions of the Schneiderian membrane and apical bone in maxillary molars referred for apical surgery: A comparative radiographic analysis using limited cone beam computed tomography. J Endod 2012;38:51–57.

82. Oberli K, Bornstein M, Von Arx T. Periapical surgery and the maxillary sinus: Radiographic parameters for clinical outcome. Oral Surg Oral Med Oral Pathol Oral Radiol Endod 2007;103:848–853.
83. Eberhardt JA, Torabinejad M, Christiansen EL. A computed tomographic study of the distances between the maxillary sinus floor and the apices of the maxillary posterior teeth. Oral Surg Oral Med Oral Pathol 1992;73:345–346.
84. Hauman C, Chandler N, Tong D. Endodontic implications of the maxillary sinus: A review. Int Endod J 2002;35:127–141.
85. Garcia B, Martorell L, Martí E, Peñarrocha M. Periapical surgery of maxillary posterior teeth. A review of the literature. Med Oral 2006;11:146–150.
86. Paula-Silva FWG, Hassan B, da Silva LAB, Leonardo MR, Wu MK. Outcome of root canal treatment in dogs determined by periapical radiography and cone bean computed tomography. J Endod 2009;35:723–726.
87. Wu MK, Shemesh H, Wesselink PR. Limitations of previously published systematic reviews evaluating the outcome of endodontic treatment. Int Endod J 2009;42:656–666.
88. Fristad I, Molven O, Halse A. Nonsurgically retreated root-filled teeth—Radiographic findings after 20–27 years. Int Endod J 2004;37:12–18.
89. Mead C, Javidan-Nejad S, Mego ME, Nash B, Torabinejad M. Levels of evidence for the outcome of endodontic surgery. J Endod 2005;31:19–24.

T Testori
L Fumagalli
F Galli

12

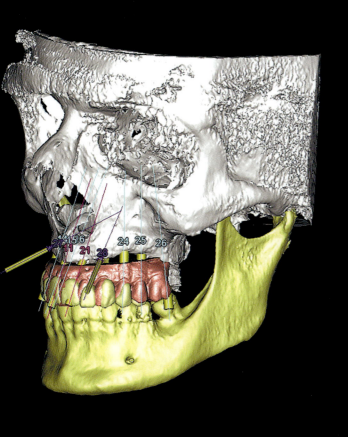

Using guided-surgery protocols allows the clinician to simplify the procedure while reducing surgical time for implant placement and the invasiveness of the surgery itself, especially if a flapless surgical approach is adopted.

The accurate preoperative planning that used to be done on working models and by other nondigital means implied that the clinician could discover the actual surgical anatomy only during the procedure, whereas today anatomy can be studied preoperatively on the computer with the utmost accuracy. The evolution of computerized planning software coupled with high-quality computed tomography (CT) and cone bem CT (CBCT) imaging techniques have contributed to providing the clinician with surgical and diagnostic tools that can be extremely valuable, especially when faced with anatomical alterations.

The purpose of this chapter is to illustrate the various guided-surgery systems available on the market and their features.

Computer-Assisted Guided Surgery: Indications and Limitations

Over the past 20 years, surgical implant placement procedures have evolved enormously, and better knowledge of bone and peri-implant tissue biology coupled with new implant designs have led to an increasingly broad range of clinical indications for modern implant dentistry with higher success rates. Apart from this evolution, achieving esthetic and functional results in implant dentistry remains the primary goal, which can only be achieved through accurate diagnosis followed by correct surgical and prosthetic procedures.

The implant position plays a key role in the final esthetic and functional result, and, once the implant is integrated, it is a (usually unchangeable) variable that may undermine the final clinical result.

Nowadays, sophisticated preoperative analytical software products are available to the implant surgeon, who can therefore diagnose, plan, and simulate the surgical procedure in an effective and minimally invasive manner. The latest analysis tools are based on 3D imaging and offer a three-dimensional view of the anatomy and of the implant site (Fig 12-1).

From 2D to 3D: Modern Imaging Techniques

Two-dimensional (2D) radiographic techniques, such as intraoral radiographs, panoramic radiographs, and lateral and posteroanterior (PA) cephalometry, were commonly used as routine diagnostic tools in implant dentistry in the 1980s and 1990s. By integrating panoramic radiographs and lateral cephalometric radiographs, the clinician tried to obtain a three-dimensional (3D) view of the patient's anatomy.[1]

However, 2D images did not provide sufficiently detailed information for an in-depth preoperative assessment, especially in cases of severe bone atrophy.

At the end of the 1980s and early 1990s, 3D radiographic techniques (ie, CT) were introduced in implant dentistry.[2-6] This late introduction of 3D imaging in the dental arena was due to the high cost of CT machines, which were available in hospitals or clinics but not in dental practices. Moreover, the radiation doses absorbed by patients were high, and the image acquisition time was very long (up to 20 minutes, as compared to a few seconds with modern CT units), which could also generate artifacts due to patient movements during the examination. CBCT, developed in the 1990s, contributed to introducing 3D imaging in non-hospital daily clinical practice.[7] The lower cost of CBCT machines, the smaller size of the equipment, and the lower doses of radiation absorbed by the patient, coupled with the possibility to reduce acquisition volume to one or two teeth, thus further reducing the absorbed radiation dose, were key factors in fostering the use of CBCT in dentistry.

Its use in other areas—in addition to implant dentistry—such as endodontics, oral surgery, and periodontics (Fig 12-2) led

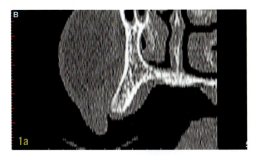
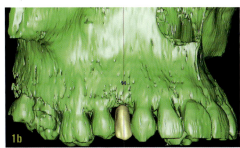

Fig 12-1a Paraxial section of an edentulous region in the premolar area.

Fig 12-1b 3D view with tooth simulation.

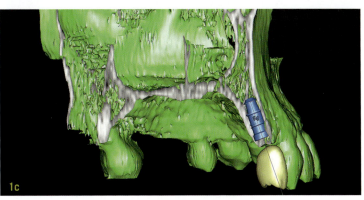

Fig 12-1c 3D paraxial section of the inserted implant with the virtual tooth.

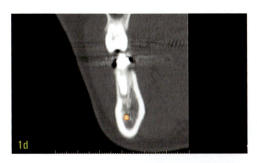
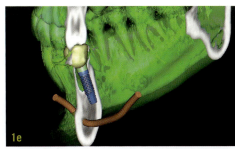

Fig 12-1d Paraxial section of a tooth with vertical fracture.

Fig 12-1e Paraxial section with virtual planning of a postextraction single implant in a mandibular premolar.

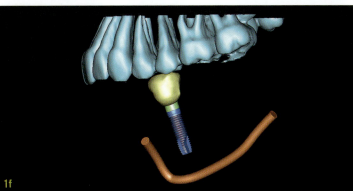

Fig 12-1f Removal of bone and dental tissues in the mandibular jaw. View of the virtual prosthetic crown, the implant, and its relationship with the inferior alveolar nerve.

Fig 12-2a Use of CBCT-based 3D diagnostics in different areas of dentistry. *(a)* Paraxial section of a tooth showing an endodontic lesion close to the mental foramen.

Fig 12-2b Paraxial section of a molar showing a periodontal lesion at the level of the furcation.

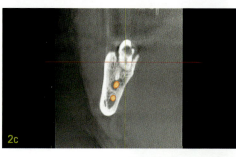

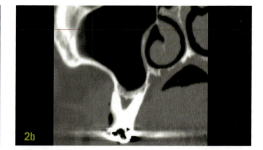

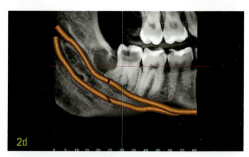

Figs 12-2c to 12-2e 3D assessment of the relationship between the root apices of third molars and the neurologic structures; *(d and e)* bifid canal.

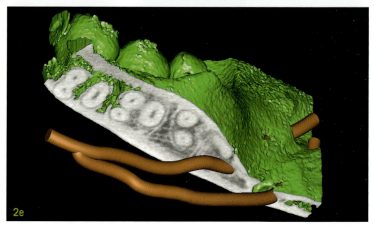

to improved diagnoses due to a more detailed analysis of the pathologic processes and their extent and to accurate monitoring of the healing process.[8–10]

Starting from the mid-1980s, the introduction of the Digital Imging and Communications in Medicine (DICOM) standard established common criteria for communication, viewing, storage, and printing of imaging information in the biomedical field.[11]

DICOM image-processing programs have remarkably improved the 3D viewing of scanned sections. Dedicated noise-reduction instruments have increased the image quality while reducing the scattering generated by highly radiopaque components (starburst), which is typical of tomography. Indeed, scattering was a major limitation of conventional CT images, as it prevented correct viewing of the scanned volume.

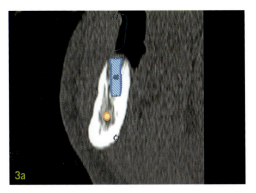

Fig 12-3a Digital planning of a case of distal edentulism. The analysis of axial and 3D sections allows evaluation of the relationship of the planned implant site with important anatomical structures. Paraxial section is shown with the virtual implant in position.

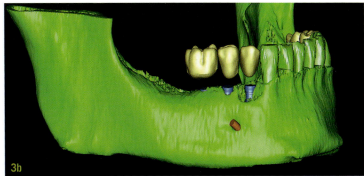

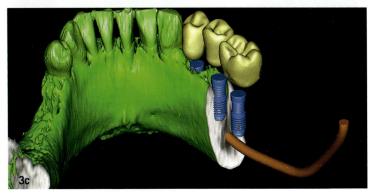

Fig 12-3b 3D imaging with virtual prosthetic teeth.
Fig 12-3c 3D axial imaging and relationship between the implants and the course of the inferior alveolar canal.

Modern CBCT has mitigated this problem, and the latest CBCT techniques have reduced the image acquisition time and thus also the error rate due to patient movements. Depending on the scanned volume, the image acquisition time is approximately 20 to 40 seconds. However, CBCT image acquisition time is a contraindication to CBCT imaging in patients suffering from Parkinson's disease, for whom a traditional spiral CT scan is still indicated.

In implant dentistry, the level of accuracy of CBCT has allowed study of the implant site with submillimeter accuracy on the three spatial planes. This allows viewing of anatomical structures that may potentially limit the implant placement space (Fig 12-3). Another useful application is the evaluation of the implant site with an accurate preoperative assessment of the residual alveolar bone in clinical cases where tooth extractions are performed (Fig 12-4).

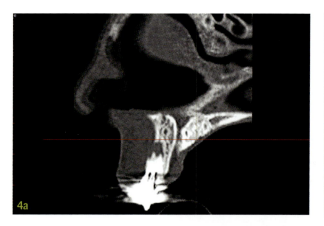
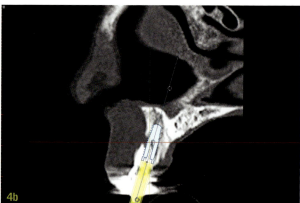
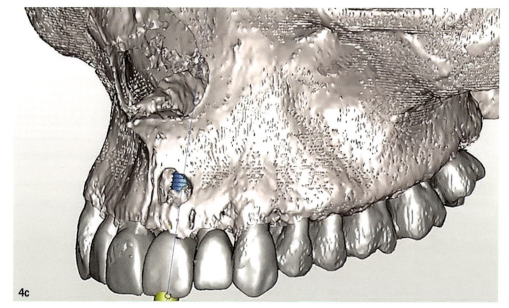

Fig 12-4a Digital treatment planning of a patient with a maxillary incisor affected by a periapical lesion and external root resorption. Paraxial section with tooth in situ. The image shows a radiolucent area on the middle third of the root and sufficient bone quantity at the apical level to stabilize the implant.

Fig 12-4b Implant planning, relationship with surrounding bone structures, and correct implant axis.

Fig 12-4c 3D imaging after virtual extraction, showing a fenestration at the level of the middle third of the root and a virtual crown in situ.

CAD/CAM Technology

Alongside the widespread use of increasingly accurate examinations, the growing interest of implant manufacturers pushed research towards computer-assisted dentistry geared towards integrating radiographic imaging and prosthetic-surgical procedures.

Computer-aided design/computer-assisted manufacturing (CAD/CAM) technologies developed in the dental area in the 1980s and 1990s, mainly in the prosthetic arena. In the implant dentistry area, their introduction took place more recently, again in the prosthetic sector, with implant abutments manufactured through industrial processes and fixtures milled with numeric-control machines instead of casting processes using lost wax. While digital information used to be obtained by scanning resin or wax models made in laboratories, now the process is fully digital. Prosthetic fixtures can be designed directly on the computer and then sent to the milling center for manufacturing.

Also, modern implant surgery is now oriented towards methods that facilitate the execution of surgical procedures.

Preparing the surgical site and positioning the implant according to the preliminary prosthetic plan has become faster and more accurate.

Combining this CAD/CAM technique with 3D implant-planning software has allowed the fabrication of surgical guides for implant placement.

Flapless Surgery

Over the past few years, the trend in medicine has been to reduce surgical invasiveness and to favor minimally invasive endoscopic procedures. Likewise, implant surgery has tried to reduce the impact of surgical procedures by limiting the use of access flaps whenever possible. The literature points out that there is limited evidence that flapless surgery offers benefits to the patients such as reduction of postoperative pain, bleeding, and swelling.[12-14] Furthermore, this approach is not risk-free, since the procedure is carried out without a direct view,[15,16] and it is crucial that the surgeon is not at the beginning of the learning curve.[17] The errors and limitations of this kind of procedure include: wrong vertical positioning of the implant, fenestration of the cortical bone during osteotomy, reduced possibility to modify hard and soft tissues.[16] Computer-assisted surgery has allowed an increase in the number of feasible flapless procedures,[18] but with flapless clinical cases the clinician must plan to open a full-thickness flap and perform bone regeneration techniques should bone dehiscence occur after implant sites have been prepared.

Computer-Assisted Surgery

The goal of implant surgery has always been to develop a presurgical plan that could be transferred to the surgical field[2,3,6,19,20] with reduced invasiveness.

It is well known that implant placement is key to obtaining good esthetic and functional results with prostheses, whose type—screw- or cement-retained—must be decided before the surgical procedure.[21,22]

To perform a correct implant treatment restoring proper esthetic and functional parameters and to allow good maintenance of the restoration, crucial factors such as a correct distribution and position of the implants are to be taken into account.

The surgical radiologic guide was the first aid for correct implant placement.[1,6,19,23] Its function was to allow for the acquisition of radiopaque landmarks during tomographic imaging, which were included in the guide on the basis of an initial wax-up of the case. The wax-up was supposed to replicate the future prosthetic restora-

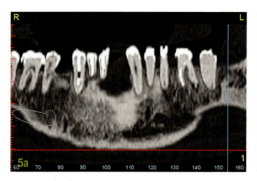
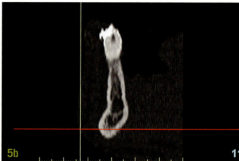
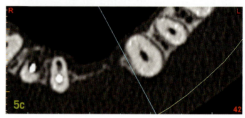

Figs 12-5a to 12-5c Examples of 3D examination without 3D images. Although the different images can be interpolated, it is hard to envision the third dimension.

tion, but the indications provided by such guides were inaccurate, especially when it came to changing the position of the landmark after the tomographic images had been taken.

Another limitation, even though these were 3D images, was the clinician's interpretation of 2D images. As a matter of fact, CT scans did not have digital support to help the end user because the image was printed on film. Therefore, the surgeon had to study a set of 2D images, usually with paraxial sections every 2 mm, to mentally visualize the third dimension (Fig 12-5).

Modern CT and CBCT machines can now work with sections of 0.5 to 1 mm, providing 3D images showing the actual clinical anatomy.

Later, stereolithographic drilling guides fabricated with prototyping techniques[24–27] allowed improvement of the 3D assessment of anatomical structures and contributed to better preoperative planning. The CAD/CAM technique contributed to developing guided surgery with reconstructions of the crest of bone on resin models in a 1:1 scale. Initially, these models were milled, but later on they were replaced by additive manufacturing processes through selective laser sintering. This also allowed reconstruction of hollow structures, such as the layout of the mandibular canal or the maxillary sinus. From the very beginning, stereolithographic models appeared to be very useful, especially in clinical cases of bone regeneration, as they allowed study of the degree of bone atrophy in more detail and identification of the most appropriate donor site for potential autologous bone grafts.[27] By mounting the model onto the articulator, the clinician could evaluate not only the variables that were strictly linked to the surgical site, but also the 3D position of the edentulous alveolar ridge as compared to the opposite arch.

The construction of stereolithographic models was a turning point in the evolution of surgical guides, which were further modified by including tubular metal guides positioned along the designed implant axis guiding the bur during osteotomy. However, different surgical guides had to be used due to the varying diameter of the burs, which required preparation of different templates for each bur. As a result of the evolution of guided surgery, a single surgical guide was developed, which permitted the passage of all burs necessary for the preparation of the implant site using manual instruments (reducers) to guide each dedicated bur (Fig 12-6).

Modern surgical guides allow the clinician to control the osteotomy on the three spatial planes and provide for guided implant placement.[28,29] A further important feature of modern guided-surgery software products is the possibility to select the volumes within a range of Hounsfield values for traditional CT scans. This allows the operator to select elements with different levels of radiopacity (bones, teeth, prostheses) and to employ a subtractive technique. For instance, you can reconstruct only the bone tissue by removing the teeth, which is very useful in postextraction implant placement (Fig 12-7).

However, current CBCT machines do not work with the Hounsfield scale but instead with a machine-specific gray scale, although in the future CBCT machines will be able to generate a 3D map in Hounsfield scale. By reducing the dose of radiation absorbed by the patient, the cone beam technology allows the operator to acquire larger FOVs and to evaluate the correct maxillomandibular relationships. However, in fully edentulous patients, the scans must be taken in centric relationship and at the correct vertical dimension of the future prosthesis (Fig 12-8).[30]

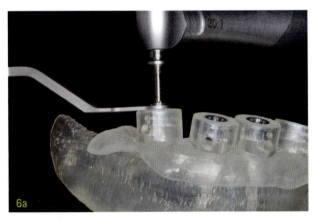
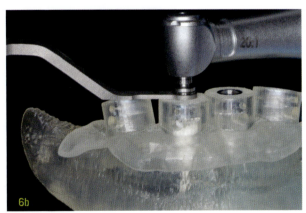

Figs 12-6a and 12-6b Example of bone-supported surgical guide adapted to the stereolithographic model. The detail shows the system of reduction cannulas and depth stops for the different osteotomy burs, using one surgical guide.

Figs 12-7a to 12-7c The process of subtracting different levels of bone density. The bone tissue can be analyzed by separating it from dental tissue. This procedure is very useful for postextraction implant placement to evaluate the amount of available bone.

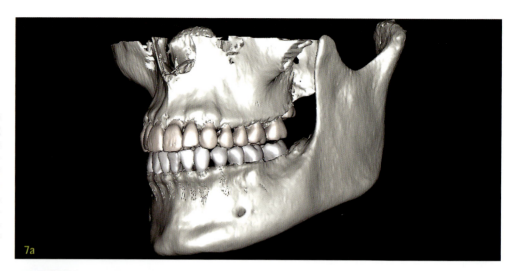

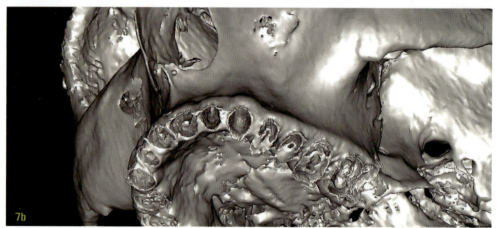

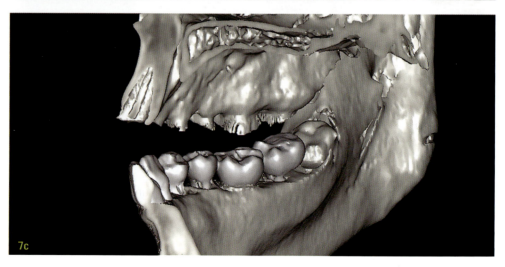

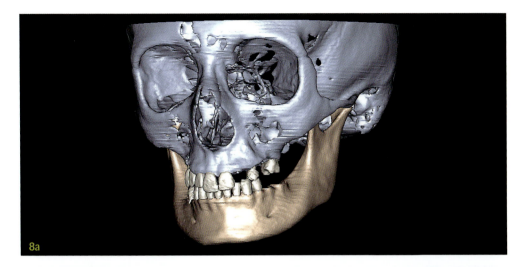

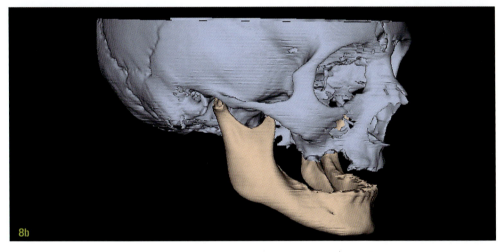

Figs 12-8a and 12-8b
Examples of wide-FOV imaging of the skull. This type of imaging allows the classic 2D cephalometric analysis to be expanded into the third dimension.

Analysis of Guided-Surgery Systems

According to Hammerle et al,[31] guided surgery can be classified into two categories, ie, dynamic and static. In dynamic surgery—also known as real-time surgery—a dynamic system reproducing the position of the patient's head and of the implant handpiece guides the clinician during implant positioning. With this system, the indications for positioning the implant are delivered in real time, guided by a viewing system. In static surgery, positioning templates are used. They are stabilized on the edentulous ridge to be treated, and they contain all the information that the surgeon needs to position the implant. The market is currently oriented towards static surgery because dynamic surgery requires expensive equipment and maintenance costs, in addition to extremely cumbersome devices for capturing the patient position, which limit their routine clinical use in all areas of the oral cavity.

Currently manufactured surgical guides for static surgery normally fall into four categories: bone-supported, tooth-supported, mucosa-supported, or mixed (tooth/mucosa- or tooth/bone-supported) guides.

From a design standpoint, bone-supported guides are the easiest to manufacture as they only require a 3D radiograph, but they do require a full-thickness flap to expose the bone surface where the guide will be placed. Tooth-supported or mucosa-supported guides, on the contrary, involve the acquisition in electronic format of the stone cast of the arch to be treated and/or the radiographic guide (scan prosthesis) during the surgical planning process. This additional step is necessary because a CT/CBCT scan cannot separate the mucosal profile of the edentulous area from adjacent soft tissues (cheeks, lips, tongue). In order to highlight the mucosal profile, a scan of the stone cast and/or of the guide is necessary to generate the soft tissue profile, through a subtraction and matching technique.

Manufacturers provide detailed instructions on the workflow to be followed depending on the selected type of guide. However, no studies have been conducted to analyze also the cost-effectiveness of planning a guided-surgery procedure as compared with conventional procedures.[32] From a time standpoint, it seems obvious that lengthier preoperative planning is required for guided surgeries as compared to freehand surgical procedures.

The Materialise Simplant System

Simplant (Materialise) is one of the most popular systems in the area of guided surgery. It is an open system that allows the clinician to use a variety of implant systems. Bone-supported, tooth-supported, mucosa-supported, and mixed (tooth/mucosa- or tooth/bone-supported) guides can be manufactured. The bone anatomy can be studied to the smallest detail (Fig 12-9a). Critical anatomical structures can be highlighted and traced in a simple manner. The software allows the clinician to design and position virtual teeth so as to make the simulation more realistic. The teeth can also be oriented as needed to simulate the future prosthetic restoration. This is very important when evaluating the appropriateness of the implant axis. If both arches are scanned using a total face approach (TFA) protocol,[26] the spatial position of the virtual teeth shows no clinically relevant differences as compared to more sophisticated protocols requiring a scan of the clinical case wax-up and its inclusion in the radiologic examination. This function is also very useful for communicating with the patient and explaining the planned treatment.

The bone volume represented on the images can be sectioned along the reference planes so as to accurately investigate the implant position, the density of the surrounding bone, and the involvement of adjacent anatomical structures.

A threshold value can be set if the implant has to be placed near critical anatomical structures or if implants are too close to each other. Implants can also be placed at predefined distances to maximize the tolerances during the

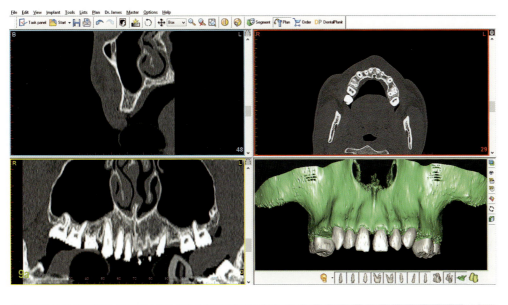

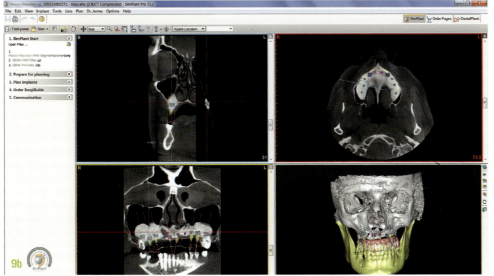

Figs 12-9a and 12-9b Example of planning executed with the Materialise Simplant system. The clinician has the three sections on the reference axial planes available at the same time, together with the 3D reconstruction. The implant axes can be studied to the smallest detail so as to plan the subsequent prosthetic stage in a simpler manner.

coupling with the prosthetic structure, as determined by a divergence between implants.
The process starts with the acquisition of the patient's DICOM data. The software version with the oral maxillofacial surgery (OMS) extension allows the operator to process both arches at the same time so as to evaluate any sagittal and vertical discrepancies even at the design stage. The software graphical engine is very fast, and the 3D model can be created in only a few steps by filtering out, if necessary, any artifacts due to highly radiopaque materials.
Once the reference panoramic curve is traced, the program summarizes all reference planes and the 3D volume on the main screen so as to allow for an assessment of the actual position of the implant on the three spatial planes (Fig 12-9b).

During the programming phase, prosthetic planning can be added to the virtual model. To do this, a radiopaque radiologic guide must be prepared according to the specific instructions supplied by the manufacturer of the navigation system.

Then, the laboratory makes an optical scan of the radiologic guide and generates a standard triangulation language (STL) file, which will be sent to the dentist. The software can automatically orientate and align the scanned volume of the prosthesis and overlay it onto to the CT image (double scanning).

This offers the operator a perfect view of the bone components as well as of the mucosal surface, allowing preoperative design of the length of the prosthetic abutments. The virtual positioning of the implant is intuitive and does not require the implant dentist to receive any special training.

Once the implants are designed with reference to their respective sites, the position can be checked—with submillimeter accuracy—against the crestal bone using a dedicated movement function (fine movements). Our school recommends using a high-resolution monitor of appropriate size (larger than 25 inches) to fully benefit from the resolution and detail features of guided-surgery software programs.

Once the implant plan is completed, the files can be sent electronically to request the surgical guide designed in this manner. Once the project is sent, the file cannot be changed. Guided-surgery implant kits include a range of burs with calibrated stops. These burs are longer than those in standard kits. This difference is due to the greater distance between the head of the handpiece and crestal bone. The thickness of the surgical guide is determined by the length of the positioning sleeves. This characteristic is a major limitation to the use of guided surgery in patients with limited mouth opening. The dimension of the surgical guide and the length of the burs may also pose limitations to the surgical procedure.

Clinical Case of Bone-Supported Guided Surgery

The patient (male, 62 years of age, physical status American Society of Anesthesiologists [ASA] 1) has a fully edentulous maxilla. The patient's desire is to replace the maxillary removable denture with a fixed prosthesis (Figs 12-10 to 12-22).

Physical examination shows severe atrophy of the crestal bone, which, over the years, has undergone severe centripetal resorption combined with coronoapical resorption. The panoramic radiograph provides an initial estimate of the available alveolar bone. To restore a correct maxillomandibular relationship, both vertically and transversally, the patient was referred to the maxillofacial surgical unit, which recommended that the patient be hospitalized to receive an surgical osteotomy treatment of the maxilla coupled with interposition and apposition of iliac bone grafts. The patient denied his consent to the recommended therapy and returned to our practice for a less invasive solution. To study the clinical case in more detail and to establish whether or not the patient's desire to receive a fixed prosthesis could be fulfilled, possibly with a prosthetic compensation for the bone deficit, before taking new radiographs we manufactured a new removable denture at a correct maxillomandibular relationship and a correct vertical dimension. Then, the prosthetic work was scanned and included in the 3D examination using the TFA protocol.[30]

After evaluating the case based on the TFA data, the patient was offered a one day–surgery solution: bilateral maxillary sinus elevation with horizontal bone reconstruction using biomaterials and resorbable membranes, delayed implant placement, and a hybrid screw-retained prosthesis compensating for the bone deficit, which this day-surgery solution cannot fully resolve. Six months after the maxillary sinus elevation procedure, we opted for a bone-supported guide due to the soft tissue deficit, which would be better compensated in the second surgical step.

Because the guide must be placed directly in contact with the alveolar crest, we decided to perform a crestal incision with distal release and a full-thickness mesial incision from the tuberosity region to the contralateral tuberosity.

The surgical guide was then positioned and affixed with two internal fixation

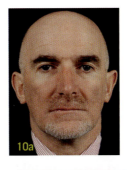
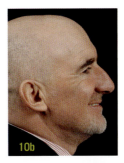

Figs 12-10a and 12-10b Frontal and lateral macroesthetic view of the patient wearing a removable partial denture.

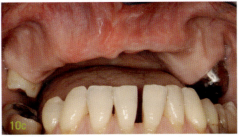

Figs 12-10c to 12-10e Frontal, occlusal, and sagittal views of the degree of atrophy of the alveolar ridge.

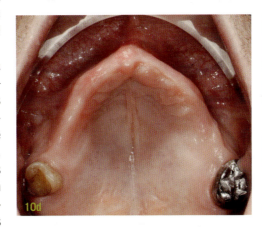
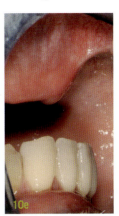

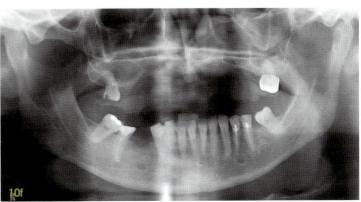

Fig 12-10f Preoperative panoramic radiograph.

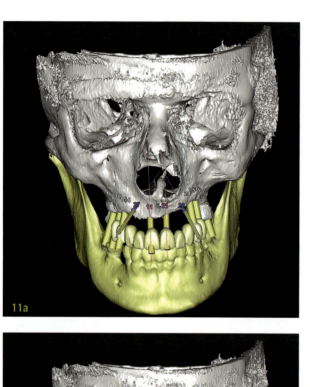
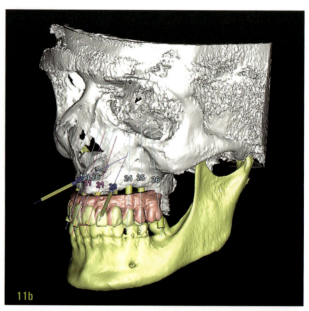
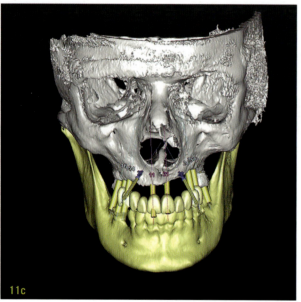
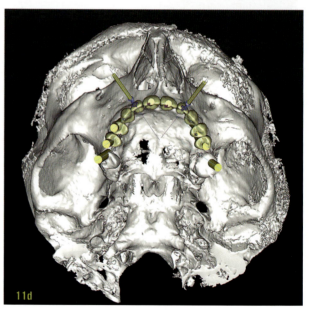

Figs 12-11a to 12-11d Virtual planning using the TFA protocol to correlate the maxillary and mandibular arches and the planned prosthetic restoration based on the patient's skeletal anatomy and facial esthetics.

screws. The implant sites were prepared using the recommended bur sequence, and 2- and 3-mm burs were used up to the recommended depth stop, irrigating with abundant saline solution.

Once all the implants were placed, the surgical guide was removed, and the positioning of the implant was checked clinically. As planned, the bone defect on the horizontal plane was restored with biomaterial and absorbable membranes, and finally the flaps were sutured. Three months after implant placement surgery, the second surgical step was performed and, once the soft tissues healed, a hybrid screw-retained prosthesis was fabricated, which effectively compensated for the bone deficit on the three spatial planes.

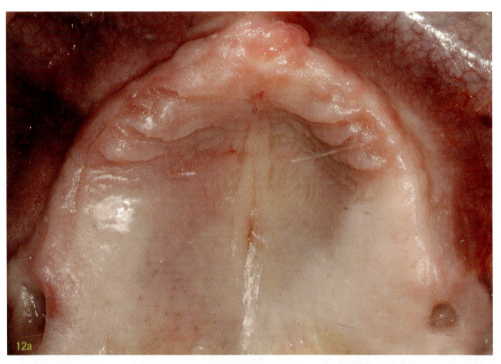

Figs 12-12a and 12-12b Surgical stage: occlusal views of the edentulous jaw and tuberosity-to-tuberosity flap design.

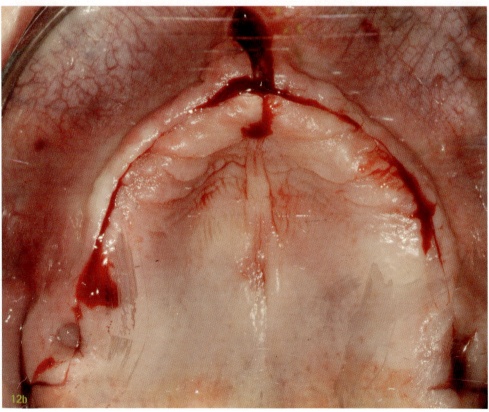

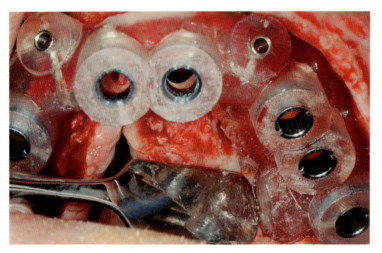
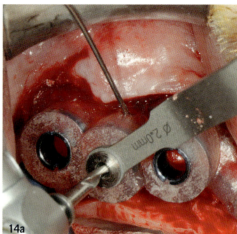

Fig 12-13 Positioning of the bone-supported surgical guide.

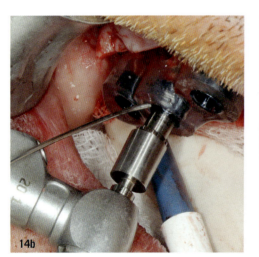
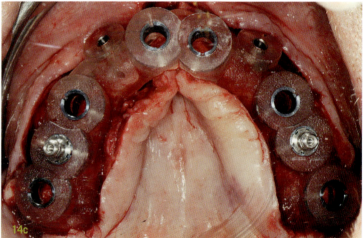

Figs 12-14a to 12-14c Preliminary steps for osteotomies in the areas of the first premolars, which stabilized the surgical guide throughout implant placement.

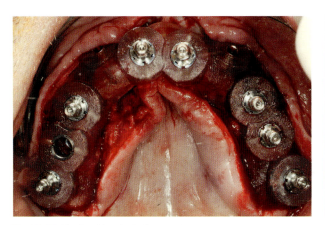

Fig 12-15 Finalized implant placement.

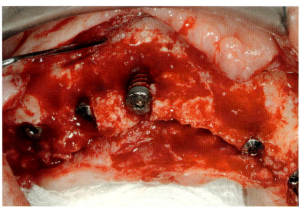

Fig 12-16 Removal of the positioning guide and clinical confirmation of the buccal dehiscence.

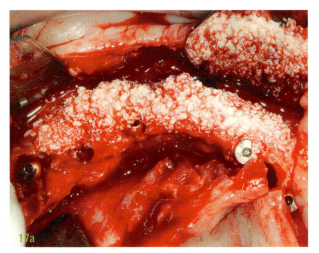

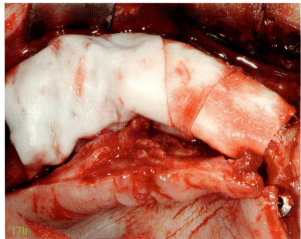

Figs 12-17a and 12-17b Reconstruction of the bone deficit with biomaterials and resorbable membranes.

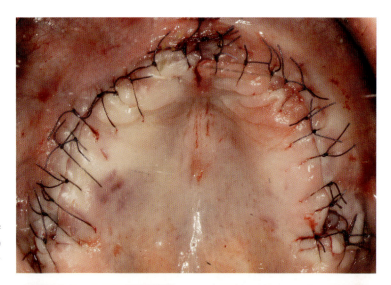

Fig 12-18 Closure of the flap with Vicryl 5-0 resorbable sutures (Ethicon).

Figs 12-19a to 12-19c Finalization of the prosthetic phase. Macro- and microesthetic views of the definitive prosthesis and follow-up panoramic radiograph.

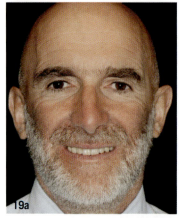
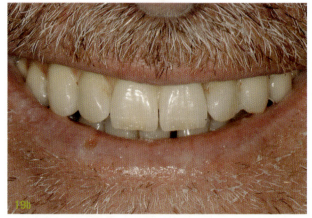
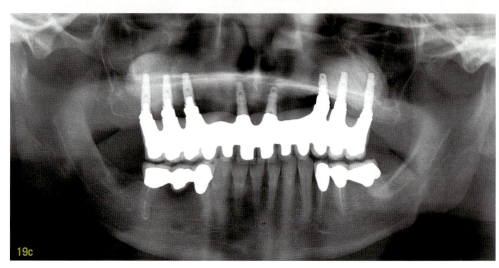

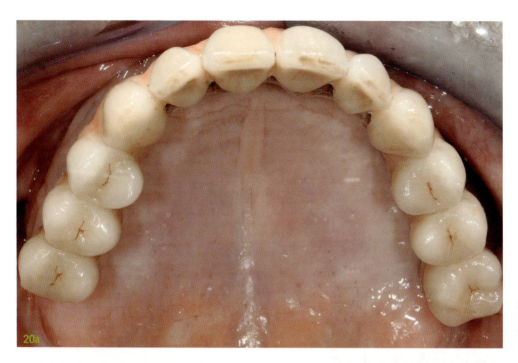
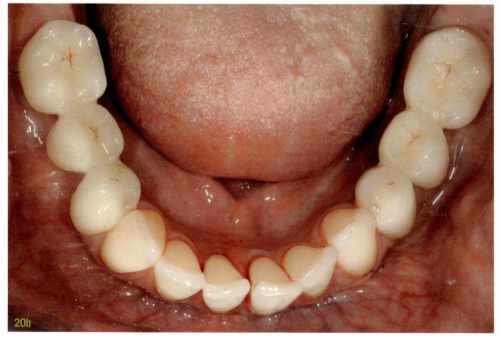

Figs 12-20a and 12-20b Intraoral occlusal view of the implant-based rehabilitation.

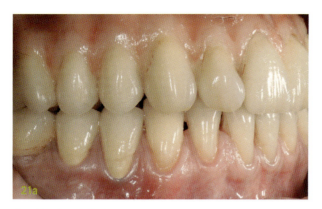
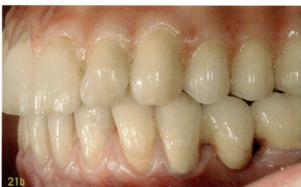

Figs 12-21a and 12-21b Lateral views of the definitive prosthesis.

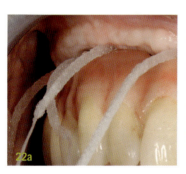
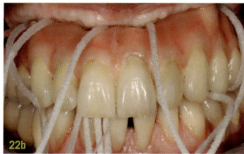
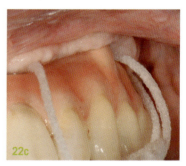

Figs 12-22a to 12-22c Assessment of adequate access for at-home dental hygiene.

Clinical Case of Mucosa-Supported Guided Surgery

The patient (male, 70 years old, physical status ASA 1) has an edentulous maxillary jaw, which had been rehabilitated with a complete removable denture. The patient's desire is to replace the removable denture with an implant-supported fixed solution (Figs 12-23 to 12-35).

Once clinical data had been collected and the radiographic data analyzed with dedicated software tools, the patient was offered a treatment plan that included a flapless approach and an immediately loaded, screw-retained fixed prosthesis. The patient's clinical examination showed a normal smile line and a Class I skeletal relationship. The volume of the complete denture in the anterior sector has caused an alteration of the facial profile in the area of the philtrum. The preservation of the bone volume in the anterior maxilla was clinically evident, with a visible canine prominence and a retroincisal papilla that was still positioned along the palatal aspect. These factors indicated moderate resorption of the alveolar ridge along the

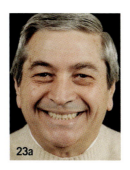
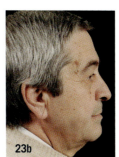

Figs 12-23a and 12-23b Extraoral frontal view. The removable complete denture featured a correct occlusal plane and good tooth exposure. The lateral view revealed excessive support of soft tissues due to the denture flange, which altered the nasolabial profile.

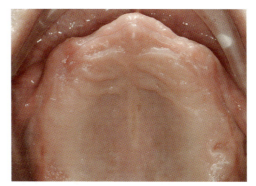

Fig 12-24 The intraoral occlusal view showed good preservation of the anterior maxillary region. The canine prominences were well represented, while the position of the retroincisal papilla indicated moderate atrophy of the maxilla. A sufficient quantity of keratinized mucosa was available on the buccal side.

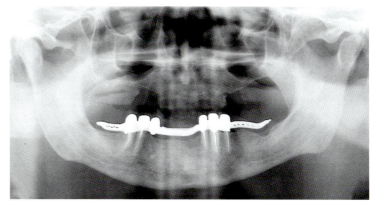

Fig 12-25 Panoramic radiograph showing sufficient bone quantity in the anterior maxillary region.

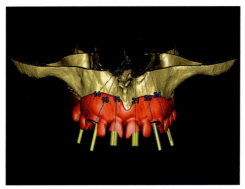

Fig 12-26 Virtual planning based on the data obtained from the 3D imaging with a radiographic template. The surgical plan included flapless surgery with four orthogonal implants and two angled implants in the lateroposterior sectors.

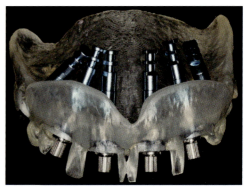

Fig 12-27 Laboratory analogs positioned in the surgical guide.

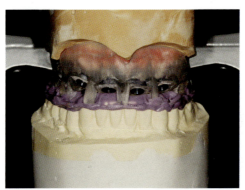

Fig 12-28 Stone casts mounted on the articulator at the correct vertical dimension and maxillomandibular relationship.

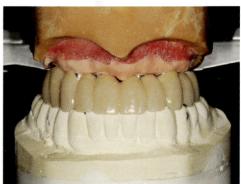

Fig 12-29 The laboratory prepared the provisional prosthesis using the information obtained from the surgical guide.

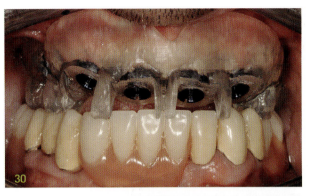
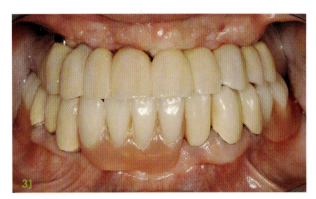
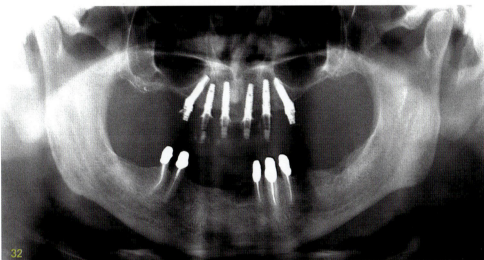

Fig 12-30 The mucosa-supported surgical guide was placed in the oral cavity to confirm the fit on the residual ridge during occlusion.

Fig 12-31 The implants were placed following the implant site preparation procedure recommended by the manufacturer. The provisional prosthesis was relined on the copings of the Quick-Bridge system (Biomet 3i) and delivered to the patient immediately after the surgical procedure.

Fig 12-32 A postsurgical panoramic radiograph showed the correct implant distribution and the angled implants positioned in such a way as to fully exploit the area under the anterior recesses of the maxillary sinus.

sagittal axis. The radiographs showed an insufficient bone quantity in the lateroposterior sectors. The implant surgical plan included six implants, of which two were, placed in the lateroposterior sectors and angled so as to avoid further regenerative surgical procedures in the maxillary sinus, which would have increased the invasiveness and the overall timing of the treatment.

This therapeutic plan needed to be confirmed after analysis of the CT data. For the surgical procedure, a radiographic template was prepared to replicate the future prostheses. The examination was carried out with the radiographic template in place so as to analyze the reciprocal position of the alveolar crest and the planned prosthesis. The analysis of the bone quantity, coupled with an assessment of the bone quality, indicated that an immediately

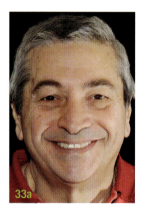
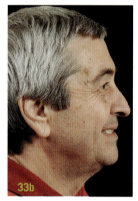
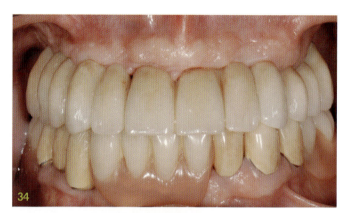

Fig 12-33a Extraoral view of the definitive implant-supported prosthesis, fabricated with a titanium bar manufactured with CAD/CAM technology and esthetic crowns, made of composite resin material, reflecting the esthetic and functional parameters planned in the presurgical stage.

Fig 12-33b Lateral view. The position of the lip is more harmonious. Because there is no labial flange, the upper lip profile had improved.

Fig 12-34 Intraoral view of the definitive prosthesis.

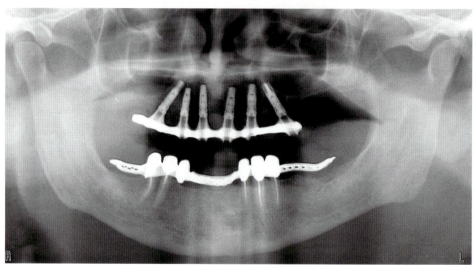

Fig 12-35 Follow-up radiograph.

loaded prosthesis could be placed. The case was then submitted to the manufacturer of the system for fabrication of a mucosa-supported guide. Next, the provisional prosthesis was manufactured in the laboratory; it would then be relined at the end of the surgical procedure so as to compensate for any discrepancy between the actual and the virtual anatomy.[33]

The surgery was carried out with a flapless approach, and the definitive prosthesis was then relined in the patient's mouth, finished in the laboratory, and connected to the implants. The extraoral clinical assessment showed a good integration of the prostheses with the patient's profile and, most significantly, an improvement of the nasolabial angle due to the absence of a labial flange. Three months after placing the provisional prostheses, the fixed prostheses were finalized. They featured a titanium bar and crowns made of composite resin material.

The 3DIEMME RealGUIDE Technique

The RealGUIDE system (3DIEMME) is an open technique that can be used with different implant systems. Similar to the Simplant System, the system supports fabrication of bone-supported, tooth-supported, or mixed (tooth/mucosa- or tooth/bone-supported) surgical guides.

Starting from the wax-up, the dental technician develops a prosthesis for an intraoral esthetic-functional try-in. Once the necessary changes are made, if any, a transparent resin duplicate is made, and an extraoral radiopaque landmark called a 3DMarker with a predefined size and shape is applied onto it. The stone model and the radiographic template are then scanned. The radiographic template is given to the patient for the CT scanning procedure.

The files generated by the scans are then sent to the manufacturer, who will integrate the two data sets. The coupling process is carried out with a technique known as "best fit," ie, an algorithm that aligns the scanned volumes based on preestablished landmarks whose size is known. Once the file with the model scans is received, the clinician will plan the clinical case (Fig 12-36). In some selected cases, the procedure can be performed directly in the dental office, which makes it faster to design and to treat the patient.

Clinical Case of Mucosa-Supported Guided Surgery

In this clinical case (Figs 12-37 to 12-47), the patient had undergone a number of extractions in the maxillary jaw, leading to total maxillary edentulism.

Before taking a CT scan, a full prosthesis was prepared with correct occlusal planes and esthetic profiles, based on a wax-up. After the esthetic-functional assessment, the prosthesis was duplicated and coupled with the extraoral radiopaque landmark.

Using the data processed by the manufacturer, the implant plan was developed. It included six implants in the maxilla, to be placed with a flapless technique and to support a screw-retained fixed full-arch

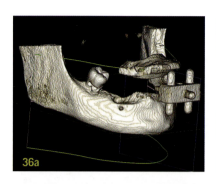
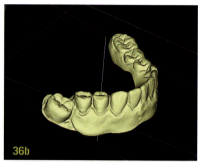
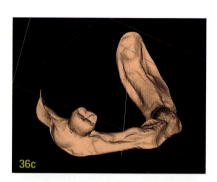
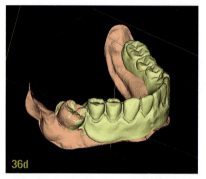
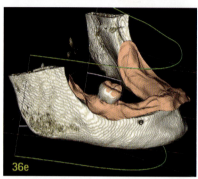
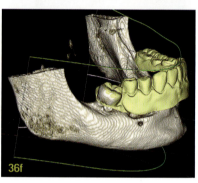
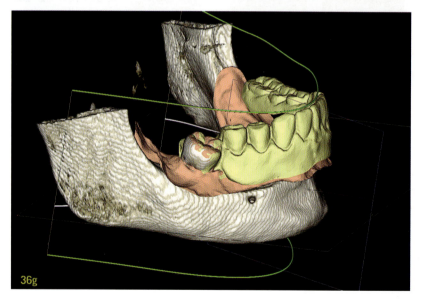

Figs 12-36a to 12-36g Scanning process and matching performed with the 3DIEMME system. The 3D bone scans are overlaid onto the digitally scanned radiographic guide (scan prosthesis).

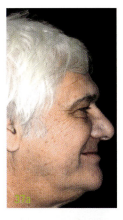 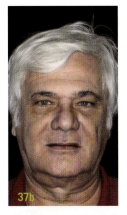 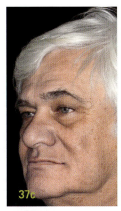 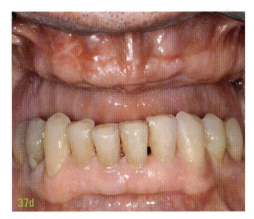

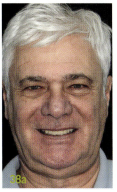 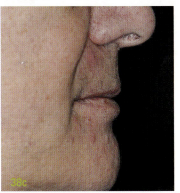 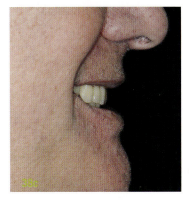

Figs 12-37a to 12-37d *(a to c)* Extraoral views of the patient, who is fully edentulous in the maxilla, showing, upon initial examination, the changes that the patient's face underwent as a consequence of losing the vertical dimension and tooth support. *(d)* The intraoral inspection shows how the maxillary jaw is affected by severe resorption involving the left and right ridges. No horizontal deficits are detected under palpation of the edentulous ridges.

Figs 12-38a to 12-38c Patient with provisional complete denture inserted, which restored the correct maxillomandibular relationship and proper esthetic parameters.

rehabilitation. During surgery, the surgical guide was tried in, and its stability on the residual ridge was tested. The accuracy of the surgical guide was also confirmed with a silicone jig that had been previously prepared on the articulator.

Following the recommendation of the authors' school, before fixing the surgical guide in place, the mucotomies were performed while holding the guide in position manually.

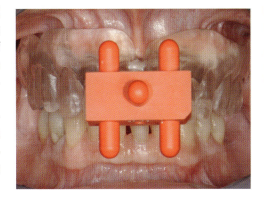

Fig 12-39 Scanning template developed from the data obtained from the full prosthesis and placement of the radiographic landmark for CT-CBCT scanning.

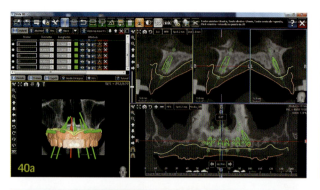
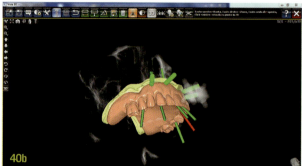
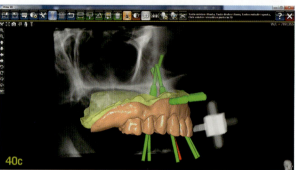
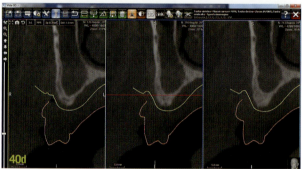
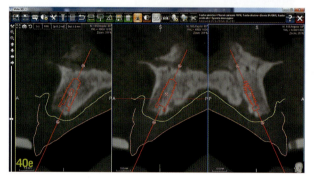
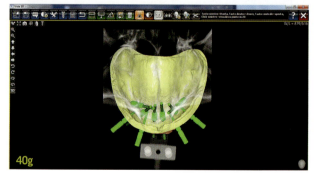

Figs 12-40a to 12-40g Design steps using dedicated software products in which the planed prosthesis is correctly included in the CBCT scan using the radiopaque landmark.

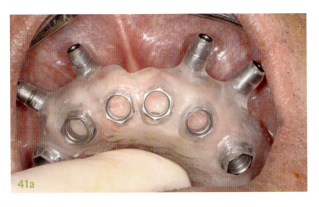
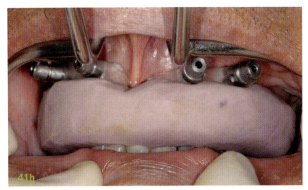

Figs 12-41a and 12-41b Surgical stage: try-in of the surgical guide and position confirmation with a silicone jig.

This allowed the surgeon to remove the guide, eliminate the mucous operculum thus created, and, if necessary, trim the edges to prevent fragments of the mucosal tissue from being introduced into the implant sites. Moreover, with angled implants it can be difficult to remove the operculum correctly.

The osteotomies for placement of the surgical guide fixation screws were then prepared, followed by preparation of the implant sites to the established depth indicated by the bur stop. The prepared implant sites were then irrigated with saline solution to remove the resulting bone fragments from the osteotomy.

The reduction guides for the cylindric burs were placed and kept under irrigation to reduce friction and, consequently, generated heat.

All osteotomy sites were prepared in sequence so as to reduce the surgical time, and the implants were placed at the preestablished depths.

Once all the implants had been placed, the surgical guide was removed and implant sta-

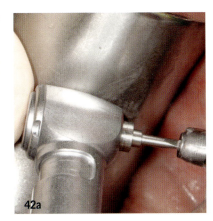
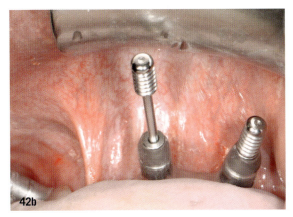

Figs 12-42a and 12-42b Osteotomies were performed for the surgical guide fixation screws, and the implant sites were prepared according to the manufacturer's instructions.

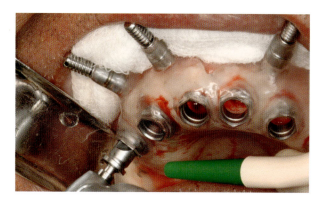

Fig 12-43 Corticotomy: Using a dedicated bur, the cortical bone of the ridge was thinned.

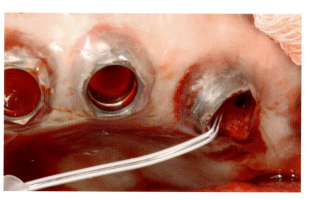

Fig 12-44 Before placing the implants, the osteotomies were rinsed with saline solution to remove any debris.

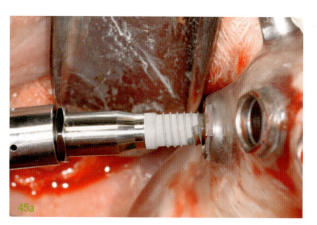

Fig 12-45a to 12-45c The implants were placed with their attached mounts, and the guide was then removed.

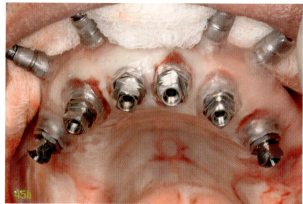

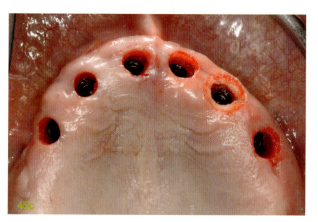

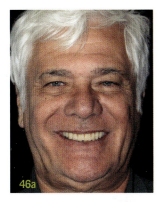
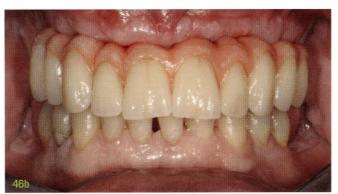

Figs 12-46a to 12-46e Clinical views of the screw-retained prosthesis. The esthetic and functional integration appeared to be good, as shown by *(a and b)* extraoral and intraoral views and *(c and d)* images during lateral excursion movements. *(e)* Access for oral hygiene procedures was also confirmed.

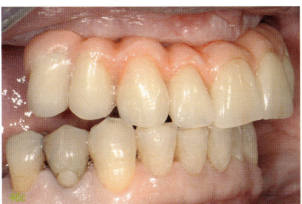
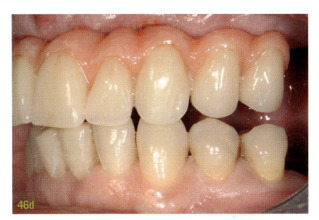
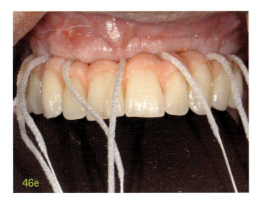
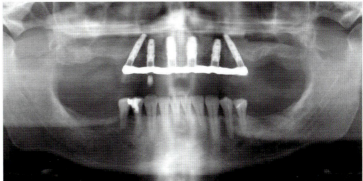

Fig 12-47 Follow-up panoramic radiograph.

bility assessed with a manual torque wrench. We believe that this step is useful because the torque measured by the implant motor with the guide in place is usually higher due to the friction generated by the various prosthetic components and by the surgical guide. After placing the implants, an impression and occlusal bite registration were taken for the fabrication of an immediately loaded prosthesis consisting of a metal bar and customized crowns in composite resin.

The Sirona Virtual Patient Concept Technique

The software developed by Sirona is a closed system that can be used only as part of the Sirona system, but it can be used with implants from different manufacturers. The virtual patient concept protocol provides for the integration of the virtual wax-up in the 3D radiograph and for the construction of a surgical guide.

The advantage of this system, as compared to others, is that all steps can be performed directly in the dental practice without relying on external radiologic centers or laboratories for model scanning.

Currently, the system requires that the tooth-supported surgical guide be fabricated at a dedicated Sirona center, but the company is working on a system that will eventually allow the surgical guide to be fabricated directly at the dental practice. However, the prosthetic abutments and crowns can be fabricated at the dental office. The operating protocol requires an optical scan of the edentulous area and of the opposing arch with the Cerec AC unit (Sirona).

The dental arches are scanned in maximum intercuspation so that the digital models can be virtually articulated using the 3D reconstruction software.

This virtual reconstruction allows the prosthetic restoration to be planned in advance to the smallest detail, including occlusal contacts, interproximal contact points, emergence profile, and thickness of the restorative materials, depending on the selected material. A CBCT scan (Galileos, Sirona) is then taken by placing an occlusal bite plate between the teeth that is relined with silicone material for occlusal registration.

The dedicated software then combines the data derived from the two acquisition systems, allowing the surgeon to plan the implant placement based on the data obtained from the simulation of the prosthetic restoration. The software offers a large implant library, and once the planning is completed, the dentist can order the surgical guide directly through the software and plan the surgical session.

Depending on the complexity of the case, the operator can take a traditional impression of the implants and send it to the laboratory for an electronic scanning of the model or perform a direct optical scan of the implant positions.

The latter procedure is fairly easy, as it simply requires that a special post called a scan body be attached to the implants; this transfers the unique implant position in the three spatial planes onto the virtual model by taking a scan with the Cerec AC optical scanner.

Once scanning has been done, the data are processed for fabrication of the customized milled posts and the prosthetic crowns.

Clinical Case of Tooth-Supported Guided Surgery

The patient presented with bilateral distal edentulism in the mandibular jaw and requested a fixed prosthetic rehabilitation (Figs 12-48 to 12-55).

An optical scan of the dental arches was taken to plan the treatment. The scans were placed in articulation through the 3D

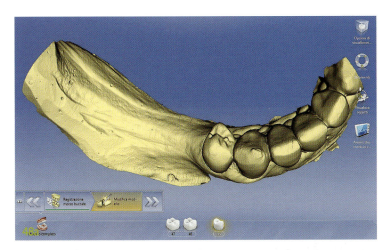
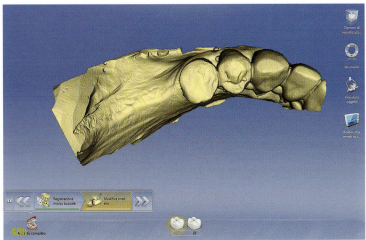
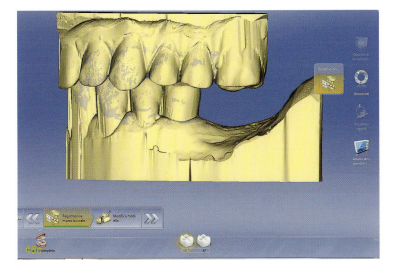

Figs 12-48a to 12-48c Optical scans of the partially edentulous arches. The virtual models were placed in articulation by the Cerec software.

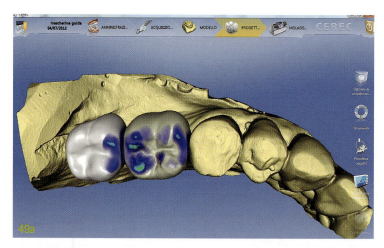
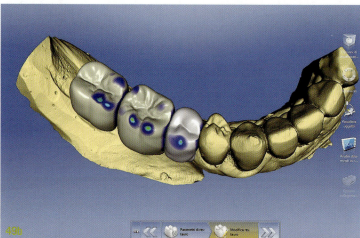

Figs 12-49a to 12-49c Steps of the virtual modeling of the prosthetic crowns.

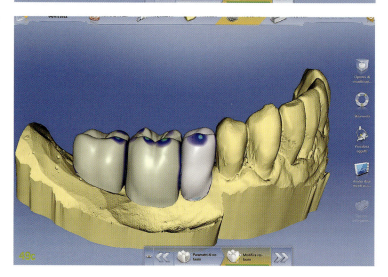

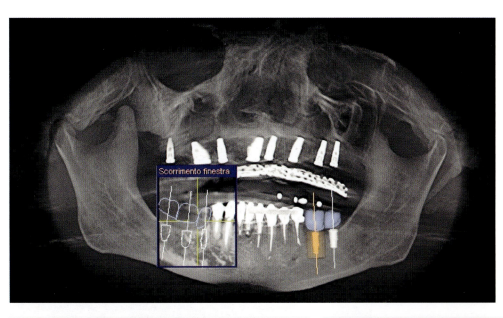

Fig 12-50 Integration of the data from the virtual wax-up of the case and the 3D examination and subsequent planning of the implant placement.

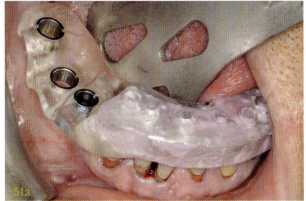
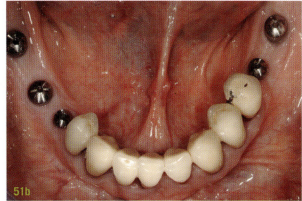

Figs 12-51a and 12-51b Surgical stage: *(a)* The tooth- and mucosa-supported surgical guide was positioned. *(b)* The implants were placed using a flapless technique, and healing abutments were attached.

processing program. A virtual wax-up of the teeth to be restored was designed on the computer. The occlusal plane was corrected to reflect the occlusal contacts of the opposing arch. Next, a low-radiation, wide-FOV CBCT was taken so that both arches could be scanned simultaneously. The software interfaced the prosthetic plan with the radiographic data before the virtual implants were placed. This allows the virtual wax-up to be viewed on the 3D reconstruction through dedicated implant-planning software.

The implant positions were designed according to the previously determined prosthetic axes. Once the prosthetic implant plan was approved, the file was sent to the manufacturing center for fabrication of the surgical guide.

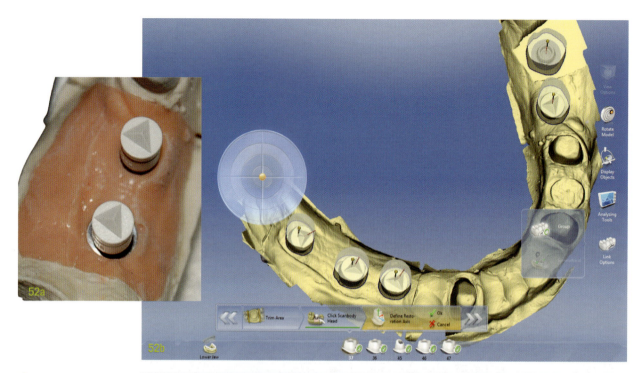

Figs 12-52a to 12-52c Once healing was completed, a traditional impression was taken. The dental technician then placed implant position-scanning devices onto the stone cast and designed the final zirconia abutments to be manufactured.

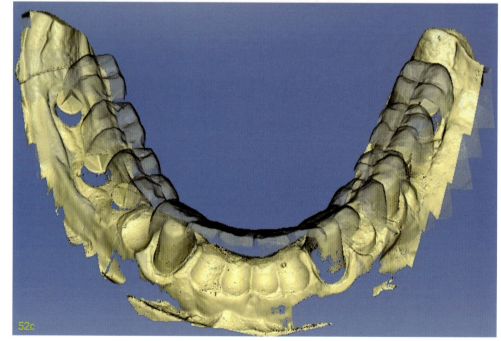

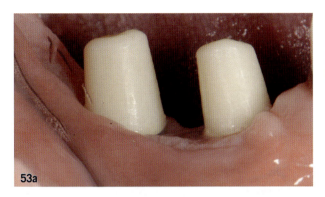
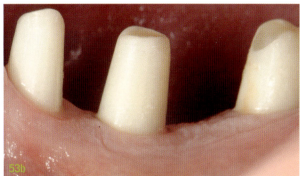

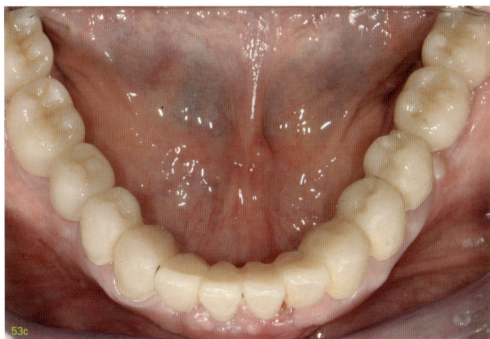

Figs 12-53a to 12-53c Placement of the definitive abutments and delivery of the provisional prostheses, both made using a milling method.

Figs 12-54a and 12-54b Intraoral scan of the definitive abutments and virtual design of the definitive crowns.

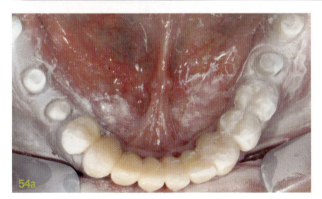
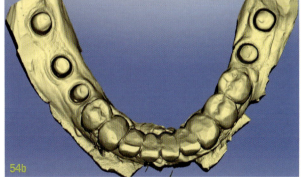

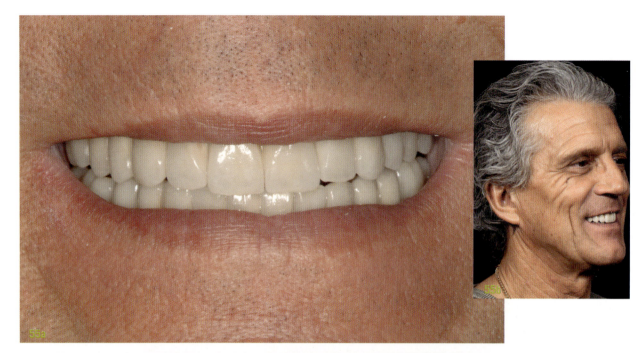
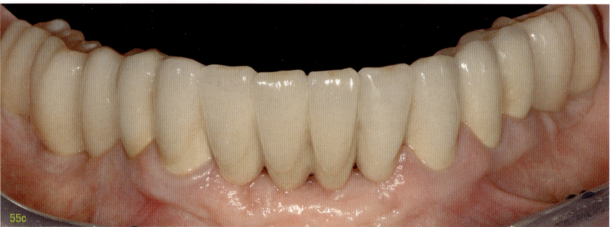

Figs 12-55a to 12-55e Delivery of the definitive prostheses: The crowns were milled and finalized in the laboratory. *(a to d)* Micro- and macroesthetic evaluation of the restorations and *(e)* follow-up panoramic radiograph.

Because no augmentation of soft tissue was required, a minimally invasive flapless surgical procedure was performed.

An impression was taken using a conventional technique after a 2-month healing period, and the laboratory prepared the cast and attached a suitable transfer coping to the implant analogs for the digital scan of the cast. The scanning could be done directly in the oral cavity without taking an impression by simply attaching the scan bodies onto the inserted implants, which transferred their positions in the three spatial planes onto the virtual model.

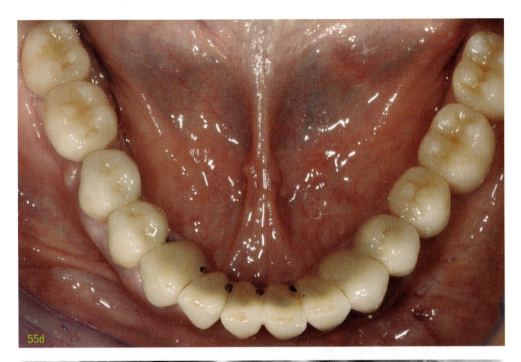

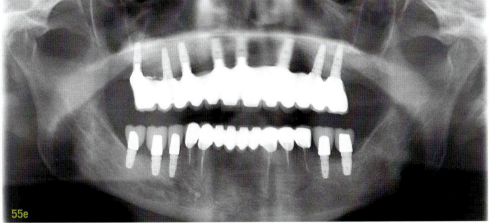

The planning software processed the data and built a virtual working model. The dental technician could then design the shape of the definitive abutments in a variety of materials (in this case, zirconia) and the provisional prosthetic restorations. The abutments were then placed, together with the provisional restorations.

The definitive crowns made of lithium disilicate were prepared directly at the dental practice after making an intraoral scan of the prosthetic abutments.

Conclusions

Guided surgery is the natural evolution of implant surgery, embracing technologic advancements with a view to delivering minimally invasive surgical procedures. The analytic capabilities of software products will continue to improve over time, and, combined with the development of increasingly sophisticated CBCT scanning systems, they will become part of routine dentistry.

The simplification of surgical treatment starts with an accurate preoperative study of the clinical case, which requires a learning curve both for the diagnostic and for the operative stages of the procedure. This is why the clinical case must be selected according to the dentist's expertise. According to our school, beginners should only treat patients with single or multiple missing teeth as opposed to those who are fully edentulous. The clinician should not be misled by the extreme simplification of the computerized decision-making process, since the clinical examination and the learning curve, as well as the clinician's expertise, remain crucial in planning and treating any implant-supported prosthetic case. It should be pointed out that the degree of accuracy of computer-assisted surgery is at the level of millimeters, but there is always some discrepancy between the actual and the virtual anatomy,[34–36] especially if the patient is treated with a flapless technique.

A multicenter clinical trial[28] assessed the accuracy of a new guided-surgery system and compared it with data in literature. In eight centers, 26 patients were treated with a total of 116 implants placed using different types of surgical guides: bone-supported, mucosa-supported, and mixed guides, depending on the type of total or partial edentulism. At the end of the surgical stage, a postoperative CT scan was taken of each patient. The study evaluated (1) the spatial discrepancy at the level of the apex and at the implant platform and (2) the angular difference between the virtual plan and the actual position of the placed

Figs 12-56a and 12-56b Images showing the overlay of preoperative CT scans (green) and postoperative CT scans (red).

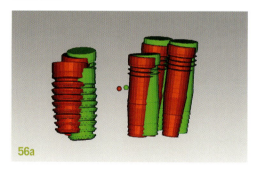
56a

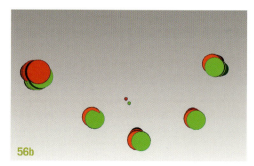
56b

implants by overlaying the preoperative CT scans of the implant plan and the postoperative CT scans (Fig 12-56).

The results show that there is a discrepancy between the actual treatment and the virtual plan, which usually amounts to approximately 1 millimeter, and an average angular discrepancy ranging from 2 to 5 degrees. However, standard deviations should also be taken into account, as the summary tables below show (Fig 12-57). This study leads one to some clinical considerations, as illustrated in Table 12-1. In clinical cases treated with a flapless ap-

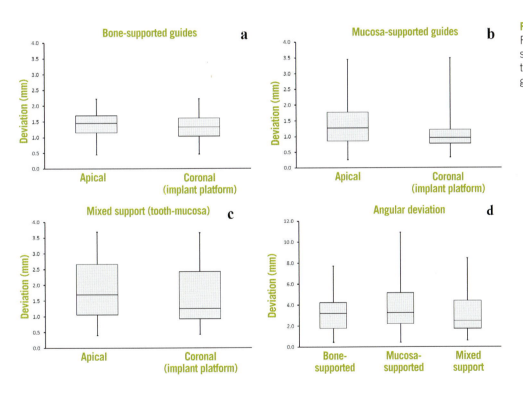

Figs 12-57a to 12-57d Forrest plots of the measurements taken using the different types of guides.

Table 12-1 Clinical considerations on navigation systems

Make an in-depth, accurate diagnosis.

Place the implant at a safe distance of at least 2 mm from critical anatomical structures.

In immediately loaded implant cases, prepare a provisional prosthesis that can be relined to compensate for any discrepancy between the virtual and the actual anatomy.

In clinical cases treated with a flapless approach, the surgeon should open a full-thickness flap and perform bone regeneration techniques if a bone dehiscence occurs after the implant sites have been prepared.

proach, the surgeon should open a full-thickness flap and perform bone regeneration techniques if a bone dehiscence occurs after the implant sites have been prepared.

While these 3D analytic programs obviously offer both advantages and disadvantages (Table 12-2), they are unquestionably important tools that can be used for diagnostic purposes and should not be considered as a useful aid only in planning implant-supported prosthetic restorations. The opportunity to reconstruct the volume along any plane allows accurate study of the maxillary area not only in implant dentistry but also in endodontics, orthodontics, and periodontics.

Table 12-2 Summary of advantages and disadvantages of computerized navigation systems

Advantages	Disadvantages
Reduction of invasiveness	Cost
Stress reduction for surgeon/patient	Limited clinical use in patients with reduced opening of the mouth
Speed of the procedure	
Simplification of the surgical and prosthetic protocols	
Patient's perception of a more professional treatment	

References

1. Testori T, Francetti L, Vercellotti T. La diagnosi in implantologia. Dent Cadmos 1998;5:13–31.
2. Mecall RA, Rosenfeld AL. The influence of residual ridge resorption patterns on implant fixture placement and tooth position. 2. Presurgical determination of prosthesis type and design. Int J Periodontics Restorative Dent 1992;12:32–51.
3. Mecall RA, Rosenfeld AL. Influence of residual ridge resorption patterns on implant fixture placement and tooth position. 1. Int J Periodontics Restorative Dent 1991;11:8–23.
4. Andersson JE, Svartz K. CT-scanning in the preoperative planning of osseointegrated implants in the maxilla. Int J Oral Maxillofac Surg 1988;17:33–35.
5. Quirynen M, Lamoral Y, Dekeyser C, et al. CT scan standard reconstruction technique for reliable jaw bone volume determination. Int J Oral Maxillofac Implants 1990;5:384–389.
6. Testori T, Barenghi A, Salvato A. La tomografia assiale computerizzata nella moderna implantologia: Reali vantaggi per una corretta programmazione chirurgico-protesica-dose assorbita dal paziente. Riv Ital Osteoint 1993;1:19–28.
7. Mozzo P, Procacci C, Tacconi A, Martini PT, Andreis IA. A new volumetric CT machine for dental imaging based on the cone-beam technique: Preliminary results. Eur Radiol 1998;8:1558–1564.
8. Ball RL, Barbizam JV, Cohenca N. Intraoperative endodontic applications of cone-beam computed tomography. J Endod 2013;39:548–557.
9. Laky M, Majdalani S, Kapferer I, et al. Periodontal probing of dental furcations compared with diagnosis by low-dose computed tomography: A case series. J Periodontol 2013;84:1740–1746.
10. Tyndall DA, Price JB, Tetradis S, et al. Position statement of the American Academy of Oral and Maxillofacial Radiology on selection criteria for the use of radiology in dental implantology with emphasis on cone beam computed tomography. Oral Surg Oral Med Oral Pathol Oral Radiol 2012;113:817–826.
11. Spilker C. The ACR-NEMA Digital Imaging and Communications Standard: A nontechnical description. J Digit Imaging 1989;2:127–131.
12. Becker W, Goldstein M, Becker BE, Sennerby L. Minimally invasive flapless implant surgery: A prospective multicenter study. Clin Implant Dent Relat Res 2005;7(suppl 1):S21–S27.
13. Fortin T, Bosson JL, Isidori M, Blanchet E. Effect of flapless surgery on pain experienced in implant placement using an image-guided system. Int J Oral Maxillofac Implants 2006;21:298–304.
14. Cannizzaro G, Leone M, Consolo U, Ferri V, Esposito M. Immediate functional loading of implants placed with flapless surgery versus conventional implants in partially edentulous patients: A 3-year randomized controlled clinical trial. Int J Oral Maxillofac Implants 2008;23:867–875.
15. Van de Velde T, Glor F, De Bruyn H. A model study on flapless implant placement by clinicians with a different experience level in implant surgery. Clin Oral Implants Res 2008;19:66–72.
16. Sclar AG. Guidelines for flapless surgery. J Oral Maxillofac Surg 2007;65:20–32.
17. Brodala N. Flapless surgery and its effect on dental implant outcomes. Int J Oral Maxillofac Implants 2009;24(suppl):118–125.
18. Arisan V, Karabuda CZ, Ozdemir T. Implant surgery using bone- and mucosa-supported stereolithographic guides in totally edentulous jaws: Surgical and post-operative outcomes of computer-aided vs standard techniques. Clin Oral Implants Res 2010;21:980–988.
19. Schwarz MS, Rothman SL, Rhodes ML, Chafetz N. Computed tomography: Part I. Preoperative assessment of the mandible for endosseous implant surgery. Int J Oral Maxillofac Implants 1987;2:137–141.

20. Schwarz MS, Rothman SL, Rhodes ML, Chafetz N. Computed tomography: Part II. Preoperative assessment of the maxilla for endosseous implant surgery. Int J Oral Maxillofac Implants 1987;2:143–148.
21. Grunder U, Gracis S, Capelli M. Influence of the 3-D bone-to-implant relationship on esthetics. Int J Periodontics Restorative Dent 2005;25:113–119.
22. Tarnow DP, Magner AW, Fletcher P. The effect of the distance from the contact point to the crest of bone on the presence or absence of the interproximal dental papilla. J Periodontol 1992;63:995–996.
23. Testori T, Zuffetti CM, Francetti L. Considerazioni cliniche e funzionali in implantologia. Linee guida. Dental Cadmos 1998;14:11–29.
24. Rosenfeld AL, Mandelaris GA, Tardieu PB. Prosthetically directed implant placement using computer software to ensure precise placement and predictable prosthetic outcomes. Part 2: Rapid-prototype medical modeling and stereolithographic drilling guides requiring bone exposure. Int J Periodontics Restorative Dent 2006;26:347–353.
25. Rosenfeld AL, Mandelaris GA, Tardieu PB. Prosthetically directed implant placement using computer software to ensure precise placement and predictable prosthetic outcomes. Part 3: Stereolithographic drilling guides that do not require bone exposure and the immediate delivery of teeth. Int J Periodontics Restorative Dent 2006;26:493–499.
26. Ganz SD. Use of stereolithographic models as diagnostic and restorative aids for predictable immediate loading of implants. Pract Proced Aesthet Dent 2003;15:763–771.
27. Capelli M, Testori T, Francetti L, Del Fabbro M, Slomp F. Modelli stereolitografici in chirurgia implantare. Grado di affidabilita. Dental Cadmos 1999;7:43–49.
28. Testori T, Robiony M, Parenti A, et al. Evaluation of accuracy and precision of a new guided surgery system: A multicenter clinical study. Int J Periodontics Restorative Dent 2014;34(suppl 3):S59–S69.
29. Tardieu PB, Vrielinck L, Escolano E, Henne M, Tardieu AL. Computer-assisted implant placement: Scan template, simplant, surgiguide, and SAFE system. Int J Periodontics Restorative Dent 2007;27:141–149.
30. Perrotti G, De Vecchi L, Testori T, Weinstein RL. Analisi facciale globale: Approccio diagnostico-terapeutico multidisciplinare alla riabilitazione implantare complessa. Ital Oral Surg 2012;11:S108–S116.
31. Hammerle CH, Stone P, Jung RE, Kapos T, Brodala N. Consensus statements and recommended clinical procedures regarding computer-assisted implant dentistry. Int J Oral Maxillofac Implants 2009;24(suppl):126–131.
32. Hultin M, Svensson KG, Trulsson M. Clinical advantages of computer-guided implant placement: A systematic review. Clin Oral Implants Res 2012;23(suppl 6):124–135.
33. Galli FPA, Fumagalli L, Capelli M, Zuffetti F, Testori T. Carico immediato provvisorio protesicamente guidato nel mascellare superiore. Ital Oral Surg 2007;6:35–40.
34. D'Haese J, Van De Velde T, Komiyama A, Hultin M, De Bruyn H. Accuracy and complications using computer-designed stereolithographic surgical guides for oral rehabilitation by means of dental implants: A review of the literature. Clin Implant Dent Relat Res 2012;14:321–335.
35. Cassetta M, Di Mambro A, Giansanti M, Stefanelli LV, Cavallini C. The intrinsic error of a stereolithographic surgical template in implant guided surgery. Int J Oral Maxillofac Surg 2013;42:264–275.
36. Cassetta M, Stefanelli LV, Giansanti M, Calasso S. Accuracy of implant placement with a stereolithographic surgical template. Int J Oral Maxillofac Implants 2012;27:655–663.

M Scarpelli

13

CBCT
Medicolegal Issues

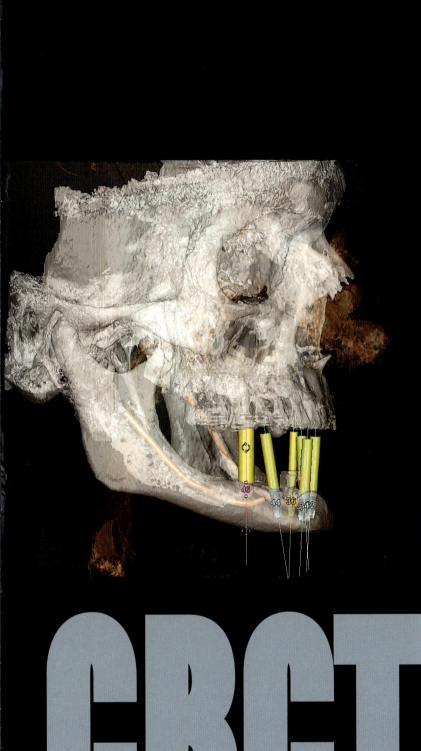

The use of cone beam computed tomography (CBCT) in the dental practice raises new issues regarding the relationship between diagnosis and treatment in dentistry, given the greater amount of information that can be gathered and used in the subsequent therapeutic process. However, this also entails problems in terms of the scope of the dentist's competence in managing critical issues, especially medicolegal aspects such as how to manage the observation of images taken for dental diagnostic purposes that show possible malformations but cannot be further interpreted by the dentist. This chapter provides some remarks on such issues, although the initial assumption is that the approach to using this method must be characterized by the usual rules of prudence and diligence that are an integral part of clinical practice, both in diagnostic and in therapeutic settings.

Informed Consent

The examination can only be performed if the patient's prior informed consent has been obtained. This is best accomplished through a straightforward, written, and understandable, document containing a clinical report detailing the reasons why such examination is required, information on the radiation dose, and the justification for the selected practice).

A copy of the informed consent shall be given to the patient, and a copy shall be kept in the patient's file.

***

One final remark: should a dentist, when performing a CBCT scan for his or her own diagnostic purposes, find himself or herself in a situation in which he/she views images that might indicate a disease of undetermined nature, for instance a tumor, the professional must refer the patient to a competent specialist (eg, radiologist or oncologist) upon recording these findings in the patient's clinical record. The authors also recommend writing a report on the findings, attaching a copy signed by the patient to the patient's clinical record to make sure that the specialist involved has actually received adequate information on such findings.

In essence, should a medical condition that does not strictly relate to the specialty domain be identified in the referred patient, the requirement is to ascertain that the receiving specialist gets all the information that the referring physician intended to deliver in the first place.

It is obviously taken for granted and considered as necessary that the dentist has received basic training that allows him or her, when performing the examination for diagnostic purposes and for a potential dental treatment following thereto, to recognize, in the viewed images, at least the most significant alterations so as to be able to cautiously refer the patient, together with the related images, to a specialist who has specific skills and abilities to interpret them. There follows the need that any dentist who is willing to use this diagnostic system in his/her clinical practice be duly trained to read and interpret the images thus obtained and to consequently manage the information generated from them that have no direct use in the treatment plan developed at the beginning.

***